Nursing against the Odds

A volume in the series

The Culture and Politics of Health Care Work
Edited by Suzanne Gordon and Sioban Nelson

Nobody's Home: Candid Reflections of a Nursing Home Aide
Thomas Edward Gass

Code Green: Money-Driven Hospitals and the Dismantling of Nursing
Dana Weinberg

NURSING
AGAINST THE ODDS
How Health Care Cost Cutting, Media Stereotypes,
and Medical Hubris Undermine Nurses and Patient Care

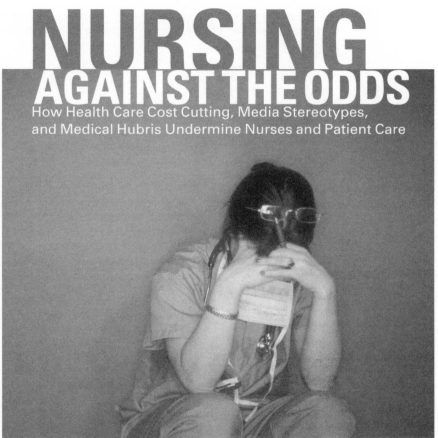

SUZANNE GORDON

ILR PRESS
an imprint of
CORNELL UNIVERSITY PRESS
Ithaca and London

First published 2005 by Cornell University Press

Printed in the United States of America

Library of Congress Cataloging-in-Publication Data

Gordon, Suzanne, 1945–
    Nursing against the odds : how health care cost cutting, media stereotypes, and medical hubris undermine nurses and patient care / Suzanne Gordon.
        p. cm.—(The culture and politics of health care work)
    Includes bibliographical references and index.
    ISBN 0-8014-3976-0 (cloth : alk. paper)
    1. Nursing—Social aspects—United States. 2. Nursing—United States—Public opinion.
3. Nurses—United States—Public opinion. 4. Nurses—United States—Social conditions.
5. Nurses in mass media. 6. Nurse and physician. I. Title. II. Series.
    RT86.5.G67 2005
    610.73'0973—dc22

                                2004028248

Cornell University Press strives to use environmentally responsible suppliers and materials to the fullest extent possible in the publishing of its books. Such materials include vegetable-based, low-VOC inks and acid-free papers that are recycled, totally chlorine-free, or partly composed of nonwood fibers. For further information, visit our website at www.cornellpress.cornell.edu.

Cloth printing   10 9 8 7 6 5 4 3 2 1

PRINTED IN U.S.A.

For Claire and Sam Fagin

Contents

Preface

The act of thanking people for their help in the production of a book so often seems to dissolve into clichés. But the truth is that only through phrases such as "there are no words to express . . ." or "I am so grateful for . . ." can I pay homage to the village it took to produce this book. The village is first of all inhabited by the many nurses, some named here, some not, who shared their stories, concerns, and hopes. Then it's made up of people whose almost daily contact and conversation inspired me and kept me going.

First I thank Carolyn Mugar and John O'Connor for their generous financial support of this project. It is very sad that John, a tireless advocate for health care reform, great supporter of nursing, and always ebullient personality, is not here today to see its completion.

I thank my agent Anne Borchardt for all her support over the years. Fran Benson, my editor and now friend, did so much more than most editors. Her editorial guidance helped me navigate tight passages, and the almost daily talks we had broke the isolation that threatens to engulf an author. Sioban Nelson's vast knowledge of nursing and health care politics—whether conveyed in face-to-face conversations or over the phone—was critical to my work. Isabel Marcus was always there when I called her—sometimes when she was in the most unexpected places—with my typical "I've just had an epiphany" (she must have wondered when the light bulb would finally go out and she could get some respite). And my long collaboration with Bernice Buresh has enriched my thinking about nursing silence.

A number of clinicians helped me understand the complexities of the x problems I deal with. Timothy McCall is, I'm sure, relieved that I won't call upon him to answer so many questions about doctor-nurse relationships, read more manuscript pages, and suggest ideas for titles. Glenn Bubley did all this too and also helped me translate medical-speak into English. Emily Lowry spent endless hours over tea thinking about the problems I write about. Margo Woods helped me understand how clinicians outside of nursing and medicine view hierarchically structured health care "teams." Jeannie Chaisson and I shared many great conversations, and her insights were invaluable.

Claire Fagin, as always, was a beacon of inspiration and a source of much-needed commiseration. Joan Lynaugh was, once again, generous with her time and advice. After he got caller ID, Alan Sager came to understand what a lie it was when I called and said, "I just have a quick question." With Julie Sochalski and Dana Weinberg I shared many hours of lively conversation that informed this book. Ross Koppel was tireless in providing advice and sending me useful articles and information. The walls in Kathy Dracup's kitchen must still reverberate with our conversations about nursing, and Charlene Harrington and I shared many dinners talking about the subject. Once again I thank Patricia Benner for all her insights and help, and Richard MacIntyre for some wonderful observations. Thanks to Tom Keighley for great chats and insights. Sean Clarke was very willing to clarify complex data. I want to thank Laurie Gottlieb and Barbara Munro for offering me an opportunity to work closely with nursing students and gain a better understanding of their education.

Andy Stern gave me initial support, as did Jamie Cohen and Larry Cohen. David Schildmeier and Anne Schott provided many useful contacts and information, and I thank Chuck Idelson for all his help and for allowing me to test some ideas in the pages of the nursing journal *Revolution*.

I can't express how grateful I am to Terry McKiernan for his editing advice and assistance. He truly piloted this book into its harbor. My assistant, Kristin Elifson, was hugely instrumental in producing this book. She did research, helped with typing, gave me moral support, and, most important, kept my work life in some semblance of order. And I want to thank Andrea Fleck Clardy for coming up with the title of this book.

I'm not sure why spouses and family always come last in the accounting of authorial gratitude. To Steve Early, my husband, what can I say? He edited drafts, provided information and wording for crucial sections, and illuminated many issues. Most of all, his constant prodding—Get back to work, When are you going to finish this? Come on, come on—is one of the reasons I did finish this book. Whenever the A.D.D. set in—which was often—he kept me on track. I have to both thank and apologize to my two wonderful daughters, Alex and Jessica. Thank you for supporting

your mother, and I beg your forgiveness for all those times when I was too
distracted by nursing to focus on you. If you don't become nurses, I'll know why.

Finally, I want to express an intellectual debt to three people. Although I've never met, never even talked to James C. Scott, his book *Seeing Like a State* shaped my thinking about the invisibility of nursing. This in spite of the fact that he never mentions the subject. Linda Aiken's work has been so important to those of us who try to give voice to nurses' work. And I thank Dan Chambliss for his support for this series, for my work, and because he gets it so right.

Nursing against the Odds

Introduction

Until February 1998, I thought I understood nursing. I had been doing research and writing on the subject since the mid-1980s, observing nurses as they cared for patients in hospitals all around the country, reading nursing textbooks, nursing journals, and histories of nursing, and collecting countless reports on contemporary nursing issues. In lectures and workshops, I had talked with thousands of nurses about how to make their profession more visible to a wider public increasingly concerned about the quality of health care.

Then, one day that winter, ever so briefly, I had to be a "nurse" myself.[1] My "patient" was my friend Kathy Dracup, herself a critical care nurse and then a professor of nursing, who had arthroscopic knee surgery when I visited her in Los Angeles. The morning of her operation, Kathy left home in a cab to be at the UCLA hospital by six thirty in the morning. At nine, a nurse called me, as Kathy's designated driver—her husband was out of town—and told me to be at the recovery room promptly at quarter of ten. We'd be out by ten, the nurse assured me. What brisk efficiency, I thought; this should be easy.

As I walked through the recovery room, I began to have second thoughts. In curtained-off cubicles, I saw woozy-looking patients who'd just emerged from surgery, and I wondered how many of them could possibly be well enough to go home. Kathy, however, seemed quite cheerful. She told me that the doctor had found less knee damage than expected. Before we left, the nurse asked Kathy if she'd ever used crutches before. "Oh, yes," she responded.

"Okay," the nurse said, "then you don't need a lesson."

2   The anesthesiologist came in to make Kathy's discharge official. Then an escort wheeled Kathy down to the parking lot where a hefty guard helped her into the car.

As we drove away, my friend's good spirits and alertness further lulled me into believing that there were no lingering effects of the anesthesia. When we pulled up in front of her house, I helped Kathy out of the car and got her standing up on her crutches without mishap. The steep walkway to her front door had a number of steps that she would have trouble climbing, but at the end of the driveway was an easier entry. Thinking that she was all right—my first mistake—I left Kathy standing alone at the bottom of the driveway while I went to open a gate. I'll not soon forget the awful feeling I had in the pit of my stomach when I turned around and saw her lying in a heap, crutches splayed out at her side. I raced back to her. Bending down, I frantically asked, "Did you hurt your leg? Did you hurt your other leg?"

Completely dazed, she replied, "I don't know what happened. I felt so dizzy. I just went down."

By sheer luck, she didn't land on her bad leg or otherwise injure herself. Nonetheless, when I bent down to try to help her up, she did not budge. I tried to pull her up, but she was dead weight. I'm five foot six inches and have a bad back. She's five feet eleven and 130 pounds. She had no mobility. I didn't have enough strength. And I had no idea how to lift a patient safely.

Looking for help, I raced over to the next-door neighbor's front door and rang the bell. No answer. I started for the house on the other side of Kathy's. "Don't bother," my patient shouted, "She's too old to help."

So I crouched down carefully between her legs and told her to put her hands around my waist and try to pull herself up. Slowly, ever so slowly, as if I were a tree trunk, she climbed me and I supported her until she was standing.

No one at the hospital had prepared me for this. But clearly, the combination of dehydration plus the lingering effects of anesthesia had left Kathy unstable at best. As we walked slowly up the driveway, I held her waist from behind. When we got to the house, there were three steps leading to the front door. Still in a postoperative daze, she lacked all kinetic problem-solving ability and simply couldn't figure out how to negotiate the steps with her crutches and a dead leg. I tried to support her, but again I just wasn't strong enough. Standing there, looking at those last three steps, I began thinking about this mountain range and the ones beyond it. Just inside the house, we faced yet another step to get into the living room and then a narrow flight of stairs up to the second floor and Kathy's bedroom. I felt like we were staring up at Mount Everest, and I knew we wouldn't make it without an assistant.

Fortunately, a truck pulled up across the street and out popped two Hispanic gardeners, ready to mow lawns and clip hedges. There was no one else in sight. Praying that Kathy wouldn't fall again, I told her, "Hold on! Please, please don't fall, I'm going to get help."

I sprinted across the street and, in Spanish, begged one of the men, "Ayuda, ayuda, help, please come, please help us." He followed me to the front door and supported Kathy under one arm while I hoisted her up under the other. As she was hobbling across the living room to the inside stairway, one of her crutches hit an unanchored throw rug. The crutch started to skid out of control. By this time I was on red alert and reached across to hold it down, narrowly averting another fall.

We helped her up the stairs, which she navigated sitting on her behind, moving upward one step at a time, until we finally managed to get her to her room and safely into bed. I thanked the gardener for his emergency services, and he left to return to his lawns.

Dripping with sweat and shaking with anxiety, I helped Kathy take off her clothes and get into her pajamas, tucked the requisite pillows under her injured leg to keep it elevated, and went down to make her some tea. It was only eleven thirty, and my nursing shift was a long way from over.

Early in the afternoon, Kathy's daughter came over and I went out to do a few errands. When I came back, there was more bad news. With her daughter's help, Kathy had gone to the bathroom. In the process of turning around to get on the toilet, she'd become dizzy again and fallen. Luckily she hadn't reinjured her knee, broken a hip, or cracked open her head, and her daughter hadn't strained her back when she came to the rescue.

I surveyed the scene of the accident to see if, belatedly, there was anything I could do. The bathroom had been designed with fashion, not illness, in mind. This was no hospital bathroom with nonskid linoleum floors, plenty of room for two people to maneuver, and grab bars near the toilet. Instead, the floor was tiled and slippery to stockinged feet. There was a treacherous throw rug near the sink.

"You shouldn't go into the bathroom without shoes on," I cautioned. The house was not safe for a person in Kathy's condition. Why bother doing an operation in the first place, I wondered, if the hospital is then going to send someone home to this obstacle course?

By ten at night, when I got Kathy to sleep and me into my own bed, the stress and worry of the day had turned my back into a spastic knot. That morning, I hadn't been the least bit reluctant to assume the caregiver role. It didn't take long to discover that home care is not a responsibility that most people (including myself) are well prepared to handle. Most of us are able and willing to offer tender loving care, but nursing work isn't just

4 a matter of TLC; it can mean the difference between recovery and complications, even life and death.

I had been given a firsthand glimpse of the nurseless future that awaits millions of us, and I saw it doesn't work.

What were, not long ago, inpatient hospital procedures are now, like Kathy's, outpatient ones. Meanwhile hospital stays themselves, when you're sick enough to be admitted, have been drastically shortened to achieve cost-cutting goals that fail to take into account patient care needs in the hospital and later at home. Wherever patients end up today—hospital, nursing home, rehab facility—they're in and out quicker and get less care, even when they're sicker. Even home care services have been radically curtailed, and the burden of follow-up care has been shifted to amateur caregivers, family and friends like myself.

Since the mid-1990s—with the advent of managed care in the United States and with different variants of cost cutting in Canada and other countries—the odds against nurses and the patients who depend on nursing care have significantly worsened. During the past decade, insurers, governments, and businesses began tightening health care purse strings, and hospitals and other health care facilities began to cut costs. Nursing, one of the largest parts of the hospital budget, was a logical target of "restructuring." Cost constraints led hospitals to lay off more experienced, and thus more expensive, nurses. They replaced RNs with poorly trained and poorly paid aides. Patients were given less time in the hospital. Nurses remaining on the wards were thus asked to care for more—and sicker—patients. As working conditions eroded, nurses began leaving the profession, and fewer recruits have entered. Why bother to go to nursing school, after all, if you can't get a decent job when you've graduated and when nurses are telling you how terrible it is at the bedside these days?

What began as just another periodic nursing shortage has turned into a major nursing crisis. The current nursing work force is aging; veteran nurses find their jobs so unfulfilling they want out; new recruits aren't entering the profession quickly enough; and those who do join the work force want to leave the bedside once they are exposed to the reality of working conditions in today's hospitals and other health care facilities.

Ten years ago, when cost cutting, restructuring, and cuts in lengths of stay emerged as health care policy, nurses, Cassandra-like, warned that patients were at risk and predicted that downsizing the nursing staff would produce a dangerous shortage of nurses. Hospital and health care administrators, some of them nurses, dismissed such concerns. Studies validating nurses' warnings are now appearing with alarming regularity. Report after report confirms the consequences of nurses' disaffection. Shortages of RNs exist in every area where nurses give direct care to the sick—in hospitals, in nursing homes, in rehabilitation hospitals, in home care, in schools, and even in hospices. In the United States, in 2002, the American Hospital Association reported that hospitals had 126,000 vacancies, or 12 percent of RN capacity.[2] The U.S. Bureau of Labor Statistics tells us that nursing is "one of the top twenty occupations to be affected by baby-boomer retirements, with employers needing to replace an estimated 331,000 RNs."[3] Reports also confirm shortages of the faculty needed to train the next generations of nurses. Policy makers and administrators no longer debate, as they did in the mid-1990s, the existence of a nursing shortage, but worry instead about its dimensions and how long it will endure. In the United States, for example, observers debate whether there will be a shortfall of 500,000, 300,000, or 200,000 nurses and whether truly catastrophic shortages will occur in 2010, 2020, or 2030.

My scary stint as an unpaid, untrained home care nurse didn't result in any patient morbidity or mortality, or a hospital readmission. Other people haven't been so lucky. Patients are now having more falls, more pneumonias, more urinary tract infections—to name only a few complications—and are also dying for want of nurses. The very hospitals that ten years ago predicted they'd have fewer patients and so would need fewer nurses have discovered that, lo and behold, people in industrialized societies aren't getting any younger or healthier. Aging patients beset with chronic illnesses are filling hospital beds, and there aren't enough nurses to take care of them.

Nurses not driven out by downsizing have voluntarily dropped out of the work force due to increased workloads, job stress, forced overtime and stagnating pay, and personal burnout. Strikes, protests, and legislative battles fought to better regulate the workplace dramatize the statistical mapping of nurses' disaffection. In spite of hospital rhetoric evincing a newfound concern for the value of nurses, nurses have had to wage bruising strikes to get modest increases in wages, safe nurse-to-patient ratios, an end to mandatory overtime, the implementation of predictable schedules, and a modicum of voice in institutional policies that govern their work. Efforts to regulate the industry or to unionize the workplace have similarly been met with hostility. In Massachusetts nurses took on the second largest hospital chain in America in a strike that was finally victorious after four bruising months. In Portland, Oregon, 2,200 RNs struck their hospital employer for over two months. In New York State, nurses have gone on strike against hospitals on Long Island, in New York City, and in Buffalo. In California, nurses have waged strikes against Catholic Healthcare West and the Kaiser system.

In 2002, in Petoskey, one of the most conservative areas of the state of Michigan, nearly three hundred nurses from Northern Michigan Hospi-

6 tal walked picket lines in subzero weather to get a first contract. The nurses wanted input into patient care as well as higher salaries. Instead of entering into serious negotiations, the hospital's board of trustees—which included powerful and wealthy representatives of the business community—hired travel nurses and other RNs to replace the veteran staff. The next year, in spite of pleas from Michigan's governor as well as a local Catholic bishop, the hospital's management and board refused to enter into binding arbitration. Instead the hospital continued to hire replacement workers and, as of September 2004, the strike had become the longest nurses' strike in U.S. history.

To further dramatize their plight, nurses, who themselves tend to be, at least in the United States, a fairly conservative group of workers, have even had to resort to the tactics of guerrilla theater. To celebrate a recent National Nurses Week and to fight for safe staffing regulations, RNs represented by the Service Employees International Union sent empty shoes to legislators across the United States to symbolize the unfilled nursing shoes that the shortage has produced. In Nevada, nurses arrived at work one day in their pajamas. They were required to work so much mandatory overtime, they said, that they might as well just sleep at the hospital. By sending letters to legislators and holding candlelight vigils, over ten thousand California nurses, represented by the California Nurses Association, generated one of the rare pieces of good news surrounding the nursing crisis. They successfully lobbied for the only piece of legislation in the United States that seriously addresses the issue of RNs' working conditions, a bill mandating safe staffing ratios for RNs. Although the California nurses were able to protect their patients, the hospital industry has increased the odds against nurses by making it more difficult for them to protect their own health. Ceding to industry pressure, in the fall of 2004 California's new governor, Arnold Schwarzenegger, vetoed a bill that would have mandated the kind of safe lift policies that would have helped nurses reduce the back, neck, and shoulder injuries from which so many suffer.[4]

RNs in the United States—who work in the world's most privatized, profit-driven health care system—are hardly alone in their dissatisfaction with their work. A 2001 study, conducted by Linda Aiken, Julie Sochalski, Judith Shamian, Anne Marie Rafferty, and several other researchers, reported on the working conditions of nurses in the United States, Canada, England, Scotland, and Germany. What is remarkable, the study noted, is the fact that nurses who work in countries with extremely different methods of financing health care share similar complaints and report "similar shortcomings."[5] Indeed they do. Nurses in Canada have held long and bitter strikes in Quebec, Nova Scotia, and Newfoundland. In British Columbia, nurses unsuccessfully petitioned their provincial legislature to give them the kind of pay increases that would keep them from migrating to other Canadian provinces or to the United States.

Nurses in Poland clogged the streets of Warsaw and other cities to protest poor pay and working conditions. In 2004 in the Australian state of Victoria, nurses risked going to jail to force the government to uphold legally mandated staffing standards. In France in 2001, nurses took to the streets of Paris militating for better working conditions. Even in Switzerland, a nation that hardly has a reputation for mass demonstrations, thousands of nurses wearing tee shirts emblazoned with the logo "Nurse Power" held a one-day protest asking for greater professional respect and remuneration.

Nurses who belong to unions and walk picket lines or who attend rallies and marches aren't the only ones going "on strike" or mounting protests. Many are members of a silent majority of burnt-out nurses who are protesting the prevailing wage and working conditions. Many are working part-time or as temporary or traveling nurses. Others are finding jobs outside hospitals in areas that remove them from the direct care of the sick. Surveys report that the vast majority of nurses who are still working in direct care are planning to quit within the next two years. In her study of the nursing work force published in *Health Affairs* in 2002, Julie Sochalski reported that eighty-one thousand of those American nurses who were not working in nursing were forty-three or younger. "The most common reasons given for working in other fields were better hours, more rewarding work, and better pay."[6]

Morale among those who remain is so low that it dissuades potential new recruits from entering the profession. Nursing school enrollments steadily declined in the mid to late 1990s. Although they started to rebound in 2003 and 2004, the number of students enrolled doesn't match the number of positions that need to be filled today or in the coming decade. There aren't even enough professors in nursing schools to teach the students that are needed, should the career suddenly become more attractive. But future nurses, like those today, would probably want to leave the bedside as soon as they experience the odds of hospital working conditions. Moreover, many new recruits to nursing exhibit a disdain for bedside nursing work. This significantly complicates the problem of nurse recruitment and suggests that one can have a nursing shortage even if the number of people who receive an RN license increases substantially.

It is now more than official. Everyone agrees, from the hospital CEO and vice president of nursing to the insurance company executive and government bureaucrat: Cassandra was right. There is a serious shortage of nurses, one that will, if it is not systematically addressed, worsen in the

8 coming decades. In fact, the nursing shortage has become a kind of mini-industry. Hospitals claim they are wooing, with every means of seduction at their disposal, the very people—expert experienced RNs—they laid off yesterday. They are also trawling the world to bring immigrant nurses from poorer countries to care for patients in richer ones. High-level summits and commissions meet to solve the "crisis" and to present the latest solution. Media and public-service campaigns have been rolled out, promising to recruit needed nurses. Large medical companies are developing and funding some of these campaigns, and health care foundations are proposing a variety of solutions. State, provincial, and federal governments are passing legislation promising to end the shortage.

Yet, when I talk to veteran nurses, they tell me that things have not changed much for the better in their workplaces. In spite of all the talk about recruitment and retention, hospitals are still restructuring and cutting nursing positions. New nurses say they want out of hospitals, and students insist that they wouldn't think of staying in bedside nursing for more than a few years before they "advance." What is worse, patients are continuing to suffer.

No matter how much public hand-wringing the latest shortage has generated, there seems to be little increase in our understanding of the three urgent questions explored in this book: Why is there an unprecedented nursing crisis? and How do we solve it? How do we change the odds so they work in favor of those delivering care to sick and vulnerable human beings?

Although this book is about the current nursing shortage, it goes beyond this shortfall to look at a long-standing crisis within nursing and to understand how the odds have long been stacked against nursing. Because this crisis and its immediate symptom, the nursing shortage, have such a broad social impact, I invite potential patients and sometime patients to explore its dimensions and causes. Most of my exploration will focus on current conditions for nurses, particularly for those in the United States. Because the nursing crisis is, in fact, global, I will also consider other countries: France, Australia, the United Kingdom, Canada, and the Nordic countries, among others. Because we can't understand the present without understanding the past, I will also briefly explore some critical historical issues, such as the development of nurse-doctor relationships, the religious origins of nursing, and class tensions within the profession. Even in discussions of contemporary issues, I'll refer to how nursing has been—as the academics term it—socially constructed.

The major focus of *Nursing against the Odds* is on conditions that affect the nurse who gives direct care to sick and vulnerable patients. She, or he, may work in a hospital as a traditional bedside nurse, in a rehabilitation or

long-term care facility, in a school or clinic or hospice, or in the home. **9**
This nurse gives direct, hands-on care and her primary mission is the care
of the sick, aging, infirm, vulnerable, and dying patient. Although there
are many people who have the letters *RN* after their names, not all of
them practice nursing, nor do they work in areas that support nursing
practice. I am not therefore going to discuss the problems of the nurse en-
trepreneur, or the so-called nurse lawyer, or the nurse who works in
health policy, or a nurse who is the CEO or COO of a hospital.

Nor will I focus on the many and significant dilemmas of what are
known as advanced practice nurses. I will not discuss the many accomplishments or problems of the nurse practitioners who provide primary
medical services, the nurse midwives who perform routine labor and deliveries and take care of routine problems in women's health, or the nurse
anesthetists who perform 85 percent of anesthesia in the United States.
Rather I am focusing on the nurses who provide direct care to the sick,
aging, chronically ill, and dying, and on those who do the critical work of
teaching and supporting nurses who provide that care.

This shortage is not primarily due to the aging of the work force. Indeed, the aging (the average nurse in America is forty-five years old) is a
symptom of the fact that there is a worldwide shortage of people willing
to put up with the conditions under which they are asked to deliver
hands-on care to the sickest, most vulnerable people in our societies.
They are tired of low pay, of poor working conditions, of doctors who
treat them like handmaids, and of hospitals and other institutions that
view them as cheap and disposable. Many say they also feel attacked or
unsupported by some nurses who are academics and managers and who
claim to be professional leaders but who work in jobs in which they are
constantly asked to "deprofessionalize"—or sometimes even disparage—
bedside nurses and fight against them, not for and with them.

Many nurses are, to use the economist Alfred O. Hirschman's phrase,
using "voice" to protest these developments. They go on strike, attend
rallies, write articles, and petition legislators for comprehensive legislation governing professional standards and behavior. Most of them are,
however, opting for what Hirschman calls "exit."[7] They are voting with
their feet, saying they want out and telling new recruits to the profession
not to come in. As birth rates continue to decline in industrial societies,
with fewer young people available to take care of sicker elderly people,
and with women having many more occupational options, nursing will
have to become a higher-status, higher-paid occupation. But long-
standing relationships and conditions that have shaped the profession,
combined with contemporary changes in health care financing and delivery, will have to be altered if nursing is to become an attractive and satis-

10 fying career in which people are encouraged to stay at the bedside for more than a few years. This means that we will have to understand how the odds have long been stacked against nurses. To do this I will consider a number of questions:

- How do doctors treat nurses, how does the medical profession view nursing, and what is the impact of nurse-physician relationships on nurses' work?
- Does the media capture what nurses really do when they are providing direct care? How are nurses portrayed in the mass media, and how does this influence the public view of nurses?
- How do hospitals and other major employers view nurses, and how is this view reflected in their treatment of nurses in the workplace? Do hospital and health care administrators understand nurses' contribution to the bottom line in heath care, or do they view nurses as self-sacrificing angels of mercy or as something candy stripers do when they move on?

I answer the first set of questions, about the relationships between doctors and nurses and between medicine and nursing, in Part One. Although most members of the public assume that doctors and nurses are all part of the medical system, do medical work, and are thus all in it together when it comes to patient care, nursing and medicine have had a long and troubling relationship. Since the late nineteenth century, doctors have been considered to be the "captain" of the medical ship. But they have made nurses—and sometimes nurses have made themselves—uneasy and sometimes unwelcome sailors on that ship. What doctors have often forgotten is the critical role nurses play in the health care system. Wherever they work, in hospitals or in homes, nurses often collect and interpret the raw data upon which medical diagnoses and treatment and nursing care plans are based. Nurses often administer or monitor medical treatments and chart the process of patients' illnesses and recovery. As Linda Aiken and her colleagues at the University of Pennsylvania have so aptly observed, nurses are the early warning and early intervention system in hospitals and many other health care institutions.

Using their considerable knowledge—and their brains, not just their hearts—they protect patients from the risks and consequences, not only of illness, disability, and infirmity, but also of the treatment of illness. And they protect patients from the risks that occur when illness and vulnerability make it difficult, impossible, or even lethal for patients to perform the activities of daily living, even ordinary acts like breathing, turning, going to the toilet unassisted, coughing, or swallowing. In the process, nurses make sure patients survive not only physically but emotionally, and **11** they help family members cope with their loved ones' illnesses and help them to assist in the process of recovery, coping, healing, or even dying. They are critical clinical educators and play an important role in prevention—helping patients learn to follow treatment regimens safely, to adjust to and recover from illness and disability, and to function in a world that disease and injury may have permanently altered.

Nurses thus follow patients as they pass through the trajectory of illness and its treatment. There are many differences and similarities between the work of doctors and nurses, but one important distinction throws additional light on the metaphor of the ship's captain. Although he doesn't specifically broach the tensions between nursing and medicine, James C. Scott, professor of political science and anthropology at Yale University, distinguishes between the abstract knowledge doctors often amass and the practical knowledge that nurses mobilize. To illuminate how the two kinds of knowledge complement each other, Scott considers the skill it takes to navigate a ship across the ocean and into port. "In seamanship, the difference between the more general knowledge of navigation and the more particular knowledge of piloting is instructive. When a large freighter or passenger liner approaches a major port, the captain typically turns the control of his vessel over to a local pilot, who brings it into the harbor and to its berth. The same procedure is followed when the ship leaves its berth until it is safely out into the sea lanes. This sensible procedure, designed to avoid accidents, reflects the fact that navigation on the open sea (a more 'abstract space') is the more general skill, while piloting a ship through traffic in a particular port is a highly contextual skill. What the pilot knows are local tides and currents along the coast and estuaries, the unique features of local wind and wave patterns, shifting sandbars, unmarked reefs, seasonal changes in microcurrents, local traffic conditions, the daily vagaries of wind patterns off headlands and along straits, how to pilot in these waters at night, not to mention how to bring many different ships safely to berth under variable conditions."[8]

The analogy between piloting and nursing is apt. What the nurse so often does is pilot the patient into the port of health, of coping, of cure—even of death. And this act of piloting takes place over the entire trajectory of illness and recovery. Unfortunately, a broad social failure to understand what nurses do, which is embedded in the medical system, often produces oppressive and dysfunctional nurse-physician relationships. Like a chronic illness, these relationships sap nurses' self-esteem, subject them to disregard, disdain, and outright abuse, aggravate class and status dilemmas inside the profession, and may end up harming vulnerable patients whose lives depend on decent nurse-physician communication and

12   collaboration. Nurses, however, are not victims of mean, callous physicians. They inhabit a system that produces poor nurse-physician relationships and often reinforces and reproduces them through nurses' very efforts to adapt to or even circumvent the limits placed on their personal and professional authority.

Public attitudes and perceptions and the media's portrayal of nursing are shaped by these relationships and by our failure to understand nursing. In Part Two I consider public attitudes—particularly as they are reflected in the media depiction of health care—which, in turn, reinforce nursing's invisibility and make it an unattractive career. As a journalist, it's been fascinating and sometimes infuriating to watch how the media depicts the health care system and the important players in it. To put it simply, doctors are portrayed as the only important players, while nurses are portrayed as little more than animate pieces of medical equipment.

As someone who has reported on nursing for years, I know these societal views firsthand. When people learn that I write about nursing, I am invariably asked, with some surprise, "Oh, I didn't know you were a nurse. Where did you practice nursing?"

What I find intriguing about this question is how nursing-specific it is. In my thirty years as a journalist I've written about coal miners, actors, ballet dancers, lonely people, cult members, rock groupies, and even football and ice hockey players. But no one has ever asked me if I'm a football player, ballet dancer, coal miner, cult member, or even lonely. I can assure you that when journalists tell people they write about medicine, few people ask them whether they are doctors. It's assumed that medicine is a subject that warrants the attention of an outside observer. Not so with nursing. Even nurses who learn I'm writing about their work approach me with wonder and ask me with astonishment why I write books and articles about them.

Their curiosity is understandable. Nurses are almost never covered in major media discussions of health care. The rare exceptions are when nurses go on strike, when there is a nursing shortage, or when a nurse kills or harms a patient. Nurses draw media attention when they walk off the job or when they are incompetent or malicious. All too often reporters, producers, and headline writers rely on shopworn clichés that paint nurses as martyrs, angels, saints, or handmaids who bask in the light of physician accomplishments. Sometimes, like nurse practitioners, they may be covered when they do "medical work" or enter into competition with MDs over medical turf. Nurses, as knowledgeable caregivers for the sick, are rarely covered when they are on the job, and their contributions, whether to the discovery of a miracle cure or to the daily care of patients, are routinely ignored.

A good example of this syndrome is the newspaper crossword puzzle. **13** Newspapers rarely mention nurses in their reports of medical advances, in which RNs play a central role. Yet newspapers frequently stereotype nursing in their crossword puzzles when, for example, they give "RN treatment" as the clue for "TLC."[9]

It's no wonder that polls report that members of the public "trust" nurses and think they're ethical and honest, yet people still don't have a clue what nurses really do and advise teenagers who want a career in health care to go into medicine not nursing.

How nursing is portrayed in the media has significant consequences for our ability to retain and recruit nurses. Some nurses protest that they don't need public recognition. All that does matter, they may tell you, is the gratitude of their patients. But years of invisibility take their toll. When nurses get no positive public credit for their work—and when most of the credit for what are referred to as "positive patient outcomes" goes to doctors—nurses' sense of professional self-worth slowly erodes. When young men and women grow up on a steady diet of medical miracle stories, doctor-focused TV documentaries, sitcoms and prime-time series— as well as movies, plays, novels, and nonfiction—it's hard to convince them that nursing is also a dynamic, interesting, evolving career. More importantly, patients don't know that when they're sick, nursing may be a critical factor in their treatment and recovery.

Nurses' dominance by medicine and their sometimes self-enforced public invisibility makes them particularly easy targets for the third player in this long-running drama—hospitals, which I examine in Part Three. Hospitals and many of the other health care institutions that employ nurses have built on dysfunctional nurse-doctor relationships and nurses' public invisibility and have used nurses as a cheap, disposable labor force. Ever since the professionalization of nursing in the nineteenth century, and probably well before, hospitals have paid nurses as little as possible, viewed physicians as revenue generators and nurses as revenue drains (today, nurses are referred to as "cost-centers"), sheltered or tolerated appalling nurse-physician relationships, and burdened nurses with untenable demands. Hospital administrators, some of them nurses, have accepted traditional female images of altruism and self-sacrifice and defined nursing as charitable devotional work, for which virtue is the primary reward. "And so, dear," some administrators ask nurses, "why are you asking for a raise?"

When nurses began to protest the latest round of layoffs that began in the mid-1990s, I routinely interviewed hospital administrators. "What do nurses want?" they wondered, throwing up their hands. Nurses, they said, are perennially dissatisfied. Nothing ever satisfies them. I beg to differ.

14 Back in the 1980s when I began writing about nursing, I heard a very different story from RNs. Although nurses back then certainly had their complaints, hospitals were trying to woo nurses and turn bedside nursing into a satisfying long-term career. Many hospitals started to give nurses higher pay, better benefits and working conditions, and greater authority and voice.[10] Most of the nurses I talked with during the early part of the decade felt positive about their current work and future prospects.

Enter cost cutting. Responding to pressure from insurers and governments, hospitals began to rescind most of the advances they had made and began to dismantle their nursing departments. Within two or three years the once-great Beth Israel Hospital in Boston—which enjoyed high rates of nurse retention because it was an international Mecca of nursing care and innovation—was transformed into an institution that was hemorrhaging RNs. Imagine then what happened to nurses in hospitals where innovative nursing practice had only just begun to be implemented or where traditional views of nursing had never been challenged.

In this part of the book, I look at the impact of cost cutting on the delivery of nursing care and the nurses who provide it. The experience my friend and I had with nurses who hurried her out of the hospital is all too typical. Under enormous pressure to enhance "throughput"—getting patients into and out of the hospital quickly in order to produce more revenue and reduce expenses—nurses are becoming facilitators of a system whose values they seriously question. Some are protesting and trying to change things for the better. Others adapt. Others want to leave. No matter what path they follow, at some point in a working day spent juggling too many patients who are far too sick, the nurse's capacity for empathy and attention often runs out.

I also explore the impact of cost cutting on the already parlous state of nurse-manager and nurse-doctor relationships. And I examine how hospitals address the nursing shortage. Are their solutions producing a happier work force or one that is more fractured, fragmented, and demoralized than ever?

The main player throughout this book are nurses themselves. How does all this impact the way nurses define themselves, describe and defend their work, and relate to one another? The odds against nurses seem to have produced a persistent and sometimes crippling identity crisis. They are deeply divided about who should be called a nurse, who should be valued and respected as a nurse, how nurses should be educated, paid, and treated, and who should shoulder the ultimate responsibility for hands-on nursing work. These divisions stem from the subjection of nursing to medical and institutional needs but also from tensions between nursing elites who educate or supervise the rank-and-file nurses. Internal tensions are evident in the conflicting solutions to the nursing crisis that elite **15** nurses and rank-and-file nurses propose.

I invite you to follow me as I talk to nurses, analyze their problems, assess popular solutions to the nursing shortage, and ultimately propose some recommendations. But before we begin, I must tell you how I identify people in the book. Because this book is a work of journalism, much of it is based on people's stories. Some of the people I interviewed spoke for attribution, and I refer to them by their real names. Others feared employer or community sanction and would speak only if I changed relevant details and assigned them pseudonyms. These names are indicated by an asterisk at first mention. To offset the conventional assumption that all doctors are men and all nurses women, I sometimes alternate between masculine and feminine pronouns when referring to medical and nursing professionals. Since nursing is still about 95 percent female, however, I often refer to nurses as "she." If a quote or paragraph is not accompanied by a note, the text has been drawn from interview material.

PART ONE

NURSES AND DOCTORS AT WORK

As the daughter of a doctor, I was steeped in the realities of "doctor-nurse relationships" long before I began to view them from the perspective of a journalist. From the time I was a young child in the 1950s, I watched how my father—a well-known ophthalmologist, researcher, and eye surgeon—related to the nurses in his office and at Cornell University Medical School/New York Hospital.

With my attention firmly focused on my father and his physician colleagues, the nurses at New York Hospital seemed always to blend into the background. I remember them as trim women who glided silently by, posture erect, faces stern, dressed in the ubiquitous starched white uniform, wearing stumpy shoes, white hose, and that forbidding yet reassuring white cap. We never mingled with "the nurses." I can't remember if they stood to attention when my father entered the room, but they were definitely not of his status. This message was conveyed by the fact that my father never seemed to greet them or stop to talk to them when I went with him to his office in the hospital. And it was underscored by the fact that, whenever we ate a meal in the hospital, we went directly to the "doctors' only" dining room. Where the nurses ate I have no idea.

When my father moved his office out of the hospital to a space just across York Avenue on Sixty-eighth Street, he of course had a nurse who

18 worked for him—but very definitely not *with* him. "My nurse" was how he referred to her. She was a middle-aged, plump, kindly figure who seemed part secretary, part technical assistant. When I overheard her calling a patient, she would, like my mother—who always introduced herself as Mrs. Dan Gordon—begin the conversation with "Hello, this is Miss Collins, Dr. Gordon's nurse."

When I was a teenager, I used to come into my father's office in Manhattan on Saturday mornings. After waiting while he saw his patients, I would get the ultimate treat—lunch at some fancy New York restaurant. While I waited for my father, I would overhear Miss Collins respond to patients' questions or requests with "I don't know, you'll have to ask the doctor." Hearing that over and over, I absorbed the idea that a nurse was someone whose knowledge was limited and who relied on the doctor, who obviously knew it all. Until I began to write about nursing, I had no idea that Miss Collins might, in fact, have known quite a bit more than I thought she did and that her demurrals were part of a carefully stitched costume she donned to play a particular role in relation to my father.

Almost forty years later, when I first began observing nurses at the Beth Israel Hospital for my book *Life Support*, I was struck by the way doctors treated nurses even in a hospital that purported to be a model of nurse influence and state-of-the-art nurse-physician relationships. Nurses consistently were denied—or denied themselves—opportunities to form productive, constructive professional partnerships with doctors. Unintentionally, physicians sent subtle messages to nurses about who was important in the hospital.

Nurses were regularly kept out of what I've come to think of as the circle of concern that doctors routinely formed as they discussed patients on a floor or unit. Each day on the clinical units, attendings or residents would stand in a circle or semicircle discussing a patient issue. If a physician walked up to the group, the circle would expand and allow him or her to enter. If a nurse walked up to this group, rather than moving out to expand the circle so it could accommodate the nurse, the physicians would continue to talk, ignoring her presence as if she did not exist. If the nurse was a woman and the physicians were women, the circle would often remain as closed as if the physicians were all males. Sometimes, if the nurse was a man (and very few were at that time), it would shift. But even this depended on the particular players, how well they knew one another, and how assertive the male nurse was. Similarly, if the female nurse was particularly assertive, she could force the circle to expand and the physicians to acknowledge her presence and patient concerns. Most often, however, she would stand outside the circle, listen to the conversation the doctors directed, and inject her views from the periphery. Sometimes she would

simply give up and walk away. This image, of doctors talking to one an- **19**
other while the nurse made her comments to their backs, became for me
a symbol of the sorry state of nursing and medical relationships.

I was also struck by the assiduous maintenance of social distance between physicians and nurses. Although the doctor's dining room of my
childhood is largely an artifact of the past, nurses and doctors seem to recreate it in hospital cafeterias all over the world. People who work together on a daily basis on the floors and in the hospital clinics rarely seem
to join one another when they have the time for a quick cup of coffee or
lunch or dinner. In hospital cafeterias, I have watched doctors sit together.
When nurses they knew walked in, they rarely asked them to join the
group. Nor did nurses tend to challenge status hierarchies by joining the
physicians. Watching this go on day after day, I became convinced that it
was a symptom of a larger problem—the professional distance that prevents doctors and nurses from consulting with one another about vital patient care issues.

When it comes to doctor-nurse relationships, what's even more interesting is how nurses themselves have adapted to—and thus reinforce—the
structured inequality of the medical system. After listening to nurses over
the years, I realize that nurse-doctor relationships are a kind of chronic
illness to which the profession may have adapted but which has nonetheless caused persistent dysfunction. Some nurses adjust to these relationships; others find indirect means to resist their imperatives or openly
rebel against them. In any event, no serious discussion of the nursing crisis can ignore the problems that nurses encounter when they work with or
around physicians.

1

Manufacturing the Dominant Doctor

It was the first week in July at the Beth Israel Hospital in Boston and a new crop of interns has just arrived in the teaching hospital. A nurse named Deborah Madison* was taking care of Ella, a forty-two-year-old woman with pancreatic cancer who was about to begin her first round of chemotherapy. Madison had worked on this cancer unit for the past five years. When she examined her patient, she found that Ella was anxious about the chemotherapy and was also in excruciating pain from the cancer.

As Ella's primary nurse, Madison had great deal of experience diagnosing and treating cancer pain. She immediately recognized that Ella needed intravenous morphine to control her suffering. But she worked in a system where doctors—even doctors with as little experience as interns beginning their residency training—were the only ones permitted to diagnose, treat, and prescribe. Indeed, for internal medicine services, newly minted doctors, under the supervision of residents, fellows, and attending physicians, were nominally in charge of hospitalized patients—and also of their nurses.

Reassuring Ella that she would do something to ease her pain, Madison walked down to the nurses' station in search of the intern in charge of the case. The young man, upon whose orders much of her work depended, was in his late twenties, tall, clean-shaven, with close-cropped black hair. He listened as Madison explained the problem and related her treatment recommendation.

* An asterisk following a name indicates a pseudonym.

22   "I don't know," the intern said nervously. "I don't think the patient is really in pain. I think she's just anxious about the chemo she'll be getting tomorrow. I'll write an order for Xanax (a tranquilizer) and that should do it."

Cognizant that she was there not only to care for patients, but also to teach novice physicians, Madison calmly repeated that the patient was having cancer pain. Xanax, while useful to treat any anxiety she might have also been feeling, would not alleviate her cancer pain. Morphine would. The intern, who like many novice physicians was extremely wary of narcotics, resisted the suggestion. No, he said adamantly, adding that he would go and see the patient.

About five minutes later, if that, he returned.

The patient, he informed Madison, was not in pain. It was just as he thought. She was anxious about her chemo.

"Did she say that?" Madison asked.

"No," he said, "the patient complained of pain." "But," he added, as he wrote the order for the Xanax, "she can't really be in pain because people who are in pain don't smile at their doctors."

Although frustrated that this young physician seemed unaware that, as one recent federal report documented, "patients may be experiencing excruciating pain even while smiling and using laughter as coping mechanisms," Madison once again tried to teach the young man about cancer pain as well as patients' responses to vulnerability and dependence.[1] Patients, she counseled, often smile at their doctors and may not be assertive about their complaints, because they don't want to bother, contradict, or potentially alienate someone upon whom they depend for their very lives.

The intern was unmovable.

Over the course of the next two hours, Madison shifted tactics. Following the appropriate channels, she paged the resident who ranked above this intern in the medical chain of command. She would try to convince him to talk to the novice doctor and secure pain medication for her patient. When the resident responded to the page, he agreed with Madison. Morphine was just what the intern should order. The two went off to find the intern and the resident repeated to the young man exactly, almost word for word, what Madison had said about the rationale for this particular choice of drug. Listening to the senior doctor and ignoring the nurse, the intern nodded and dutifully wrote the order for the narcotic.

Madison went back to the patient and told her that the doctor had ordered the drug. She then administered the medication and monitored its effectiveness. Ella was finally able to relax. Although Madison diagnosed the patient's problem and recommended the correct treatment for it, when the interaction was recorded in the patient's chart, the intern was

given credit for both making the diagnosis and ordering the medication. **23**
When Ella was about to leave the hospital several days later, she wrote
notes to thank her caregivers. Although she jotted a short thank-you note
to her nurses, there was no mention of what the nurse did to help relieve
her pain. In fact, she saved most of her gratitude for her doctors. "Thank
you so much," she told the intern, "for all you did for me."

Risky Business

When nurses go to work in a hospital or other health care institution,
they expect to confront a certain number of predictable risks. They may
injure their backs if they try to turn a patient without help, or lift a patient
who's fallen in the cramped space of a hospital bathroom. They may stick
themselves with an infected needle because another hospital worker has
failed to dispose of it correctly or because some hospital administrators do
not purchase safe needles. They may contract a new and mysterious disease like SARS. They may be verbally or physically attacked by a mentally
ill patient who becomes violent or by a patient or family member frustrated with an increasingly impersonal health care system. Through a variety of workplace and legislative measures, nurses try to minimize these
risks.

Other less publicized risks that nurses encounter jeopardize their patients. On a daily basis, nurses work with physicians who fail to communicate with them about critical clinical issues, deny them access to needed
information and resources, subject them to verbal abuse when they try to
do their job, and misinterpret collegial disagreements about clinical issues
as challenges to medical authority and hierarchy. Some physicians rudely
overrule nurses' clinical concerns and subject nurses to verbal abuse and
humiliation. In rarer cases, some physicians physically abuse RNs. Added
to this is the fact that the medical system often gives physicians credit for
nurses' contributions. This means nurses have little experience with positive credit but have a great deal of experience with negative accountability. All of these patterns of communication and behavior make nursing a
very risky job, and not only for the so-called uppity nurse who refuses to
couch her questions and concerns in the demure rituals of medical dominance.

Even nurses who work hard at staying in their assigned place by observing the accepted rules of deference may find that MD-RN relationships can be hazardous to their professional self-esteem, as well as to their
personal health and well-being. The incident I described above, for example, happened at a hospital in which nurses received a great deal of
credit for their work. It occurred during the heyday of nurse empower-

24 ment in the early 1990s. But no matter how much institutional support nurses had—support that has, we shall see, largely disappeared today—they were still stuck in a medical system characterized by rigid inequality. While there is increasing attention to the problem of "disruptive physicians"—who often bully those they consider to be inferiors—little systematic attention is paid to the fact that the medical system as a whole is a disruptive, sometimes toxic environment for many who work in it.

Relationship Interruptus

Over the past thirty years, many articles have been written about this structured inequality. Two of the most famous—"The Doctor-Nurse Game" and "The Doctor-Nurse Game Revisited," published in 1967 and 1990 respectively—were written by the psychiatrist Leonard Stein.[2] The original article analyzed why doctors failed to consult with nurses and why nurses adopted indirect or even passive-aggressive strategies to deal with doctors. Then in 1990, during the last nursing shortage, Stein and two other physicians reexamined the state of nurse-physician relationships. The authors argued that the women's and civil-rights movements had fomented a rebellion among nurses. More nurses, the authors insisted, were socialized outside the old hospital schools, had advanced degrees, and wanted to be viewed as "autonomous," "independent" professionals. The "new" nurse was more than willing to make direct recommendations. In fact, many bluntly challenged physicians. Others exhibited outright hostility to MDs. Some seemed to want to replace physicians and claim, as their own "domain," disease prevention, patient education, management of chronic illness, and holistic care or "treatment of the whole person"—things which doctors should do but too often ignore.

The "Doctor-Nurse Game Revisited" suggested that nurse-physician relationships were improving, because nurses were no longer tolerating medicine's traditional dominance. Twelve years later, however, one of the only systematic, quantitative studies of the impact of physician-nurse relationships on nurse retention painted a much more sobering picture. The principal investigator on the study, which was published in the *American Journal of Nursing*, was Alan H. Rosenstein, a physician and vice president and medical director of the VHA's West Coast hospitals.[3] He and his coinvestigators sent out surveys to RNs and MDs in the VHA, which runs a quarter of the community-owned hospitals in the United States and is the largest employer of RNs in the country. The survey was designed to determine how physicians and nurses in the VHA system "viewed nurse-physician relationships, disruptive physician behavior, the institutional response to such behavior, and how such behavior affected nurse satisfaction, morale, and retention." The article reported on preliminary findings from the first 1,200 responses analyzed. Of these, 720 were from nurses and 173 from physicians from eighty-four different hospitals.

Respondents reported that nurse-physician relationships, which seemed less of an issue to physicians, were extremely important to nurses. Almost all nurses had experienced or witnessed some form of "disruptive physician behavior," which included screaming, berating of colleagues or patients, use of abusive language, and other instances of disrespect or condescension toward nurse colleagues. Nurses believed that disruptive physician behavior had a serious impact on morale and nurse retention. Many respondents cited examples of nurses who had, because of such problems, left a hospital or asked to be switched from a unit or shift because of them. Nurses also felt that physicians did not give them enough respect or understand the impact of their behavior. Most nurses stated that their institution did not deal effectively with the problem.

The psychologist Larry Harmon is the codirector of the Physicians' Development Program in Miami, which evaluates, educates, and monitors physicians and nurses and other health care providers. Harmon defines "disruptive behavior" as "any behavior which results in diminishing team members' ability to do their best work." He classifies such behavior as verbal, physical, and indirect behavior.

"Disruptive verbal behavior," Harmon explains, "includes sarcastic comments, snapping at others when frustrated, or talking down to people. Physical disruption occurs when doctors throw small objects when angry, raise their fists at someone, give someone the finger, or actually strike or assault someone." Indirect disruptive behavior includes things like criticizing people behind their back, spreading rumors, or pouting or intentional selective ignoring. "For example," Harmon says, "the physician won't talk to one particular nurse as a way of punishing him or her."

This kind of behavior has become such a problem that, in its 2002 alert about the nursing shortage, the Joint Commission on the Accreditation of Health Care Organizations (JCAHCO) also raised the issue of nurse-physician relationships. "Incidents of verbal abuse of nurses, typically by physicians, are unfortunately well known, even commonplace," the report stated.[4] It called for a voluntary policy of zero tolerance in the workplace and suggested that medical societies develop guidelines to deal with abusive physicians.

In Canada, the Status of Women Sector of the Quebec Federation of Nurses conducted research to ascertain the level of violence against nurses in Quebec. Nurses told of being humiliated, screamed at, and subjected to temper tantrums as well as physical abuse. Ninety percent of the

26 union's members said they'd been "victims of at least one act of assault or aggression during their career."[5] Among abusers of nurses, doctors figured prominently. The number of incidents, the union said, indicated "that doctors can express their anger against their closest workers as they see fit."[6]

In my interviews with nurses, their most common complaints were that physicians do not understand what role nurses play in the health care system, misunderstand whom nurses serve, do not value the knowledge and skill that nurses have amassed during their careers, and fail to appreciate that collaborative, cooperative, collegial relationships between physicians and nurses are central to quality patient care. Most nurses feel that although nurses work closely with doctors and respect their training, skill, and expertise, doctors do not reciprocate.

In his study of the hospital workplace, the sociologist Daniel Chambliss recorded similar complaints. "If there is a single dominant theme of nurses' complaints about their work, it is the lack of respect they feel, from laypersons, from coworkers, and especially from physicians. It is nearly universally felt and resented. 'The docs never listen to us,' they say, 'you don't get any recognition from doctors'; doctors don't read the nurse's notes in the patients' chart, don't ask her what she has seen or what she thinks, they don't take her seriously." Chambliss, who spent over ten years observing nurses and physicians interact, agreed with the nurses. The "daily evidence" of physician disregard, he wrote, was "truly pervasive; I was genuinely surprised at how common the obvious disrespect is."[7]

When I was recently in Adelaide, Australia, a nurse manager of a cardiac unit related an illustrative incident. Because of the closure of an oncology service in the area, cardiac nurses were being asked to treat oncology patients at a cardiac unit that was being prepared to take on an extra load of cancer patients. The nurses were given a quick course to teach them how to deal with oncology patients. Before their hasty tutorial was even complete, an oncologist in the hospital admitted a patient to the unit. When the nurse manager told the physician that the RNs didn't yet know how to deal with chemotherapy drugs, and had not mastered the complexities of inserting needles into porta catheters (devices that are surgically inserted into the subclavian vein to allow easier, and over time less painful, access for chemotherapy and blood tests), he became irate. No oncologist would ever imagine that a cardiologist could simply stroll in and replace him. Nonetheless, this physician insisted that a cardiac nurse could easily replace an oncology nurse. "Surely someone around here can manage this. You are nurses after all," he fumed.

See One, Do One, Teach One

In medical schools, doctors in training are taught to do procedures through the process of "see one, do one, teach one." That also seems to be the way novice physicians are taught to look down on nurses. Listen to John E. Heffner, MD, medical director of the Medical University of South Carolina, "complimenting" nurses in the introduction he wrote in 2002 to a brochure about nursing that the hospital distributed for Nurses Week:

"We physicians at MUSC have much to appreciate in working with our nursing staff. Nurses amplify by their extended bedside presence the value of our brief daily patient encounters. The expertise and personal touch of our nurses drive much of the community's perception of our health care facilities. And the vigilance and judgment of our nurses permit us to travel to our daily duties yet still respond to any sudden clinical event."[8]

One hopes that nurses can recognize whether a doctor is competent or not before they "amplify" his actions. Imagine, for example, what would have happened to the cancer patient we met at the beginning of this chapter had her nurse "amplified" the inexperience of the intern.

In the eyes of many physicians, the title "Registered Nurse" often diminishes the bearer. Even the RN who graduates from a top program or who has a list of initials trailing her name is defined as someone who is not a member of the medical club, who does not have much medical knowledge, and whose concerns can be discounted because she doesn't know medicine. Denise Webster, in her 1985 study of medical students' views about nurses, writes that "one of the challenges facing medical students entering the clinical phase of their education is to ascertain who does what. As the role of the physician became narrower and more specific in the student's mind, i.e., the diagnosis and treatment of illness, the answer regarding the nurse's role became no clearer as a consequence of exposure to nurses and nursing in clinical settings." Webster explained that few medical students had "an awareness that nurses had legitimate roles that were independent of physician's orders and expectations."[9] "Many doctors (and many nurses)," Daniel Chambliss writes, "regard nursing as a sort of 'lesser' medicine, with the subordination of nursing dictated by the shorter period of training."[10]

Laurie Gottlieb, a nurse who holds a PhD and is a former director of the McGill School of Nursing, once told me an illustrative story. A physician with whom she worked complimented her on her skill and knowledge by exclaiming, "You're so smart. You could be a doctor." For him,

28 this was the highest compliment he could bestow. For her, it reflected his disdain for nursing. It would be like a male colleague telling her, "You're so smart. You could be a man."

Even male nurses are subject to this kind of disregard. As Dave Latham* explains, "No matter how much experience a nurse has, doctors still consider us to be second-class citizens." The doctors' attitude, says Latham, a nurse in Illinois, is: "I have a medical degree and you don't."

Where and how do doctors learn to devalue nurses and nursing? Is it in the classroom, in their apprenticeship training, or both? More than most professionals, doctors gain a sense of professional self (and self-regard) during a protracted period of apprenticeship training.[11] The first two years of their schooling is spent in the classroom. In the past, schools of medicine rarely mentioned the role of the nurse in classroom training. Today some schools of medicine invite the occasional nurse in to give a lecture to medical students. But most younger doctors report that they learned next to nothing about nurses during their medical school years. Few medical students are taught alongside nursing students. Most don't know about the various kinds of nurses, nursing programs, or nursing research as a field.

After the first two years of medical school, doctors-in-training spend little time in formal classroom work. In their third year, medical students move directly onto hospital wards. Once they graduate from medical school, they spend between three and six years (or sometimes more) as residents in internal medicine, surgery, pediatrics, or psychiatry. Doctors who choose to specialize further will extend their training in, say, oncology, vascular surgery, pediatric cardiac surgery, pediatric psychiatry, or endocrinology.

Throughout their years on the wards, doctors attend daily lectures and study a great deal to pass a variety of exams. But most of their years in training are spent in a system in which they are mentored by older, more experienced physicians. "Tribalism is encouraged," write D. C. Aron and L. A. Headrick, "by the apprenticeship style of medical education in which students learn to be doctors as part of tightly knit physician teams, especially in the hospital."[12]

During their long training, what doctors learn about nurses—or for that matter about most other members of health care "teams"—is shaped by the behavior and attitudes of their seniors and mentors. Some of these mentors are residents who have only a few more years on the job than they have. Some are attending physicians who are vastly more experienced and who clearly convey that the physician is the captain of the ship.

"In medical training," says Dr. Timothy McCall a forty-seven-year-old internist, journalist, and author of *Examining Your Doctor: A Patient's Guide to Avoiding Harmful Medical Care,* "most of the socialization of the doctor **29** happens between the cracks in the third and fourth year and beyond, when you come into contact with clinicians in the university teaching hospital. That's when the values carefully inculcated in you by your well-meaning public health professor in the first two years are basically blown off in five minutes. In the first couple of years you learn that primary care and prevention are important, for example. Then when you get into third year, you are surrounded by specialists and you learn what they think of primary care and prevention. Which is not much."

"There is no formal training for medical students on how to interact with other medical professionals," writes Robert C. McKersie, a Chicago family physician who recently finished his training. "How doctors relate to and interact with nurses, nutritionists, other members of the medical team, and even patients, is learned by following the example of the senior residents and attending physicians. Medicine has a strict pecking order, in which one does not question superiors even if they have been disrespectful to a patient or a fellow health care worker. This system often leaves the more sensitive and caring medical students and residents feeling that they are in the minority and powerless."[13]

Senior doctors may never specifically tell medical students, interns, and residents that nurses are their inferiors. But by innuendo or example they are taught that most nurses are probably not that bright to begin with, are minimally educated, and are meant to work for doctors and make it easier for them to take care of patients.

When she was still an intern at Lincoln Hospital in the Bronx, says Alice Rothchild, she and her fellow trainees were taught nothing about nurses and had little or no significant contact with bedside nurses. Dr. Rothchild is now a fifty-five-year-old obstetrician/gynecologist at Boston's Beth Israel Deaconess Medical Center. "We went on rounds with the chief resident," Rothchild recalls. "Residents would present each case. The head nurse would follow us and then stand at the back of the cluster taking notes on medical changes and orders."

"If a nurse asked a clarifying question, it was just background noise," Rothchild says. "It didn't reflect her curiosity, her need to do her job. She was asking a question to help us do our jobs by better following our orders. The nurse was not viewed as someone who had important information about a patient, but as a scribe whose job was to take notes."

In my book *Life Support,* I borrowed Lillian Rubin's term "intimate strangers" to describe the relationships between most doctors and nurses.[14] The parallel universes that doctors and nurses have long inhabited make it difficult for doctors to see nurses work. "What nurses did," Rothchild says, "was pretty much a mystery. You wrote the orders, and

30 then they happened. But how did they happen? We didn't think about that. You don't think about whether nurses are thinking about their work as opposed to just doing it. The reigning idea was that the doctor understood what was going on and the nurses just did a bunch of pretty mindless tasks."

"Nurses were, in some ways, below notice," agrees Emily Lowry, a fifty-six-year-old internist. "When nurses were good and helpful, they were like a good tool or a sharp pencil. When they were bad, or made a mistake, they were a nuisance. But nobody would try to figure out why. They were just there. They either gave you a hard time or helped you out. You, as the doctor, were what mattered. Nurses were there to maintain the *doctor's* orders, or to carry out *your* plans."

"Most medical students are simply thrown on to the floors with no explanation about the other clinicians they will be working with," says Margo Woods, a nutritionist and researcher who teaches medical students, interns, and residents at Tufts Medical School. "Medical training is extremely unsupportive," she continues. "The doctor-in-training quickly learns that he or she is constantly being judged. He quickly learns never to put himself in a one-down position by admitting that he is insecure about his knowledge or that he does not know something." Physicians, she says, are discouraged from asking for help, because they are reluctant to admit to feelings of insecurity or vulnerability, or to expose gaps in their knowledge. This will make doctors even unwilling to listen to or attend to nurses.

In some medical schools and hospitals, medical students or interns are told that nurses can be useful assets in their education and that they may actually learn something from nurses. But again, this depends on the mentor. A female resident at Boston Children's Hospital told me she didn't learn anything about nurses during her years at Harvard Medical School. In her residency, she picked things up as she went along. She learned that there is a nursing hierarchy, that there is such a thing as nursing research, and that nurses too had their specialties. Because the resident who mentored her told her never to see patients without stopping in and checking with the nurse who was taking care of them, she did what she'd been advised to do and always talked to the nurses. From the nurses' reactions, she learned that this practice was unusual. "You're practically the only one who consults with us," they told her.

Most of the physicians in training I have interviewed tended to define the nurse in negative terms. "If you're not nice to the nurse, she can make your life hell." "Better not get in bad with the nurses, they can be a real pain if you do." This negative description reflects not only a view of the subordinate as a potential problem but also a view about how subordinates are likely to feel about their subordination. Nurses may not appreciate that they are expected to train doctors how to be their superiors, and some may respond in a passive-aggressive manner, which of course just reproduces the cycle of dysfunction.

"One of the things that happens when interns are introduced to a rotation in our hospital is they're warned about rotations when nurses are tough on them," explains Bonnie O'Connor, an associate professor and researcher in the Department of Pediatrics at Brown Medical School / Rhode Island Hospital and a folklorist and ethnographer who has worked in medical education for fifteen years. "Interns can't understand why this would be. What they don't understand is that experienced nurses are supposed to put up with the fact that interns slow up the process of care, that they're clumsy, and that they have authority over a nurse with years of experience."

These tensions are an inevitable result of working in a teaching hospital where you are confronted by a constantly revolving set of learners. But for nurses these tensions are different from the ones physicians encounter. Unlike physicians who teach new classes of medical students, nurses don't get paid to teach medical students and residents. Their teaching load is usually not factored into their patient load, and they get little recognition and no status as teachers in a teaching hospital. In spite of the fact that they constantly teach doctors-in-training, there is no formal acknowledgment of this fact. Quite to the contrary, doctors-in-training are usually not taught to view the nurses as formal or even informal instructors. Instead, as we've seen, they're generally taught to worry about how hard nurses will be on them. For most doctors, the teaching hospital has one set of teachers and one set of learners—physicians. Most physicians are unaware that nurses also learn in teaching hospitals.

Several years ago, I gave a workshop for nurses at the McGill University Health Center. Several of the RNs from one of the MUHC hospitals were frustrated because they constantly had to explain what they did to each individual intern or resident who rotated into their unit. To simplify their working lives, they decided to write a description of their role in caring for patients and helping to teach doctors-in-training. The material never saw the light of day. The nurses said the physicians in charge of the unit wouldn't let the nurses print and distribute it. Nurses, they seemed to feel, should not have the temerity to teach doctors-in-training.

Rather than teach residents, nurses are constantly asked to reproduce their own subordination to each new generation of doctors. Listen to conversations that veteran nurses have with junior doctors and you con-

32 stantly hear them list a set of signs and symptoms in catalogue fashion and then ask the doctor, "What do you think?" "What do you want to do about this?" "Would you like to get this or that lab test?"

The nurse may know what's wrong and what to do about it. Yet, year after year, she's supposed to teach interns and residents how to exert their authority in spite of their lack of knowledge. Not surprisingly, given their socialization, many doctors ignore nurses' concerns. They may even fail to read the nurses' notes, which form a critical part of the chronology of the patient's progress as recorded in the patient's chart.

The Issue of Nurses' Notes

"Did I read nurses' notes when I was in medical school or training? I'm not sure I even knew they existed or if they were even in the charts," says Rothchild. And McCall confesses that "of course we were never taught to read nurses' notes. I don't even remember if they were written in the charts in my years of training. But even when I did read them, I was always struck by how silly they seemed." McCall says that if, by some accident, he found himself reading a nursing note, he like many other physicians found them a baffling, incomprehensible, and sometimes ridiculous parody of the physician's progress notes. Nurses would use terms like "alteration in skin condition, and alteration in bowel function." They would mobilize complex circumlocutions that would, in his view, dance around the problem rather than define it. This simply confirmed the doctor's view that nurses and their notes had nothing to add to the clinical picture.

Mardge Cohen, an attending physician and director of Women's HIV Research at Cook County Hospital in Chicago, explains her frustration with how nurses in her institution write their notes in the patient charts. "We say a patient has congestive heart failure. In our progress notes—or SOAP (Subjective, Objective, Assessment, Plan) notes—we document that the subjective phenomenon is that the patient complains of shortness of breath. The objective phenomena we collect include vital signs, like the results of a chest X ray or lung exam on which rales were found. Then comes the assessment, which is that CHF is still present, exacerbated, or worsening, and the plan is that we will say, 'increase diuretics or search for other reasons for the decompensation.'"

Rather than connecting her activities or concerns to the medical diagnosis, Cohen says that, no matter what the medical diagnosis or patient's condition, nurses always write notes on two categories: injury prevention and knowledge deficit. "This just appeared a few years ago. It seems incomprehensible to me or not particularly helpful. The patient may be in a coma and the nurse is told to talk about 'knowledge deficits.'"

Cohen says she understands that nurses need to be able to discuss what **33** they do and chart their contributions to care, but she feels that this particular way of doing it does not allow the physician or other members of the team to understand what the patient is experiencing, what the nurse is concluding, or what the nurse is encountering in dealing with the patient. "We obviously need a way to communicate with one another, but if this kind of charting makes doctors not want to read the nurses' notes, I don't think this is the right way."

What many modern doctors find so baffling is the "nursing diagnosis." As we'll see in a later chapter, nurses have been, in their view, chained to medicine, medicine's descriptions of diseases, and medical orders, while feeling simultaneously restricted in their use of the language of medical diagnosis and opinion. Like other oppressed groups, they have struggled to find a way to communicate to one another and to explain the work they do. Nursing diagnosis, which was developed in the 1950s, was their attempt to professionalize and liberate themselves from these peculiar restrictions and give language to their work. In modern systems of financial reimbursement, doctors, for example, have numerous descriptions of their treatments and procedures, which are then translated into health insurance billing codes. Nursing activities have been bundled with the sheets and blankets in a patient's room charge. Nursing diagnosis, many academic nurses believe, allows them to describe their specific contributions and activities. Doctors find some of this language confusing. Nurses, as they see it, are trying to say or describe the same things doctors say and describe, but in an unnecessarily roundabout way.

"You have a conversation with a nurse that's great, and then you look at the nurse's note and all you can get out of it are the vital signs or things like 'alteration in comfort,'" says Emily Lowry. "But of course the nurse doesn't say that in conversation to you. They say, 'He hasn't had a bowel movement in three days,' 'He's not eating,' or 'His wife is sick,' and then you look at the note in the chart and it says 'alteration in nutrition,' . . . and it doesn't say anything useful except for the vital signs."

Dress and Address

Nursing's subordination to medicine is also reflected in modern modes of address. Linguists, anthropologists, and sociologists who study power and authority in the modern workplace and in relationships of dominance and subordination have developed a sophisticated analysis of how "discourse" reflects either power or solidarity. "The key to power is asymmetry," writes Deborah Tannen. "Power governs asymmetrical relationships where one is subordinate to another; solidarity governs symmetrical rela-

34 tionships characterized by social equality and similarity." In many languages power and deference are embedded in forms of address, notably in the use of personal pronouns, like the French *tu* and *vous* or German *Sie* and *Du*. "In English the closest parallel is to be found in forms of address: first name versus title-last name," Tannen writes. "In Brown and Gilman's system, power is associated with nonreciprocal use of pronouns; in English the parallel would be a situation in which one speaker addresses the other by first name but is addressed by title-last name."[15]

This is precisely what occurs in medicine. In many modern workplaces, differences of power are muted by the fact that workers, even of different social classes and professional categories, tend to be on a first-name basis and remain so when people from outside their workplace enter it. Medicine is an exception to the increasing informality and egalitarianism of modern culture. When they talk to nurses, many physicians tend to call RNs by their first names, while they expect to be addressed by their last name and title, as in "Hello, Jane. I'm Dr. Smith. Would you hand me the patient's chart?" Nurses are expected to refer to physicians as "Dr. Smith" while they introduce themselves as "Joan" or "Jim."

Of course, a nurse and a physician may be on a first-name basis. But in the presence of a patient, the same doctor will usually expect that a nurse will refer to him as "Doctor—." He will continue to refer to the nurse by her or his first name.[16] In some countries, like France, doctors use similar means to assert even more authority over the nurse. Though they may use the formal pronoun when talking to the nurse, they will call her by her first name, while they are called by their last name and title.

Dress is another workplace "language" and similarly indicates power or solidarity. In her book *Of Two Minds*, the anthropologist T. M. Luhrmann explains that modes of dress are very important to doctors. Doctors want to signal unambiguously that they are not nurses. "Every hospital I was in had an implicit dress code in which doctors looked like one another and emphatically not like the nurses."[17] To indicate the fact, physicians in the medical workplace usually dress in business clothes, sometimes protected by a long lab coat, or in the case of the doctor-in-training by a short white coat. Surgeons wear dark-colored scrubs (so do surgical nurses). In the past, nurses dressed for status as well as comfort with the starched white uniform and cap. Today, physicians still dress for status as well as easy identification, while nurses have jettisoned the starched whites for—well, anything goes. Particularly in North America, nurses today tend to dress in pajama-like outfits with heart, flower, and angel designs or in pastels. Only nurse practitioners, clinical specialists, or other advanced practice nurses routinely don white lab coats. In fact, since nonnursing personnel also wear the same kind of outfits as bedside nurses, it is often hard to tell by dress alone who is a nurse. Nurses blend into an undifferentiated mass of people whose outfits signal an asymmetrical power relationship with **35** wearers of lab coats or business suits.

As a rule, deference and subordination lead people to overlook the concerns of others and even to justify abusing them physically or verbally. This is true in medicine. "You watched older doctors scream and yell at nurses, and it was pretty appalling," says Alice Rothchild. "When we were in surgery, a few doctors threw things at medical students and at nurses. There were a lot of compassionate docs but there were also the yellers in the ORs and on the floors. They yelled at med students and at nurses. That was the way doctors had been taught to express authority—to yell at people below them. It's part of the pathology of the system."

Doctors who verbally abuse subordinates often do so because a system in which they are superiors and nurses subordinates allows doctors to avoid accountability. If a nurse makes a mistake and the physician yells at her, this behavior may be reinforced if the nurse doesn't complain, as Larry Harmon explains. "If a physician yells at a nurse because she makes a mistake and then no mistakes occur for a month, then that's reinforcing. The physician unconsciously feels, 'Well, if I yell, that will improve behavior.'" As Harmon observes, some of the most disruptive physicians are highly perfectionistic, which adds to the pattern of abuse. "Some physicians demand the best. They want the best. But they may be so overextended that they don't have the time or communication skills to express their expectations clearly. As a result they feel an omnipotence that enables them to expect something without communicating it. When they don't get it, because they're very high-strung, they overreact."

If the physician uses verbal abuse as a tension-releasing strategy, this pattern of behavior may be similarly reinforced. The doctor feels stressed. She yells at a nurse. He doesn't complain—which means the doctor doesn't have to deal with the added stress of responding to that complaint. The hospital doesn't act to curb the behavior. So the physician feels his tactics worked: "I got it off my chest. It felt good." Harmon continues, "Many physicians do feel guilty, but they're on to the next thing. They may never get around to expressing their regrets to the nurse."

On the other hand, some doctors are unable to apologize for their disruptive behavior because they are emotionally incapable of taking responsibility for their conduct. They have, as Harmon puts it, no self-insight. "All they focus on is the mistake the nurse made, not the way they reacted to it," Harmon says. "Their attitude is 'she made me do it. I would never have done that if she had filled my request properly.' This is the response of the typical batterer: 'she drove me to it.'"

Whether doctors abuse nurses because they are too stressed, are too perfectionistic, or have more serious emotional problems, their behavior is aided and abetted by institutional attitudes and assumptions. Doctors

36 often get away with abuse because, Harmon explains, "the most disruptive physicians are sometimes the best and the brightest. They're hardworking. They're high-volume and high-revenue producers and they're highly perfectionistic and high stress, which often comprises the profile of a disruptive physician. Physicians enjoy a unique role in that they don't often work for the hospital, so they have no direct boss to reprimand them."

By failing to reduce the long workdays of medical training, hospitals have encouraged the doctors' tendency to berate or belittle. Chronic sleep deprivation makes matters much worse. Physicians-in-training have been traditionally used as cheap hospital labor and worked nearly to death—between eighty and a hundred hours per week. Timothy McCall wrote an important early article on the impact of resident hours on quality of care. He referred to the case of patient Libby Zion, who died in a New York hospital. A grand jury investigating the case found that long resident hours were involved.[18] A number of studies on sleep deprivation in medical training have documented that it "has a significant effect on human functioning."[19] While there seems to be some debate about whether and how chronic sleep deprivation affects the actual performance of physicians' work, there is little debate about the fact that it severely affects their moods.[20] Chronic sleep deprivation makes them irritable, angry, and resentful.

Some doctors-in-training understandably develop a sense of entitlement. They must give up a normal life for years, often postponing marriage and family; they end up saddled with huge medical school debts that delay their ability to enjoy their earning potential; and they are often screamed at and abused by their physician mentors. "Doctors go through this terrible training," McCall explains, "and cope with a great deal of insecurity. Many doctors end up feeling like everybody owes them something. The public owes them a very good living, their patients owe them respect and deference, and nurses owe them obedience and assistance and should tolerate their outbursts."

Painful as it is, the hazing period the doctor-in-training is expected to endure has a definite end point. Once the boot camp of residency is over, the apprentice doctor who was ritually abused can look forward to freedom from such abuse. Or, like some abused children, he can in turn become an abuser.

Health Care Team—"Plus ça change . . ."

Today the metaphor of the captain of the ship is increasingly being supplemented by the more fashionable notion of the physician as leader of the "interdisciplinary health care team." The problem is that doctors are not taught how to work in teams or manage them. "Doctors are now taught a bit about how to cooperate more with other doctors. Which is an important step forward," says Margo Woods, speaking from long experience. "As for interdisciplinary teamwork, there is little practice in this." Doctors are also taught more about patient communication. But communication instruction tends to focus on dyads—doctor-doctor, doctor-patient—not on members of the health care team.

International studies of medical errors and injuries in various health care systems point to a medical culture in which rigid hierarchies, fear of vulnerability, and the lack of understanding of the interdependent nature of patient care make effective team work and communication difficult. "Few newly qualified physicians have the skills necessary to improve care and patient safety," D. C. Aron and L. A. Headrick write. "These include the ability to perceive and work effectively in interdependencies; the ability to understand work as a process; skill in collecting, aggregating, analyzing, and displaying data on processes and outcomes of care; skills in designing healthcare processes; the ability to work in teams and in collaboration with managers and patients; and the willingness to examine honestly and learn from mistakes."[21]

There is even less incentive for doctors to collaborate with nurses, whom they consider to have an inferior education. "Doctors simply never learn how to say to someone—like a nurse—'Have you noticed anything that would be pertinent to this problem?'" Woods elaborates: "They don't learn how to say, 'What do you think about this? I'm thinking about doing such and such?' If doctors have a hard time doing this with other doctors, then to admit gaps in knowledge or really consult with people like nurses, whom they think of as subordinates, is positively embarrassing."

Since conflicts between team members have usually been resolved by a doctor giving an order that a nurse is supposed to obey, doctors acquire little skill in negotiating or consulting with nurses. When I asked the resident at Children's Hospital how she was taught to deal with conflicts that arise between nurses and physicians, she said that she received no training at all. Medical training, she said, didn't teach people how to handle conflict. The young woman also added that during training, health care professionals are rarely complimented for their successes and mastery. It's just assumed that you'll do it right, she said. So when you do it right, no one praises you.

When members of the University of Texas Human Factors Research Project compared physicians and airline pilots in their study of medical errors and injuries, they noted how socialization of workers can affect teamwork. Pilots—hardly known as a group of sensitive New Age guys—

38 have been recently taught to view their own work realistically and genuine teamwork favorably. They were, for example, far less likely to deny weakness (the effect of fatigue, stress, or personal problems on performance) than were surgeons and anesthetists. "Most pilots (97%) and intensive care staff (94%) rejected steep hierarchies (in which senior team members are not open to input from junior members), but only 55% of consultant surgeons rejected such hierarchies." Surgical nurses, anesthetic nurses, and anesthetic residents gave their teams rather poor scores for teamwork. On the other hand, surgeons and surgical residents rated their teams very highly. Not surprisingly then, 70 percent of the respondents in the study "did not agree that junior team members should not question the decisions made by senior team members." Consultant or attending surgeons were the least likely to tolerate real intrateam discussion around critical issues or disagreements.[22]

Bonnie O'Connor describes a common attitude: "When it comes to collaboration, doctors tend to view collaboration as 'Why don't you come over to my house and see what I'm doing? Then we'll work together.' It's not seen as 'Why don't I come and spend some time in your neighborhood and see what I can learn there?' The assumption is that there's nothing of interest to the physician going on in your neighborhood or that what is going on is wrong."

The definition of teamwork, O'Connor elaborates, is very medicocentric. O'Connor, who proudly calls herself a "card-carrying pluralist," believes that to have a real team people must value each other's independent contributions and recognize that the team has an identity of its own. "This doesn't mean that everyone can do surgery, or have the skills a nurse has to help a patient recover, or the social worker has to do discharge planning. It does mean that people recognize that the whole is greater than the sum of its parts and does not exist to support just one of its players—that is, the physician."

Today, changes in the health care environment may actually be making physicians less eager to participate as members on a team in which they share knowledge and control. "I notice a lot of resistance and defensiveness about interdisciplinary teamwork among doctors today," O'Connor notes. "Physicians feel very assailed by nonphysicians and even nonclinicians. There are now patient activist movements. Ethicists are trying to tell them what to do. So are hospital and insurance company administrators, who are business people. People like me are coming in and saying: Here's how you pay attention to cultural stuff. You're not doing it right, here's how to do it. So there's a lot of discomfort about being on an interdisciplinary team without asserting that the physician is going to be the boss."

"Because doctors are always operating on the edge of their knowledge," says Woods, "they become very uncomfortable venturing into unfamiliar territory. They don't have enough information about what the different members of the team know and do. If something another member of the team recommends doesn't work right away, the doctor's tendency is not to find out why, but just to cut them out of the loop. Whether it is discussing a patient's nutritional status or wishes at the end of life, the doctor has neither the time nor training to deal, nor does he or she learn the psychological or communication skill to deal with these things, so what happens is it simply doesn't get done, or is done poorly."

This is a particularly acute problem in the area of palliative and end-of-life care. When patients are not doing well and it is time to initiate DNR (Do Not Resuscitate) orders or discuss palliative care, nurses are often the ones with a more accurate read on patients' and families' willingness or ability to confront these issues. They may also have valuable insights about the clinical appropriateness of discontinuing treatment or shifting to more aggressive pain and symptom control. Doctors, on the other hand, may be reluctant to stop futile aggressive treatment, tend not to be well schooled in conducting discussions with patients, and are not well remunerated for taking the time to do so. Doctors, in the United States at least, are paid for performing procedures on patients, not spending hours explaining the ins and outs of palliative care and how to manage chronic illness.

Nurses may be in an optimal position to confront these issues and hold such discussions with patients and families. But to discuss these matters is to step on the treacherous territory of patient prognosis. "It all goes back to power and authority," says Cynda Rushton, assistant professor at the Johns Hopkins School of Nursing and an expert in pediatric palliative care. "It has been one of the sacred cows of medicine that physicians own the patient's prognosis and that 'medical' judgment is the only judgment that counts in this area."

In 1995 the *Journal of the American Medical Association* (*JAMA*) documented the extent of the problem of nurse-physician communication around end-of-life care in a highly publicized study of patients' suffering at the end of life.[23] To help patients die with less aggressive treatment and in greater comfort, doctors were provided with up-to-date information on patient prognoses. Expert nurses communicated with patients and families and relayed information about patient wishes to physicians, and great attention was paid to pain control. Yet the results were abysmal. Physicians did not understand or heed patient's wishes or nurses' concerns, and too many patients spent too much time in ICUs, and too many died in pain. In media interviews following the release of the study, and in

40 a *JAMA* editorial by Dr. Bernard Lo,[24] none of the physician commentators talked about the problem of physician-nurse communication, which was, in fact, one of the major problems uncovered in the study. Instead they focused almost exclusively on doctor-patient communication, which can't really be remedied if doctors won't listen to nurses who are trying to convey important patient information to them.

Eight years after that study, too little has changed. Nurses, Rushton says, still get a lot of "negative responses when they even venture tentatively into that area [communicating with patients and doctors]. I've seen some really ugly encounters, where the doctor will become very emotional and really threaten the nurse. 'I'm going to take you off this case.' 'I don't want you talking to my patient.' 'You have no role to play here.' Sometimes, it borders on verbal abuse," Rushton adds.

If doctors spent more time meeting with nurses, all those involved in a patient's treatment might share similar views about its potential course and outcome. That doctors don't take that time—and increasingly, in the world of managed care and cost cutting, don't have much time to spend with either patients or nurses—means that nurses risk rebuke if they talk to patients about pain and symptom management or other aspects of their condition. This is a particular problem for nurses trying to do end-of-life care, because they feel that many doctors want to *own* the patient's prognosis. Such an attitude makes it difficult for nurses to initiate conversations about the patient's wishes and to effectively manage their pain and symptoms. As Aron and Headrick put it, "Improvement in health care delivery (even one's own practice) is almost always an interdisciplinary process, requiring the expertise and collaboration of everyone who works in the system to be redesigned. The professionals involved must be ready to contribute their own knowledge and skills and be willing to learn from the expertise of others."[25]

Teamwork, thus defined, requires spending time and energy to meet with others on the health care team. Just as doctors take little time to consult informally with nurses to clarify issues or work through differing opinions, they don't tend to take the time to meet formally with the team.

Ten years ago, when I observed doctors and nurses at the hematology/oncology clinic at the Beth Israel Hospital, they seemed to communicate in what I've come to think of as hit-and-run conversations. They would talk briefly before going into an exam room or when exiting. They would converse during a patient meeting. Doctors would meet with doctors to discuss clinical issues. Nurses would meet with nurses. Nurses and social workers also set aside time each week to meet and talk about patients. Apart from their conversations on the fly, doctors, nurses, and social workers never met together. When I asked a physician friend who still works in the clinic if things had changed in the past ten years, he told me **41** that, unfortunately, they had not.

Although they are involved in surgeries and have insights into surgical mishaps, nurses are often excluded from one of the most venerable traditions in medicine, the morbidity and mortality conference, or M&M. In teaching hospitals, this is when surgeons conduct a weekly review of mistakes made in the operating theater. The problem with these discussions is that they include only one set of the players, the physicians.[26]

"Discussions in the M&M conference can be very direct," says Robert M. Wachter, professor of medicine and epidemiology and associate chair of the Department of Medicine at the UCSF Medical Center, "but part of the problem is that there aren't the other people in the room who need to understand these problems and need to make necessary changes happen." Some of these key players, Wachter says, are hospital administrators and people who control the budgets, "but a very big piece of this is that only one species of team members is sitting in the room." Wachter points out that this "species," if left alone to discuss problems, has a tendency to "trash" the people who have been left outside. "If doctors are talking about an error, it's easy to point fingers at anyone who is not in the room and who can't defend themselves. '*If only* the nurses had just done this. *If only* radiology had done that. *If only* the ER knew what they were doing.' That's what you hear. When there's a major failure of communication and teamwork, the other people on the team and other parties in the communication are not there to be part of the conversation."

Not having all the relevant players take part in the discussion, Wachter says, also means that the job of conveying information about what actually happened during the M&M conference can become a cumbersome exercise in second- or thirdhand reporting. "From time to time we would come up with an error in the interaction between our service and others. Yet these others were not in the room. So my job as chief of service was to find them, tell them what went on, get their take on it, and come up with a robust solution—which, of course, involves after-the-fact secondhand recounting of what should have gone on with the entire group."

These after-the-fact ways of dealing with problems are meant to prevent future mishaps, but prevention is stymied by the absence of mechanisms that allow a nurse, or even a junior physician, to leap over status hierarchies to save a patient in immediate jeopardy. Medical hierarchies, of course, aren't designed to silence and intimidate only nurses. They also silence doctors who are in or have recently completed residency. These new folks on the block may be afraid to rock the boat or challenge those upon whom their careers depend. Similarly, doctors may play the "knowledge game" with doctors who challenge them. "You're an anesthetist,"

42 an incompetent surgeon says, "What do you know about cardiac surgery?" "You're an internist. What do you know about OB?" The difference between the discounting of doctors and of nurses is that doctors may be told they don't have enough knowledge about a particular medical field. But "not enough" is quite different from "none at all."

Should a nurse thus have an urgent problem with a doctor's actions, he or she can call in the nursing manager or an administrator on call. The higher-up can then address the problem. In some instances, this mechanism works. Sometimes they don't. Sometimes it appears that formal mechanisms to address problems aren't used because they are poorly advertised, or because no one knows that such an administrator or senior clinician is available. They may also be ineffective because the people that nurses rely on to state their case—nurse managers—may themselves be as disempowered as staff nurses. The nurse manager may not feel she has the power to go over the doctor's head. She may have witnessed senior doctors scream at junior doctors or other nurses or have experienced a browbeating herself, which would discourage her from standing up for the nurses whose interests she is supposed to represent. Often neither nursing nor medical higher-ups are any better at interdisciplinary communication than their so-called subordinates.

Similarly, nurses may be discouraged from appealing to higher-ups because such efforts have fallen on deaf ears. "Nurses who speak out, particularly in a manner that is critical of doctors, are still seen as committing an act of disloyalty, regardless of the legitimacy of the concern," Justice Murray Sinclair wrote in a provincial inquest report on pediatric deaths in Winnipeg, Canada. "Alternatively, the hospital may not be interested in investigating the issue, perhaps for reasons of legal liability."[27]

Have Things Really Changed?

"But now that women are doctors, haven't things changed?" That's a question I'm often asked when I talk to friends or other members of the public about nurse-doctor relationships. Surely, many people think, since so many women have given up the white cap for the white coat, gender stereotypes are a thing of the past and female physicians eagerly exhibit solidarity with their nursing sisters. Thus when I mentioned doctor-nurse relationships to a sociologist studying women and medicine, one of his first questions was, Did I find any touching examples of solidarity between female doctors and female nurses?

Occasionally I have observed female doctors who are more egalitarian with nurses they worked with, but I confess that I have never observed a joint endeavor to overcome male status and privilege. In my observations of doctors and nurses at work in the postfeminist workplace, female **43** physicians were neither much more nor less supportive of nurses than male doctors. When efforts were made to prevent pediatric surgery deaths in Winnipeg, female anesthetists and intensivists were supportive of nurses who tried to raise the alarm about a dangerous surgeon, but both, to varying degrees, were put down by male surgeons. In Massachusetts, when female nurses in labor and delivery tried to warn female residents and a female obstetrician that a baby was getting into serious trouble, female doctors apparently refused to listen to female nurses.

I have heard female surgeons complain that they have to dress in the same room as the nurses. And even now, in the twenty-first century, some medical women are joining medical men in fretting about the dangers of the "overtrained RN." In her book *PC, M.D.* the physician Sally Satel attacks "a growing cabal of feminist nurses" who are fueled by "a fiery resentment of the medical establishment, the so-called male medical elite," and whose "antipathy represents a thoroughly postmodern rejection of the prevailing medical culture wherein doctors direct the patient's treatment and nurses carry out many of those directives." Like nineteenth-century physicians who worried about nurses who wanted to venture from the practical to the theoretical, Satel cautions against nurses who dare to dally in alternative therapies, consider the spiritual side of patient care, or study the philosophies of French intellectuals like Michel Foucault and Jacques Derrida.[28]

Claire Fagin, dean emerita of the University of Pennsylvania School of Nursing, who has studied nurse-physician collaboration, sums up the situation, "What's been the biggest disappointment is women in medicine. It's not surprising to us when male doctors are abusive and disregard nurses. Because of their conflicted situation in the field, some female physicians can be just awful. As nurses, we get used to the disappointment, which is even sadder."

Traditional male-female dominance and oppression sometimes erupts into violence against nurses. Although there are no statistics confirming this, most of the incidents of slapping, hitting, pulling, and throwing of objects I have heard about involve male physicians and female nurses. I have observed and heard about female physicians who are rude or humiliating or who have even thrown things at nurses. But no nurse I have spoken to has ever reported that a female doctor hit a female nurse. Nor have I ever heard about a female doctor hitting a male nurse.

Ironically, traditional gender expectations and stereotypes may impel some female doctors to treat nurses badly or adopt negative attitudes toward them. Such demeaning attitudes may also reflect their anxieties in the workplace. Insecure about their status, they find that "lording" it over

44   nurses is a way to prove that they're part of the medical boys' club. It also ensures that no one confuses the female doctor with a nurse—which is a significant problem for women in medicine. That's because while women have moved into medicine in far greater numbers over the past three decades, nursing has remained overwhelmingly female. Female doctors thus enter a medical workplace in which patients can realistically expect that most of the women who enter their exam or hospital rooms to care for them will be nurses. Which means that the female doctor may be routinely mistaken for a nurse.

"I would walk into a room," Alice Rothchild remembers, "and the patient would say, 'Can you get me a bedpan? Can you take my tray?' 'Goddamn it,' I would think. 'I've worked really hard for this MD. Can't you just get it? I'm a doctor. Can't you understand that women can be in positions you don't expect them to be in?' The challenge is to figure out a way to make it clear who's who without ever belittling nurses."

"When you're in training and you're insecure, those moments when you're taken for a nurse are off-putting," says Emily Lowry. "As you gain more confidence and you mature, you take it in stride and it's easier to make it clear who you are with grace and good humor. I say, 'No, I'm not a nurse. I'm just a useless doctor.'"

Tension between female doctors and female nurses arises out of a lack of grace and good humor at just such moments of role confusion. Nurses have long complained about the physician who considered himself too busy and important to take the seconds needed to give a patient a glass of water, or shift the position of a pillow. When asked, the male physician would tell the patient that he'd get the nurse to do it. Some nurses expected, perhaps naively, more of women doctors.

Some female doctors, on the other hand, feel that female nurses ask things of them that they would not ask male doctors. They are right: the female nurse may indeed have a double standard—one born of oppression and frustration. Lowry recounts a scenario. "I'll ask the nurse to do something, and she'll say, 'Why can't *you* take them to the bathroom?' I doubt they would have ever said that to a male physician." Similarly, nurses are also much more likely, Lowry says, to tell her about a male doctor who was a jerk and expect that she would commiserate in a sisterly fashion, which, if the complaint is justified, Lowry says she usually does.

Some nurses may greet the arrival of a female doctor with sullenness or passive aggression. This may be due to their own personal problems or insecurities, but it may also be due to their disappointed expectations. The way some female physicians not only reproduce status hierarchies but also choose less-than-optimal ways to distinguish themselves from nurses has produced some very disgruntled nurses.

Both physicians and nurses say that relationships are best when mutual respect is shown. Most nurses don't want to be doctors, but they do want to be respected by doctors. Female physicians who recognize this fact display an understanding of the importance of nursing. They also understand the complexities of the gender and status politics of the doctor-nurse relationship. "When a nurse tells me in nurse-speak that a woman has painful urination and frequency instead of saying she has dysuria, I know she thinks that the person has a urinary tract infection," Rothchild says. "When she uses classic nurse talk and asks me, 'Would you like to get a clean catch and send a culture to the lab?' I know she's making as much of a diagnosis as I am. I also know that some nurses know a lot more than I do. When I go into the ICU, I always talk to the nurses first. When I'm in a high-tech environment like that, I don't know the drugs, the tubes, and alarms and machines. Why is that blinking? Why is that alarm going off? That's not my turf. I realize I need help so that I can help participate in the care of patients."

Female physicians who have mentors like Rothchild might reproduce this collaborative behavior. But this is not how all female doctors have been mentored and thus seem to feel or act.

Young female physicians today seem no more likely to recognize the complex role that nurses play in diagnosis and treatment than were their forefathers. Denise Rich* is a thirty-two-year-old fellow in hematology-oncology at a Boston teaching hospital. She did her undergraduate work at Harvard, finished an MD/PhD at another prestigious medical school and went on to train in Boston. When I spoke to her, she was in her first year of a fellowship.

Rich explained that her first lessons about nursing came in her third year of study when students moved onto the hospital floors. Unlike many doctors in training, Rich says, "Our mentors repeated to us that you need to learn from nurses, that nurses are the people who are going to be taking care of the patients most of the time. They know more than you, as medical students, in most cases. Learn from them when you can."

As she advanced in her training, Rich described a subtle and important shift in her perceptions and tutorials. "In internship you learned: Don't abuse them, because there is more danger or potential for that. Don't yell at them, treat them well. But as residents it changed. It was harder because you know more than they do, and so it's more like teamwork than learning from them. You work with them, be respectful when you ask for things, be respectful of their time and energy. But you no longer learn from them. They don't have as much knowledge."

Rich's language is instructive and reflects the values of the system in which she is being trained. She does not say that the nurse has different or

46 complementary knowledge. She believes the nurse has less knowledge (and, one suspects, inferior knowledge).

If "knowledge" means the knowledge of disease processes that is gained in medical school or from medical journals, then of course few bedside nurses can compete with four years of college, four years of medical school and an MD/PhD and years of residency and fellowship training. If, however, one includes an in-depth knowledge of nursing and the practical know-how gained from piloting a legion of patients through cancer treatment to the shore of remission, then the nurse may know more than the doctor about any number of things. Similarly, if the nurse has extensive "local" knowledge of how one particular patient is coping with nausea, cancer pain, and the impact of chemotherapy, or how much social support she receives, then the nurse has quite a lot to teach the doctor.

Rich also faithfully mirrored male physicians in their attitudes toward the nurses' role in diagnosis and treatment. I asked Rich whether she considered nurses' suggestions about patient problems and what should be done about them as part of the diagnostic process.

"No," she replied adamantly. "I think they give us advice and their opinion. In general the diagnosis is left to us doctors."

What's the difference between opinion and diagnosis, I asked.

"A diagnosis means I tell you what it is," she answered. "Nurses don't do that. They tell you what they think it might be, give us a few options, and sometimes they say, 'Maybe you should consider this, or do you think it could possibly be this. Usually they are asking our opinion or bouncing things off us and seeing what we think as far as the diagnosis is concerned.' They'll say, 'Should I send a urine sample to the lab to get a culture, because maybe they have a UTI? Do you want to give them this?' They tend to ask and let us make a decision. We're the ones who have to come up with the diagnosis and what the patient has and write the prescription."

To Rich the game seems to be the reality. Unlike Alice Rothchild, she seems unaware that the nurse actually has judgments, not just advice and opinions, but that she is perhaps reluctant to share them for fear that the doctor would take umbrage.

To see if she would be offended, I ask Rich what she would do if a nurse directly stated what she thought was wrong and what treatment was needed. "If they said it in a nice, respectful way, I would do it. If they did it in a respectful way," she repeated, "and I agreed with them. But it's never happened to me. They've always asked me for my opinion."

Differences of status between female doctors and female nurses appear in even more subtle measures of hierarchy and deference. A number of the female physicians I spoke to referred to nurses as personal posses- sions, as "my nurses." Even some of my most progressive female physi- cian friends, who wouldn't tolerate a secretary or worker being ill-treated or dealt with as personal property, didn't seem to have a clue that they were doing the same to RNs. A friend didn't seem to find it disturbing that her nurse used to answer the phone with "Hello, this is Dr. Smith's nurse." When I talked to her about nursing, she constantly described the nurse as her object—there only to serve her.

The pediatric practice where I take my kids is pretty much a female- run show, with first-generation feminist docs and second-generation postfeminist ones. The practice has a fairly steady group of nurses. But the list of clinicians on a plaque in the waiting room includes only the names of doctors. No nurses. No nurse practitioners. Just docs.

Except for the most elite nurses, the social distance between female physicians and nurses sometimes seems even more pronounced than that between male doctors and female nurses. In the past, female nurses and male doctors may not have socialized much, but they did tend to date and sometimes marry. Now, with more women in medicine, male doctors often marry female ones. And female doctors don't seem to cross status boundaries by socializing much with female nurses. The resident at the Harvard teaching hospital said she is quite friendly with nurses at work. They share a superficial workplace camaraderie. She chats them up. They ask her questions about how she's doing. But it would never occur to her to suggest to a nurse with whom she has such amicable conversations that they go for a drink or cup of coffee after work.

Would she go for a drink or cup of coffee with a fellow doctor-in- training? "Of course," she said.

In many cases, this social distance reflects class differences. More nurses come from working- or middle-class backgrounds, while more doctors are from the upper middle class. But it also reflects the status hi- erarchies that don't seem to shift much, no matter what nurses do, at least in conventional ways, to challenge them. A number of the nurses the res- ident works with have bachelor's and master's degrees. Some may even have doctorates. Some are of the same class and social background. They have husbands who are professors, lawyers, and doctors. They may be pa- tients of the doctor in question. While this may translate into polite so- ciability at the dinner party or courteous treatment in the exam room, once the two disciplines share the same occupational space, traditional patterns of behavior reassert themselves.

When I talk with both younger female and male doctors, I am struck by the peculiar problem women's liberation has created for nursing. Doc- tors trained in earlier periods, when there were few women physicians

48 and women had few professional options, may have been taught not to expect much of nurses, but they probably didn't blame women for becoming nurses. In an era when women's employment choices were so narrow, a woman who wanted or needed to work generally became a nurse, teacher, social worker, or secretary. To doctors-in-training today, there is nothing unusual about a woman in medicine. What is unusual to them is the woman who chooses nursing rather than medicine.

"I sometimes wonder why someone would choose nursing," a female pediatric resident said. Echoing her, many of the younger doctors I interviewed seemed unable to understand why a woman who can become a doctor would voluntarily choose to become a nurse. If you wanted a career in medicine, why wouldn't you become a doctor instead of settling for something so much less challenging, knowledgeable, ambitious, and important?

Creating the Invisible Nurse

The medical system consistently entangles nurses in a series of Catch-22s. The female nurse who is bright and ambitious should have become a female doctor. If she actually chooses nursing—particularly bedside nursing—how could she be bright and ambitious? If she isn't bright and ambitious and has no medical knowledge to boot, why should doctors consult with her and attend to her concerns? Even more significantly, when a nurse makes a contribution to patient care—one that could illuminate what she really knows and really does—the system often gives the credit for her action and contribution to the physician. This means that the nurse is stuck in the most pernicious Catch-22 of all: whatever the nurse does confers credit on the physician. The only credit the nurse is sure to get is discredit, which may be rapidly assigned if he makes a mistake or is "insubordinate" or "uppity."

"Every night, a thousand times a night, all over the country, nurses are calling doctors reporting that a patient has a fever and asking doctors what they should do about it, or asking the doctor whether they should give the patient Tylenol," says Gordon Schiff, an internist at Cook County Hospital in Chicago. "And every night, doctors are berating nurses for calling them up and bothering them, because they are reporting a fever, and the doctors are thinking to themselves, 'Why are you so stupid that you are asking me whether you should give Tylenol? Of course, you shouldn't give Tylenol. Everybody knows you shouldn't mask a fever. You need to do something about why the patient has the fever.'"

But that, Schiff points out, is the conundrum. Nurses are severely restricted in what they can do for patients without a doctor's order. "We have structured the system in a way that gives the bedside nurse such a limited repertoire that she can't order a chest X ray or a urine culture. She can't order labs on her own. She can't get antibiotics. In a lot of places she can't tell the doctor what she really thinks and what she really knows and what she knows should be done. She can only make suggestions. And all of this then reinforces what the physician was likely taught either through formal or informal lessons and socialization, which is that the nurse is really stupid, because she uses dumb language, makes dumb suggestions, and doesn't know anywhere near what the physicians knows."

This doesn't only create problems between nurses and doctors, it creates problems and reinforces status hierarchies between nurses. When I was lecturing to a class at a prestigious nursing school, a student in the advanced practice cohort told me that she'd been at a dinner party at a physician's house. The physician received a call interrupting his dinner. It was from a nurse asking for clarification of an order. He was irate at being disturbed and his wife was even more so. "How can she be so stupid?" the wife exclaimed. The student relating this story, who was planning to become a nurse practitioner, was not at all disturbed by the doctor's reaction. She seemed to identify more with the physician than with the bedside nurse. "I have a real problem with the nurse part of being a nurse practitioner," she confided.

To avoid an endless series of late-night phone calls and interruptions, some institutions give nurses greater latitude. They create unit- or institution-wide protocols that grant nurses the temporary authority to undertake a specified range of actions. Similarly, physicians may write standing orders such as "Don't call me unless the patient has a fever over 100.5." Or "two Tylenol 650 mg. PO. Q 4 hours. PRN Pain" (i.e., give the patient two Tylenol by mouth every four hours as needed for pain).

In some institutions, nurses simply do a number of things on their own and the doctor rubber-stamps them afterward. On ICUs nurses put in catheters or even an arterial line and then tell doctors later. On oncology services, nurses may order antiemetics for patients with chemotherapy-induced nausea, or pain medication to relieve cancer pain. The doctor will then write an ex post facto order to legitimate the action the nurse has taken.

"Nurses are always ordering things that they consider to be pro forma when the doctor is unavailable," says Emily Lowry. "When I was recently on vacation, I came back and found that I had ordered a whole bunch of things from South Africa. They ordered Tylenol, lab tests—urine and culture for urinary symptoms. They ordered physical therapy when it was needed and it was too much trouble to call the on-call doctor. And they

50 felt it was all quite pro forma, which it was. And of course I signed them all when I got back."

Why do doctors tolerate these private "liberties" when their organizations are so vociferous in publicly denouncing nurses who want more authority? It's simple. If nurses "work to rule" by calling a doctor for every little thing, refusing to give medications, move patients, or change diets until they actually reached a physician, the system would grind to a halt. The sociologist Andrew Abbott calls this bypassing of onerous and extensive restrictions "workplace assimilations." "Boundaries between professional jurisdictions . . . tend to disappear in worksites, particularly in overworked worksites," Abbott writes. "Subordinate professionals, non-professionals, and members of related, equal professions learn on the job a craft version of a given profession's knowledge systems. While they lack theoretical training that justifies membership in that profession, they generally acquire much of the diagnostic, therapeutic, and inferential systems. . . . If the public knew the extent of workplace assimilation, it would profoundly suspect professionals' claim of comprehensive jurisdiction," Abbott concludes.[29]

A great deal of effort, on the part of both doctors—and, ironically, nurses—is spent making sure the public doesn't know how much medical diagnosis, treatment, and prescription nurses actually undertake. Doctors do this by attributing a nurse's action to the physician. The nurse isn't really acting on her own knowledge and judgment when they take the actions described above, doctors argue, they are acting on the physician's. They don't really have any agency of their own; they are just temporarily borrowing the doctor's agency. They know "my own preferences," doctors tell me, and would never knowingly violate them or exceed their authority.

Credit for the judgments and knowledge guiding these actions still goes to the doctor or to higher-ups in the institution. The nurse is still seen as an agent without knowledge and judgment—and ultimately not an agent at all.

What is worse is that physicians often take credit for a nurse's knowledge, judgment, and action. Recall Deborah Madison's experience with the intern in charge of her patient. The very structure of the medical system conceals nurse's activities while giving credit for them to a physician who initially opposed her recommendations. The elimination of nursing's contributions to the complex story of medical decision making and treatment is so routine that most doctors do not consider it to be problematic. Patients don't know what nurses really do. And nurses view it as the very air they breathe.

This failure to account for nursing's contributions has been integrated **51** into the formal process of medical accounting, both financial and reportorial. Hospitals, for example, account for the cost of medications, medical tools, equipment, and supplies. Before the bundling of charges under DRGs (diagnostic-related groups), you could find out what an aspirin cost, what a scalpel cost, even what a pencil cost. And physicians, of course, have always billed for their services. But hospitals did not include a financial accounting of nurses' services in any hospital bill or invoice. As if they were a sheet or pillowcase, nursing services were the original bundled service, integrated into the room charge. This, erroneously in my view, has led some American nursing elites to insist that the way nurses will finally make it onto the radar screen is to set up their own agencies and sell their services back to the hospital, just as physicians do.

In their discussion of how medical education, training, and work so often preclude a recognition of interdependence, Aron and Headrick explain that doctors have a limited ability to "understand work as a process."[30] Given the accounting structures of medicine, it is difficult for nurses' contributions to be included in the meetings, conferences, reports, and charting of medical care.

Medicine also routinely claims credit for nurses' work in the chronicling of medical care in books, articles, columns, letters to the editor, or comments from doctors describing their work to a broader public. An interesting example is a letter to the editor printed in the *New York Times*. Physician Arthur M. Magun, director of quality assurance at Columbia University, is opposing efforts to reduce the grueling schedules of interns and residents, which range from eighty hours per week to over a hundred. Doctors should remain at the bedside as long as possible, Magun argues, because "experienced doctors realize that long hours at the bedside of a sick patient watching the drama of illness unfold and being there to understand the results of one's intervention or lack of it are the best route to becoming an outstanding doctor."[31]

A year later, surgeon Steven G. Friedman wrote an op-ed for the same paper on the shortage of candidates for surgical programs. Echoing Magun, he cited shortened resident hours as one of the causes of the crisis. "Will patients now be better off with shift workers (i.e., doctors who work shorter shifts) who have never seen the complete progress of an illness than they were with tired doctors who cared for them throughout the night?"[32]

For anyone who has actually tallied how much time surgeons spend at the patient's bedside after they leave the OR, this image of the surgeon hovering at the patient's bedside is almost laughable. Who actually spends

52 long hours at the bedside of a sick patient watching the drama of illness unfold or caring for patients "throughout the night"? Is it really the doctors? In most of the hospitals I've visited in my fifteen years as a health journalist, doctors typically spend only a few minutes at each patient's bedside, and when surgeons are in the hospital, whether for 120 hours or 80, most of those hours are spent in the operating room, not in the recovery room or patient's room. I recently met an Egyptian surgeon who had moved to the United States. Unable to transfer his medical license easily, he was working as a nursing assistant in a hospital and studying to become an RN. He said he was shocked at how little time doctors in the United States spend with their patients, particularly surgeons. "They come in the room for five minutes and the nurses do everything, and then they bill and make big bucks." In Egypt and Saudi Arabia, where he practiced, doctors were there all the time and did the bulk of care that nurses do in the United States.

So if anyone truly has "a front-row seat to the spectacle of illness" and can assess the results of treatment interventions, it is nurses. And as we shall see, even they are rarely able to watch the drama of illness unfold. Today, as soon as patients are stabilized, they're likely to be transferred to a nursing home or other subacute facility, or go home. In which case it's nursing staff and family members who learn the most about the wisdom and efficacy of medical interventions, not physicians.

Even some of the most ethical and progressive doctors seem to take credit for nurses' work without understanding the consequences. Consider, for example, the group Médecins sans Frontières—Doctors Without Borders—which won the Nobel Peace Prize in 1999 for its courageous international work. What is less well known is that the majority of its members are not doctors but nurses. Yet the organization is not called Doctors and Nurses Without Borders, or even Medicine Without Borders—names that would more correctly convey the role nurses and other nonphysicians play in the group.

On its international homepage, MSF includes a link to stories that have appeared about the group in the British paper the *Guardian* and posts a number of recent press releases. Most of the press releases have physicians as spokespeople and define the group as a medical group providing medical services. Given the group's name and spokespeople, most readers would assume that the staff and those teams are made up of doctors.

Several years ago, I was talking with one of the leaders of the organization. When I politely asked this female physician leader about the choice of name, she became extremely annoyed. The organization now had "name recognition," she insisted. I suggested that a small change in its title would hardly jeopardize its renown. She responded angrily, "Well, I certainly hope we would never do anything that stupid." This medical confiscation of nurses' contributions assures, as one nurse put it, that "doctors get all the credit when something goes right. We get credit only when something goes wrong."

Ann Williamson, a nurse executive at the UCSF Medical Center (University of California, San Francisco) recounted an example of this problem of discredit. As happens every day in hospitals across the country, a nurse was working with doctors who were involved in the tricky maneuver of placing a feeding tube in the stomach of a patient on the intensive care unit. During the insertion it's easy to mistake the trachea for the esophagus and to insert the tube into the lungs rather than stomach or small intestine. To do so means that fluid and nutritional matter will go into the lungs, where it could cause a pneumonia or potentially drown the patient. So nurses and doctors use a variety of mechanisms to assure correct placement. Sometimes an X ray is taken to make sure the tube is correctly inserted. The nurse will also pump air into the tube and listen with a stethoscope placed over the abdomen to listen for gurgling in the stomach.

In this particular case an X ray was indeed taken, but the nurse wasn't confident that the X ray technicians had read the right film or read it correctly. When he pumped air into the tube, he was certain that he couldn't hear any gurgling in the stomach. On the other hand, he felt he could hear air moving through the tube when the patient breathed, a sign that the tube was misplaced.

The resident placing the tube disagreed. He insisted that the tube was correctly placed, that the X ray verified placement, and that it was safe to feed the patient through the tube.

Understanding the significance of a potential mistake, the nurse continued to object, insisting that another X ray be taken or that X-ray technicians verify that this X ray was read correctly. Again the doctor objected. But the nurse stood his ground.

Ten minutes into the debate, the X-ray department called. "I hope you haven't started the feedings yet," the technician said. The nurse was right. The tube had been placed incorrectly.

Although the tube was finally placed correctly and the mistake avoided, the nurse never got credit for his call. The doctor never came back to the unit to express appreciation for his persistence. What happened was not noted in the chart. Did the resident mention it in his discussions with his colleagues? Probably not. Was it used as part of a case study to teach medical students about the role nurses play in the hospital? Not that Williamson knew. The nurse saved the patient's life, but from the medical point of view, his action simply didn't exist.

54   Williamson invited me to think of what would have happened, had the nurse not fought with the resident and instead started tube feedings. He would have been blamed for what happened. Why didn't he listen harder, question further? In this instance, he received no credit for success. But had he remained silent, he would have shouldered lots of blame.

Dave Latham describes an even more interesting situation. While he was working on the neurological unit at an Illinois hospital, a patient came in to be diagnosed. The patient was just staring into space, almost catatonic. The nurse who was taking care of him told the doctor she thought that the patient was having seizures and suggested that they give him Valium. After much discussion, the doctor finally agreed. The patient got the Valium and woke right up. Instead of thanking the nurse, the doctor said, "I hate it when the nurses are right."

2

Designing the Doctor-Nurse Game

I met Kimberly Hahn in the spring of 2001 at a lecture I gave for nurses at the hospital at the University of Virginia. Hahn, who has been a nurse for eight years, has worked for the past three on the vascular surgery floor of the teaching institution for the university's medical school, which means that she works with a rotating crop of interns and residents. As part of my talk I asked nurses to tell a story that illustrates how their routine daily work makes a difference to patient care. Hahn volunteered and came up to the mike to relate a recent experience.

She was caring for a patient who, four days earlier, had undergone surgery for an abdominal aortic aneurysm—what's known as a "Triple A." The patient had a weakness or thinning in the wall of his abdominal aorta, the artery that feeds blood to the lower half of the body. If, under the constant pressure of blood flow, this thin wall ruptured, the patient would almost certainly bleed to death.

When the intern in charge of the case saw the patient earlier that morning, the patient appeared to be stable and was thus scheduled to go home a few hours later. When Hahn walked into the room to check on him, she found that he was sweaty and pale. When she listened to his heart, she found it was beating much too fast. She did an EKG—an electrical charting of the heart's rhythm—and found that, as she suspected, he was in "atrial fibrillation." He had an irregular heartbeat that could compromise his heart's ability to pump blood. She put the man on oxygen and checked the results of previous lab tests. Was an imbalance in his electrolytes—various salts in his blood such as potassium and magnesium—causing the problem?

56   Hahn also consulted with an intern. The intern told Hahn to give the patient a drug called Lopressor, a beta-blocker that controls blood pressure and heart rate. But Hahn knew this was the wrong call. Aside from having had an aneurysm, the man also had chronic obstructive pulmonary disease (COPD), that is, lung disease. Lopressor is dangerous for anyone with COPD. If this patient took Lopressor, he might end up in the intensive care unit with serious breathing problems. Hahn explained all this to the inexperienced doctor and suggested he prescribe another drug, called diltiazem, which could safely deal with the patient's elevated heart rate without aggravating his COPD. She also suggested that they use Lasix, a diuretic. During surgery, patients are often given a great deal of fluid. Sometimes it takes days for the body to eliminate this extra load. The patient had put on weight, which indicated that he might be "fluid overloaded."

The intern followed her advice. When the medication began to have an effect on the patient's heart rate and blood pressure, the intern decided he could be discharged. Hahn, however, recognized that the patient was still unstable. Even though he seemed to be awash in his own bodily fluids, inside his circulatory system there was actually not enough fluid. The edema, or swelling, he was experiencing was a result of fluid collecting outside of his bloodstream in tissues and between cells. As the medication helped his body eliminate all the excess fluids, it could put him at risk for low blood pressure, shock, or low blood supply to the heart, which could cause a heart attack. Even though his heart rate was steadier, Hahn knew he could still have a potentially fatal blood clot. If any of this happened at home, the patient could die. She wanted the patient to stay in the hospital, where his changing condition could be closely monitored and cardiologists could consult on his care.

With little experience handling this kind of patient, the intern, Hahn knew, was dealing in snapshots. In his sporadic contacts with the patient, he saw a man whose condition was improving, whereas Hahn anticipated a more complex trajectory of recovery that included not only highs but many potential lows. Finally, after she had discussed the matter with the intern, he concurred. The patient stayed in the hospital. When the cardiologist finally came to check his status, he agreed with Hahn. In order to be safe, the patient needed close monitoring.

As they listened to their colleague recount this experience later, nurses in the lecture hall nodded knowingly. When I suggested that Hahn's story illustrates how nurses routinely diagnose problems, making lifesaving prescription and treatment recommendations and helping physicians avoid potentially fatal mistakes, Hahn agreed. "Yes, that's true. We do that every day. But why," she asked, her voice dropping in sadness rather than anger, "do physicians know this when they are interns and residents and **57** so quickly forget it when they become attendings and are too busy to round with the nurse, or even bother to talk to us to get critical information about their patients?"

To answer that question we have to go back to the nineteenth century, when nurse-doctor relationships were established in the hospital. Most hospitals in the early nineteenth century were not devoted either to medical teaching or practice. They were charitable, philanthropic institutions dedicated to caring for the sick poor and sometimes simply to housing the destitute.[1] Indeed, with the exception of physicians trained in the large medically run hospitals in Paris, Edinburgh, Berlin, and other cities in Europe and North America, most doctors had no formal institutional training. "Medical training varied from classical university education and the study of Greek and Latin medical texts, on the one hand, to broom-and-apron apprenticeship in an apothecary's shop, on the other—and sometimes involved no recognizable education at all," according to M. Jeanne Peterson.[2] Doctors enjoyed little prestige and suffered from a rather poor public image. Competition for patients was cutthroat and doctors trying to eke out a living in the countryside or large cities were attacking each other rather than seeking to bolster the public's trust in the profession.[3]

With only a few exceptions, doctors didn't run hospitals. Church- or community-run hospitals gave doctors space to observe and treat the sick, but clerics or community authorities controlled them. Physicians, as the nursing historian Joan Lynaugh has described them, were "welcome visitors in these hospitals," with the operative term being "visitor." While nurses were sometimes actual live-in residents of these hospitals, some physicians never even set foot in them.[4] They cared for their patients in the patients' homes or in their offices. (When possible, surgeons did use hospital facilities for obvious reasons). In Protestant countries, hospital boards of trustees or governors—made up of affluent or influential laymen—employed physicians. The lay boards made all the major decisions about how the hospital functioned and chose which poor patients were worthy enough to be admitted. As Lynaugh vividly explains, "the town drunk couldn't necessarily get admitted, but a productive working man could."

In the late nineteenth century, all of this began to change. Scientists and physicians were gaining more knowledge of anatomy, physiology, and chemistry. They were learning more about contagion and how to relieve pain. They developed more accurate diagnostic equipment and devised treatments that actually did less harm than good. The hospital started to view patients through a different lens. To the new, scientifically minded

58 physician, the hospitalized patient was no longer a charity case to be warehoused or cared for, but a focus of objective scientific inquiry. Other doctors, patients, and members of the public began to judge doctors on the basis of their clinical know-how more than their bedside manner. Doctors began to be less interested in worthy people than in worthy cases—that is, interesting ones.

Physicians soon believed that the hospital could furnish them with a steady stream of medical subjects and would be the perfect place to teach future generations of doctors. They needed the hospital as their practice workshop. They also wanted to wrest hospital decision making from lay or ecclesiastical boards and turn the hospital into a laboratory and classroom. They were also determined to marginalize irregular practitioners. Persona non grata included "jealous midwives, doctor-women, and busy neighbors" as well as hydropaths, natural healers, members of healing sects like those that flourished in America, and doctors educated outside of the hospital.[5]

While scientific medicine was in its infancy in the mid-nineteenth century, nurse reformers like Florence Nightingale viewed the hospital as a target of reform and a potential employer of a growing number of women who needed, or wanted, work outside the home. In Britain, nurse reformers planned to mold the character of these new nurses and give them a rudimentary education. Then they would operate in a separate female sphere—managed by a lady-nurse matron—of their own inside the hospital. While most physicians were happy to get more helping hands in the hospital, for a variety of reasons, many physicians worried about a group of people—in this case women—who also wanted (at least some) knowledge, power, and control and who could potentially challenge their burgeoning authority. While they generally supported the idea of training schools for nurses, many physicians associated nursing reform with the movement for the education and emancipation of women—and the even more terrifying prospect of the female physician.[6]

Negotiating the Education and Authority of Nursing

Physicians' fears weren't entirely unfounded. Women in the nineteenth century were seeking the right to vote and legal reforms that would make it easier for women to divorce. They wanted to gain legal status and identity separate from that of their fathers and husbands. They also wanted higher education and access to professions like medicine. With only a few notable exceptions, like Lavinia Dock in the United States, reformers such as Nightingale were not outright feminists. In fact, some bent over backward to reassure doctors they weren't trying to compete **59** with them for financial resources or social status. All they wanted, they insisted, was to have their own female sphere of action and authority. But many male physicians believed that giving women a serious education and authority, even in that separate sphere, was a slippery slope. While many physicians recognized that a trained cadre of nurses could prove useful, the question was how to make use of nurses without creating a source of competition for money or status—one that might encourage even more women to try to become doctors.

Peterson argues that gaining control over the nursing profession was a test case in physicians' efforts to shift control from lay boards to physician leaders.[7] This battle and others were played out on hospital wards and in hospital boardrooms as well as in the pages of medical journals and daily newspapers. The articles, letters, and editorials that were published in the *Lancet* and the *British Medical Journal* (*BMJ*) and in publications like the *Times, Blackwood's Magazine,* the *Guardian,* and the *Fortnightly Review,* as well as in a variety of medical and lay publications in the New World, showed how radical the nurses' demands were.

When medical men defended their control of the hospital, they grounded their arguments in the notion that they had "special knowledge" that no one else—patients, lay public, or anyone else in the clinical setting—possessed.[8] But if that knowledge was to be "special"—accessible only to physicians—it could not be shared by anyone else. Since nurses had become competitors in the hospital, doctors made very sure medical knowledge was off limits to them. Couched in terms of what was best for the patient, the female sex, and society as a whole, physicians talked about the dangers education posed to women and to patient care. The *Lancet* warned that, for women, adding the strain of intellectual work to the "drain on the general system" that menstruation imposed on the female body and spirit would exacerbate the "physical deterioration induced by the menstrual functions." It would, the *Lancet* opined, lead not just to "serious damage to the general health," but "to the undoing of the female constitution."[9]

"What is wanted," the *Lancet* argued, "is a better system of education adapted to the capacity and requirements of woman, and not an entire revolution involving the annihilation of those sexual distinctions which have existed from prehistoric times."[10] Doctors were also certain that if some women became doctors, no women would want to be nurses. These doctors established a clear moral dichotomy between women who wanted to learn about doctoring and those who were content to stay in the female sphere of nursing. The *Lancet,* among other publications, insisted that "if

60   those women who are seeking, at an extravagant cost of time and money, to enter the medical profession, were content to work in the only department of medical practice which is properly open to them—namely, as midwives and nurses—no objections could fairly be raised, provided that they always practiced under the supervision of qualified medical practitioners."[11]

Because of their "feminine folly or feebleness," nurses could never be entrusted with drugs in the dispensary or gain any medical knowledge, the *Lancet* wrote. Instead, they should be tutored only in subject matter that would make them "useful to physicians."[12] In a letter to the *Times*, physicians presented a clear expression of medicine's view of nurses. "The medical argument is . . . that nursing is merely one of the means of cure, like the administration of medicines or the performance of operations; and that, like these, it can only be rightly carried out under absolute and unconditional subjection, in every principle and detail, to the doctor who is responsible for the case."[13]

This view of nursing precluded even elite lady nurses' control over the nursing work force. Doctors contended that because they were women, nurses—although constitutionally designed to cooperate with men—were constitutionally unable to cooperate with and thus manage or lead other women. Many prominent physicians weighed in on this subject, including John Braxton Hicks, who identified the contractions that are often confused with the advent of labor.

At the thought of nurses having control over nursing, Hicks must have experienced his own spasms. In an article in the *British Medical Journal*, he painted a dire portrait of power-mad nursing superintendents who failed to grasp that the nursing staff is "naturally the handmaid" of physicians. If she worked in a nursing hierarchy controlled by an independent matron or superintendent, the ordinary bedside nurse, he warned, would look "to the matron more as her centre" and would be "less interested in pleasing the medical authorities."[14] Such a system, Hicks contended, could not be tolerated.

Sir William Gull, consulting physician to Guy's Hospital, asserted that "there is no proper duty which the nurse has to perform, even to the placing of a pillow, which does not or may not involve a principle, and a principle which can be only properly met by one who has had the advantage of medical instruction. It is a fundamental and dangerous error to maintain that any system of nursing has sources of knowledge not derived from the profession."[15]

In a fascinating study of the secularization and professionalization of nursing in France, Katrin Schultheiss describes the debate about the laicization of nursing under the Third Republic. Politicians attacked clerical **61** power in the hospitals and schools and wanted to laicize teaching and nursing. Although many medical men supported the nursing reforms championed by well-bred women reformers like Nightingale, the effort to laicize nursing stumbled on the rock of one critical question: which nurse, religious or lay, would be cheapest and demonstrate the appropriate deference to physicians? "As long as nursing was clearly understood to be a custodial, maternal, or charitable occupation, and as long as the nurses were regarded as the social, economic, and educational peers of the patients, rather than the doctors, there would be no ambiguity about who held medical authority within the hospital."[16]

In Lyons, for example, medical men supported a kind of hybrid religious nurse. These *hospitalières* were not cloistered and did not take annual vows. They "undertook a lifelong commitment to serve the sick and poor under harsh physical conditions and with virtually no monetary compensation," yet they "remained under the direct authority of the secular administration."[17] These nurses were useful because their devotion was easily exploited by civil administrators who didn't want to pay the real cost of nursing care.

Those physicians who wanted to replace religious nurses with lay nurses believed that "the very existence of an autonomous community of women called into question the hierarchy of power within municipal institutions." One medical reformer of nursing happily reported that lay nurses were "infinitely more subordinate than the religious nurses and more scrupulous in the strict execution of doctors' orders."[18] Moreover, lay nurses would be cheaper than the religious variety because they didn't expect lifetime security.

Both English and French physicians also resisted the introduction of a better class of women into nursing, because educated upper-class women, they argued, would be more demanding. In France, "as long as nursing was understood to be a natural attribute of womanhood, it was deemed useful and important, yet subordinate and unthreatening. Once reformers demanded rigorous training as well as substantive authority for nurses as medical professionals, politicians, administrators, and doctors alike balked."[19]

In the United States, doctors were just as concerned about nurses invading their territory. In 1876, in an article entitled "On the Training of Nurses for the Sick," John Packard, MD, made the case perfectly. The nurse, he felt, needed only practical not scientific knowledge. "What we want in a nurse is an attendant for the sick, one who has practical familiarity with what is to be done and the best way of doing it."[20] Nurses,

62 Packard argued, needed to know what they were doing but not why they were doing it. Teaching a nurse to place a bandage on an eye, to administer an antidote to a poison, to collect a patient's urine, or to make observations that were promptly reported to the physician was one thing. Teaching a nurse about the anatomy of the eye, or about the properties of "poisons and their antidotes, the examination of urine," or how to take "accounts of cases" would be too expensive. More to the point, it would create "a person with theories of her own, or with a smattering of other people's theories."[21]

The nurses didn't agree. Over a decade later, nurses were still clamoring for what physicians deemed to be unnecessary knowledge, and the editors of the *Boston Medical and Surgical Journal* were reiterating their objections. They emphasized that in order to intelligently cooperate with the physician, the nurse should not be an utterly empty vessel. Although the editors admitted that "the day has gone by when physicians could afford to keep their nurses in utter ignorance of what medicine they were administering," they were quick to add that "we do not mean that he (the physician) should *consult* with his nurse; we only insist that the latter should know the nature of the drugs which she is administering, what they are designed to effect, and how to meet any untoward and unexpected, though possible, symptoms which may arise in consequence of possible idiosyncrasies."[22]

Nurses continued their struggle to gain the kind of education deemed necessary for professional work. But doctors continually objected because, they insisted, nurses could not possibly consider themselves to be professional workers. Laying the groundwork for the sociological theories that would exclude nurses from the ranks of professionals, Dr. W. Gilman Thompson brought nineteenth-century notions of women's possibilities into the twentieth. A profession, he wrote in 1906 in the *New York Medical Journal*, " 'implies professed attainments in special knowledge, as distinguished from mere skill.' The work of a nurse is an honorable calling or vocation, and nothing further. It implies the exercise of acquired proficiency in certain more or less mechanical duties, and is not primarily designed to contribute to the sum of human knowledge or the advancement of science."[23]

Earlier, doctors wrote a new character into the medical/nursing drama—the "overtrained nurse"—and used her to justify their restrictions on nurses. Doctors argued that theories and ideas from the well-meaning but ultimately enfeebled female mind—the mind of a child unable to distinguish her own limitations—would cause actual harm. They were, thus, quick to publicize and pillory nurses who made mistakes due to their lack or surfeit of medical knowledge, as well as any nursing school that dared to introduce "medical" subjects into their sparse curriculum. "Subjects of purely medical and surgical concern are beginning to be included in the 'studies' of the nurse," the *Lancet* warned.[24]

Almost thirty years later, doctors were waging the same crusade. Thompson's article "The Overtrained Nurse" took aim at schools of nursing that operated without "medical control or supervision" and produced nurses who "are absurdly overtrained and wrongly trained."[25] In some schools of nursing, he wrote, examiners had the audacity to ask students questions like "What are the following operations: colpoperineoplasty, cholecystectomy, myomectomy, colpocystotomy? What is immunity? Does the presence of albumen necessarily indicate disease of the kidneys?" Thompson insisted that nurses did not need to—and indeed should not—know the names of the operations their patients were to undergo. Nor did they need to understand why their patients might be susceptible to infection or how to identify specific signs of pathology. These things, he insisted, did not concern nursing but "first, second, or third year medicine."[26]

Creating the virtuous, knowledgeless, self-sacrificing nurse involved not only intellectual restrictions but also behavioral prohibitions. The activities of doctors became sacrosanct domains, assiduously protected from such dangerous creatures as overtrained or undertrained nurses. Enshrined in law and statute—acts governing nursing and medical practices—medicine was narrowly defined as something only physicians practiced. The nurse who ventured into "medical" territory could be prosecuted or persecuted for practicing medicine without a license. If a nurse observed her patient and came to a conclusion about his or her problem, the term "diagnosis" could never be applied to that process. If she arrived at a plan of care, it could never be called a "treatment." If she suggested a medication to a doctor and the doctor agreed, that was not called prescribing. What was far more important was that nurses, in their own practice, could only function if they had a doctor's orders, which did indeed cover everything from the positioning of a pillow to helping a patient go to the bathroom.

Although they were instructed to reach doctors for orders day or night, interrupt them during surgery, or wake them up at home when necessary, nurses were socialized to sound sufficiently apologetic. If they knew what was wrong with the patient and what medications or actions were needed to remedy it, they often ensured that the course of action appeared to be the doctor's idea. "The problem might be this or that," the nurse would suggest. "Would you like to get this or that test?" "Would you like to order this or that medication?" she would hint, maneuvering through the obstacle course of deference. Nurses were expected to stand up when a

64 doctor entered a room or to open a door for a doctor if they were passing through it together. And, of course, they were never to directly challenge a doctor's judgment or authority. They learned how to clothe any concern or caution—like the fact that the doctor was giving the wrong drug or operating on the wrong limb—in suitably circumlocutory garb.

Finally, the hospital, which had formerly been a nursing institution in which physicians were welcome visitors, became a medical institution where doctors maintained direct control. Of course, the efficient nursing of the patient influenced hospital organization, design, and development. But the nurse's working day was often structured for the convenience of the physician.

In her book detailing the battles about control over nursing at hospitals in London in the 1870s and 1880s, Judith Moore discusses the problems nurses had when the famous surgeon Joseph Lister moved from his hospital in Edinburgh to take up residence at King's College in London. Lister demanded that thirty more surgical beds be added to the hospital. He also insisted that the operating theater that had been used only twice a week be used everyday. In addition, he introduced antiseptic technique into the operating theater.[27] This meant that nurses cared for more patients. The introduction of antisepsis, although critical to patient care, was also an added burden on the nursing staff. It was not doctors but nurses who washed sheets and scrubbed the floors, tables, basins, and surgical equipment. Nurses were neither consulted about these changes nor about how they could best adapt to them.

In the nineteenth century serious conversations between nurses and patients about their medical conditions were off limits. Nurses today talk almost obsessively about their role as patient educators or advocates and celebrate their commitment to "patient-centered care." Their almost exclusive focus on this role may stem from the fact that medicine has long envisioned the nurse as the physician's advocate and nursing as physician centered. Even in the hospital where she was employed, doctors believed that the nurse worked for the physician, not the patient. Nurses could communicate to the patient only what the doctor wanted or allowed. Answering questions about a patient's condition, updating information about a patient's status, and educating the patient about his or her illness were the physician's job.

Thus, if the patient was dying and the doctor didn't want the patient to know, the nurse could not reveal it. If the patient had a serious illness, more serious than the patient or his family recognized, the nurse could not correct this misconception. Since patients, of course, constantly asked questions of their nurses, nurses were often in the peculiar position of having to assert their ignorance and reinforce their subordination by replying, "I don't know. You'll have to ask the doctor."

In some instances, the nurse may have been able to answer the question **65** better than the physician. In other cases, because of the limited education a nurse received, she may not have had enough knowledge to do so. But then why should she bother to gain that knowledge when she wasn't allowed to put it to use?

Although nurses and doctors depended on a shared language, it was a language many nurses felt they were not allowed to use. If a nurse used a medical term, it would suggest she had medical knowledge and could thus intelligently form a medical opinion. How, one might wonder, could nurses "intelligently cooperate with the physician" and report to him without using medical knowledge? Only by engaging in a fascinating game of hide and seek. The nurse had to hide her conclusion in a sea of verbiage, describing the diverse aspects of what she saw, bit by frustrating bit, while never reaching a conclusion about the phenomenon she observed or reported.

Faced with a patient suffering what we commonly call diarrhea, the nurse could describe "loose stool" but not use the "medical" term that would more concisely name it. Rather than telling or writing that the patient had a suspected heart attack, the nurse could describe the signs and symptoms without using the sacrosanct term "myocardial infarction." Rather than explaining that a mentally ill patient was hallucinating, the nurse could describe the content of his or her fantasies.

As I noted earlier, in the mid-twentieth century nurses ultimately embraced these linguistic circumlocutions by creating "nursing diagnosis," now taught in many nursing schools. This proved to be a double-edged sword. It was a clever way of getting around medical restrictions so that nurses could account for their work. But many have argued that it was also a self-defeating discourse that ghettoized nurses, even while women's liberation was creating opportunities for them to make their work visible to a broader public.

As nineteenth-century medical servants, doctors did want nurses to be assertive, take initiative, and communicate with patients. They wanted nurses to reinforce the physician's authority and take the lead anytime they detected that a patient might not demonstrate, through word or deed, the requisite respect for their doctor.

Interestingly, this preoccupation with physician authority and respect stemmed, in part, from the recognition of nurses' potential to undermine it. Both in the hospital and in private duty nursing in the home, nurses were with patients twenty-four hours a day. Just as doctors worried that the bedside nurse supervised by the lady nurse would almost certainly form an alliance against the doctor, doctors imagined that the patient supervised by the bedside or private duty nurse could form an equally dangerous liaison. Dumb as they were supposed to be, nurses were apparently

66 smart enough to recognize whether a doctor was competent, greedy, or knowledgeable about the latest treatments. Nurses could thus sway patients toward physicians they enjoyed working with or whom they felt were skilled and up-to-date, and away from physicians with dubious credentials. This could have a serious impact on a doctor's ability to get patients and make a living.

The nurse, according to the editors of the *Boston Medical and Surgical Journal*, should "not allow herself, by word or look, to impair the confidence of others in him, though he be not her favorite physician; he is there not by her choice, but by that of the family, and any attempt to excite prejudice against him in favor of another (who may really be far less worthy) must be characterized as mean and mischievous meddling, if not dishonorable intriguing."[28] The nurse must make sure patients "respected their doctor."

These concerns followed nurses into every arena in which they practiced, even public health, in which physicians showed little interest. Karen Buhler-Wilkerson cites numerous incidents where doctors tried to limit nurses' practice in home care because they feared that nurses would successfully compete for social respect and resources. In Boston in the 1890s, for example, doctors "confided to lady managers of home care agencies that 'the constant danger with trained nurses is that they shall usurp the doctors' position and prescribe for patients.'"[29]

At the turn of the twentieth century, with the founding of the Henry Street Settlement on the lower east side of Manhattan, Lillian Wald and her colleagues developed public health nursing "to improve the standards of living" of the sick poor. One of the great innovations of the Henry Street Settlement was the establishment of a "First Aid Room," a kind of community clinic where immigrants could gain easy access to nursing care for routine health problems. Although this innovation was wildly successful and of great help to poor patients, doctors soon complained that "nurses were carrying ointments and even giving pills outside the strict control of physicians."[30] If nurses weren't supposed to have knowledge, they were supposed to have virtues. Lots of them, in fact: "In the economy of nature," the *Lancet* explained, "the ministry of woman is one of help and sympathy. The essential principle, the key-note of her work in the world is aid; to sustain, succour, revive, and even sometimes shelter, man in the struggle and duty of life, is her peculiar function."[31] Women were supposed to be "efficient providers of care," who pursued "higher incentives to activity, zeal, and faithfulness than the mere earning of wages."[32] The French reformer Bourneville extolled training schools that taught moral refinement and "feminine tenderness of spirit" and that "furnish personnel with the same guarantees (as religious orders) of aptitude and devotion."[33] What better way to obtain cheap labor than to instill in the nurses the view that they should sacrifice their material needs to a higher mission or calling?

And indeed, this was the role that was recommended to them. Nurses were supposed to cheerfully or solemnly, as the case warranted, play the role of the ultimate agent of the divine—the ministering angel. As the bishop of Rochester explained in the *Times* of London, nurses were to make of the hospital not only a "place of pain" but a "place of joy . . . where there were angels in human form earning happiness and giving happiness."[34]

The Nursing Response

Given the rules of the period, most nurse reformers accepted this definition of the nurse's role. Some agreed with the basic gender assumptions, others acquiesced to a patriarchal authority they did not have the power to successfully challenge. In Bordeaux, the nurse reformer Anna Hamilton, inspired by Nightingale, was able to gain support for her project of a training school for nurses from Paul-Louis Lande, a physician who became mayor of Bordeaux, only because she "rejected all aspects of reform that expanded the nurses' autonomy or authority beyond the narrowest limits." Hamilton reassured Lande that "it is extremely ridiculous for a nurse who possesses neither the knowledge nor the rights nor the sex of the doctor, to try to imitate his way of interacting with the patient and to try to use his language."[35]

Some nurses openly preached the virtues of silence and invisibility (much as my mother did in the late 1950s when she advised me, "If you show a boy how smart you are you'll scare him off"). On the American frontier in 1889 a mother superior of the Sisters of the Incarnate Word advised a sister, "Remain hidden, Alphonse. I cannot recommend this as much as I would like to, and beg you to give this spirit to our sisters. It is better that people take us for imbeciles, in no matter what, than to consider us clever and intelligent, agreeable to popular or worldly opinion."[36]

Even some of the most outspoken nurses, like Lillian Wald's colleague the socialist Lavinia Dock, were understandably nervous about any public confrontation with powerful physicians. Thus after the spat about the First Aid Room, Dock and Wald began to insist that "the real Henry Street Settlement nurse will make the doctor feel that she is exerting every effort to have his treatment, not hers, intelligently followed."[37]

Because they were women, even the most educated or well-to-do nurse reformers, like Isabel Hampton, Adelaide Nutting, or Ethel Bedford Fenwick, had no legal or social power with which to oppose the medical dom-

68 ination of their profession and of the delivery of health care in general. "Nurse reformers," Joan Lynaugh elaborates, "had to accept the medical view of how health care should be conducted, of the hospital and how it should be run and of who should take care of the sick and how they should be taken care of. That cost nursing a great deal because it was set in a framework of subjugation and authority."

Nurse reformers won the fight to feminize nursing. In many countries in the nineteenth century—in France, Spain, and Italy, and in the United States during the Civil War, for example—men did nursing work. Reformers were so successful in their feminizing mission that by the later part of the nineteenth century men were pushed out of nursing as the field was professionalized. In the United States men were not admitted to most training schools except for those especially set up for the training of men. The more nursing became associated with the stigmatized feminine, the easier it was to dismiss it as a profession.[38]

The scope of nursing education was strictly limited and largely delivered to nurses by physicians. Indeed, to call early hospital schools "schools" would be an exaggeration. Nursing students were far more servants than students and spent most of their time providing cheap labor for hospitals. Courses were squeezed in when pupils had a moment off the ward, but then they were generally too tired to absorb anything they were taught. Once they graduated, most weren't employed in the hospital but had to find work in private duty in people's homes. A new set of indentured students/servants were recruited to do backbreaking labor in the hospital.[39]

Nurse reformers engineered an enormous accomplishment, the first mass profession for respectable women working outside the home. Because of the period in which they worked, however, the stage was set for nurses to be viewed as an endless source of cheap, disposable labor for hospitals, as servants to doctors, and as angels, saints, and martyrs to the public and the media.

Concealing the Nurse's Medical and Technical Mastery

Rather than being viewed as interdependent with medicine, nursing was turned into a dependent, subordinate profession. This view of medical dominance and nurse deference was maintained through the construction of what has been considered an almost unbreachable divide between the "medical" and "nursing" forms of knowledge and practice. The nurse, on one side of the divide, was not supposed to engage in the practice of medicine even though she was constantly practicing it. Meanwhile the doctor, on the other side, gained his reputation for scientific and technological mastery, absent the nurse but constantly depending her knowledge, judgments, and actions.

In *Say Little, Do Much: Nursing, Nuns and Hospitals in the 19th Century*, Sioban Nelson describes a little-known fact: about half of the hospitals established in the New World in the mid to late nineteenth century were founded, built, staffed, and administered by nurses—women from religious orders who traveled to Australia, New Zealand, Canada, and the United States. These women set up the only health care available in many areas. Although we pass by the hospitals every day—the Providences, the Deaconesses, the St. Vincents, and the St. Francises or Mercys—few people know that they were founded and administered by nurses.[40]

In another critical study, Margarete Sandelowski describes how medical advances were, and still are, dependent on nurses' ability to manipulate technology, interpret its results, and explain technological interventions in a way that encourages patients to accept these interventions and "comply" with medical treatments. From the discovery of the thermometer to the development of intensive heart and fetal monitoring, "The key to accurate medical diagnosis and patient recovery," Sandelowski writes, "was the close observation of the trained nurse."[41] As observing patients became far more than a matter of a short daily visit, but rather required checking, monitoring, recording, and reporting over a period of days or weeks, doctors could not possibly care for a full load of patients without the assistance of skilled observers. These skilled observers had to record and rerecord and report symptoms and signs throughout the patient's hospitalization or illness. Treatments had to be given, then repeated, then given yet again. While all this was going on, the patient had to be fed, washed, clothed, and helped to get through the day.

Doctors had neither the time nor the inclination to engage in this kind of educated observation, treatment administration, and monitoring. To effect a successful cure or to amass the data that would "contribute to the sum of human knowledge or the advancement of science,"[42] physicians depended on nurses, who, Sandelowski writes, had "to differentiate between subjective and objective symptoms, between symptoms and signs, between real and feigned symptoms, between leading and misleading symptoms, and between symptoms and signs significant for nursing care and those significant for medical care. . . . Nurses were to appraise the condition of every visible portion of the body, using parameters appropriate for that part. . . . What could be discerned from outside comprised virtually all the information available to the general nursing or medical practitioner."[43]

Nurses' observations and activities became more important as medical

70   technology advanced, and nurses utilized many of the diagnostic tools we have come to associate with medical progress. Consider the thermometer, one of the first and most interesting examples of this process. From the moment that the first thermometers replaced the hand on the feverish brow in the mid-nineteenth century, physicians relied on nurses to take and interpret the patient's temperature. Physicians expected nurses to "know what caused various temperatures to occur and the nursing measures that would lower or raise temperature to normal levels."[44]

Manipulating this early diagnostic technology wasn't easy. Early thermometers were hardly the sleek, digital devices that slip into a patient's mouth. Made of glass, they were unwieldy, foot long instruments. They did not retain the temperature reading once removed from the patient but had to be read when they were in contact with the patient's skin. Fragile devices that could present a danger to the patient, they had to be carefully used to prevent injury.

Clinical thermometry, Sandelowski argues, allowed "the labor of diagnosis to be separated into unequal parts, with nurses increasingly assuming what were perceived as the largely mechanical tasks of taking and recording temperatures and of maintaining thermometers, and physicians taking on what was considered the higher-order interpretive task of evaluating what the temperatures meant. By placing the tasks of diagnosis in a hierarchy and reserving the label of diagnosis only for physicians' acts of interpretation, physicians could deny that nonphysicians played any part in thermometric diagnosis."[45] While physicians were the ones to insert the first intravenous devices, nurses were the ones to make their utilization possible, since patients' arms had to be immobilized once the needle was inserted into their vein.

Oxygen therapy was also an instructive example of this invisible collaboration between physician and nurse in both diagnosis and treatment. While physicians were supposed to be the ones who possessed the theoretical knowledge of the scientific properties of oxygen, it was nurses who delivered the therapy to patients and who thus had what Sandelowski calls the "practical knowledge of enactment and application."[46]

Doctors similarly depended on nurses to do the job of "educating patients about new devices, getting patients to accept and comply with their use, and alleviating patients' fears about them."[47] If medical treatment is frightening today, when many of us are born and die in hospitals, and watch television shows like *ER* or read about the medical breakthroughs in newspapers and magazines, imagine how terrifying medical technology and treatments appeared to people who had never set foot in a hospital and whose only contact with medicine was herbs and poultices. The nurses' ability to approach and reassure terrified patients, to keep them quiet, and to help them agree to treatment was critical to the doctor's capacity to introduce many new technological developments.

Nurses, however, were not allowed or invited to formally cross the threshold from handmaid to collaborator and colleague. Indeed, even as nurses advanced in the skills of data collection and interpretation, physicians maintained the fiction that they did neither. Sandelowski cites one typical physician comment: "Outside of correct reports, the nurse has nothing to do with diagnosis or prognosis. And, beyond executing orders, and recording bedside notes, (she) has no part in the treatment." "On one hand," she continues, "many physicians saw nurses as Baconian data collectors whose only job was to obtain the 'raw data' the physician required. On the other hand, nurses were not just to report whatever they saw without interpretive comment; they should also discern the likely reason for a symptom, know what a symptom meant, and take the required action."[48]

Nurses have continued to play a central role in the development and use of the technology of medical cure and treatment. In the 1950s, 1960s, and 1970s nurses were instrumental in the creation of the intensive care unit, which, in Julie Fairman and Joan Lynaugh's words, arose because an "increasingly complex hospital population" was suffering from "acute episodes of chronic diseases such as heart and vascular disease." Although advances in medical treatment led these patients to have higher expectations for their survival, it was also clear that only intensive nursing care could mitigate serious complications—or death. As operations became more complex and treatments more sophisticated, patients were at risk for a variety of complications such as shock, airway obstruction, systemic infections (sepsis), infection, wound hemorrhage, and potentially fatal heart rhythm irregularities. Nurses quickly recognized that something needed to be done to allow them to care for such sick patients. "The units were invented because of the problems that came from a patient being desperately ill and needing *one* nurse. . . . Finding a way to respond to that situation multiplied by thousands of times forced us to change the hospital," an early critical care nurse explained.[49]

As new technologies were developed, nurses have been some of their primary users. They are often more knowledgeable about the functioning and use of such equipment than doctors. Indeed, "the benefits of machine monitoring could not be fully harnessed without nurses who understood and could act immediately on the information monitors generated," Sandelowski writes.[50] While the public does not recognize this fact, medical equipment manufacturers certainly do. Equipment makers understand that nurses are the primary users of certain types of medical technology. They have consulted nurses in the design of the technology, used

72 them as salespeople for the technology, and employed them to educate doctors and nurses about its use.

While, at physician's behest, nurses clearly played an increasing role in the diagnosis and treatment of patients, their on-stage activity was hidden behind an opaque scrim of physician agency and control. As nurses became more expert at things like IV therapy or the taking and interpreting of vital signs, they always did so under the guise of being the "physician's agent," or borrowing his agency.[51] While nurses were given legal permission to perform more medical tasks and became more expert than medical men, doctors held on to control even in areas where nurses attained the highest level of technical mastery. Moreover, as Sandelowski explained to me, rather than upgrading the nurse who performed tasks that doctors used to do, medicine downgraded the tasks. Doctors were relieved from activities they considered routine and transferred those activities to nurses. Now that nurses have advanced into nurse-practitioner roles, many members of the public consider them to be cheaper doctors who do the routine, less complex tasks of medicine. "Nurses," Sandelowski says, "get the responsibility without the authority."

Making Nursing a Semi-profession

For well over a hundred years, doctors have fought for—and society has granted—what sociologist Eliot Freidson has described as an "organized monopoly" over all of health care. This, along with advances in public health, delivered tangible benefits. Medicine, Freidson has written, was thus able to gain "command of the criteria that qualify men to work at healing, of exclusive competence to determine the proper content and effective method of performing medical work, and freely consulted by those thought to need its help." This organized monopoly gave doctors state control and thus the right to control the work of other clinical disciplines, like nursing. "Legally and otherwise the physician's right to diagnose, cut, and prescribe is the center around which the work of many other occupations swings, and the physician's authority and responsibility in that constellation of work are primary," Freidson explains.[52]

Nurses gain great skill in manipulating medical technology. They often interpret the meaning of the results gained from the use of medical technology, act on it themselves, and convey it to doctors. They administer medications, monitor patients' responses to treatment, protect patients against the side effects of those medications, help patients live their lives while they are ill and are being treated for an illness. They are critical to patient education and, they claim, are particularly adept at listening to and advocating for patients. But the performance of all of these activities is dependent on the orders of, and "knowledge" of doctors and is under girded by decades of deference to the concept of "medically necessary care" and the absence of any parallel concept of "necessary nursing care."[53]

This is why Freidson argued that "an aggressive occupation like nursing can have its own schools for training, can control licensing boards in many instances, and can have its own 'service' in the hospital, in this way giving the appearance of formal, state-supported, and departmental autonomy, but the work which its members perform remains subject to the order of another occupation." Given this state of affairs, Freidson goes on to say, nursing "cannot gain occupational autonomy no matter how intelligent and aggressive its leadership."[54]

Medicine's monopoly has also helped to deny nursing the legitimating title of a "profession." Over the course of a hundred and fifty years, sociological definitions of professions have withheld this prestigious title from nursing. Nursing has instead been consigned to the limbo of a "para-profession," "semi-profession," or "allied" profession.

In a famous *New Yorker* cartoon map of the United States, Manhattan occupies a vast foreground while the rest of the country recedes into a miniaturized background. In a similar manner, sociological cartographers depict what is essential to medicine and what and is marginal. High school and elementary teaching, nursing, and social work have often been found wanting. An essay by Fred E. Katz in *The Semi-Professions and Their Organization: Teachers, Nurses, Social Workers*, edited by the sociologist Amitai Etzioni, is a prime example. Katz explains that hospitals "harness both scientific and non-scientific resources for the care and treatment of patients." Medicine represents the former while nursing represents "nonscientific caring." Hospitals do nurses a great favor, Katz asserts, by allowing the nonscientific, care-minded RN onto the premises. "In return for the right to practice nonscientific, nurturent care that has no clear place in the medical textbooks, the nurse accepts a low place in the hospital's status hierarchy." Nurses are "cheerful and loving," because "nurturence" is the "fundamental ingredient of traditional nursing, far more so than the harnessing of rational knowledge."[55]

The doctor, on the other hand, is expected to be the "rightful knower," the proper "guardian of knowledge." Doctors are involved in dynamic, creative work in which there is, apparently, never a dull moment. Nursing involves the performance of a series of tedious, "clearly delineated tasks, tasks that can be written down on an assignment sheet and checked off when they are done." While doctors deliver serious diagnostic and treatment services that are of enormous consequence, Katz repeatedly reminds us, nurses mobilize the "knowledge of the heart" in the delivery of TLC.

74 So devoted are RNs to this mission that they willingly conceal any contributions they themselves make to medical treatment. With the exception of some malcontents in nursing leadership, the ordinary nurse is committed to "knowing her place."[56]

These medical and sociological descriptions illustrate the trap that was set for nurses and sometimes by nurses. Nurses have rarely been given public credit for their technical skills. These skills clearly demonstrate that nurses have the intellectual capacity not only to perform "mere practical skills" but also to master complex concepts and processes and to participate actively in diagnosis and treatment. Nurses have successfully used this technological and medical knowledge and know-how to upgrade their status within their own profession and to create intraprofessional status hierarchies. Their technical/medical roles have not, however, lifted the profile of the rest of the profession either with the public or with medicine.

As we shall see, while nurses congratulate one another on their "expanded," "enhanced," or "advanced" practice roles, many members of the public or policy community believe that the new nurse is no longer "just a nurse" (read just a servant). She has become someone and something else—a sort of almost doctor. Nurses who are left doing "just nursing" remain prisoners of a nineteenth-century dichotomy. The Catch-22 is complete. The caring, nurturing side of nursing with its ability to deliver efficient care and make order out of chaos—so connected to femininity—seems to be the only uncontested space for nurses, yet it is simultaneously devalued. As Rosenberg has argued, nursing's claims to legitimacy, like the emphasis on female sensibility, have always been a double-edged sword. To fit into the spaces allocated to them, "discussions of nursing's intellectual content often turned on its unique ability to provide order and efficiency in the ward and sick room, and not on discipline-specific cognitive skills."[57]

Today nursing is viewed as passive and static, while medicine is active and dynamic. Nursing is mired in tedium, while medicine advances toward wide horizons of progress. While she is practical, hands-on, and has little intellectual curiosity or scientific ambition, he is "heads on," needs intellectual stimulation and a consistent sense of challenge. When it comes to remuneration and reward, the same either/or's apply. She is supposed to be self-sacrificing, altruistic, and content with the virtues that are their own rewards. But if we don't pay him—or now her—enough, we will never get the best and the brightest. (When was the last time you heard someone say that about a nurse?) Which is why she's never supposed to go on strike, whereas when he threatens to withdraw his services, politicians and insurers hop to it. For her, the gratitude and love of the pa- tient is always enough, as is the fact that she is loved because she is ethical and honest. For him, to be loved is never enough. Even if scorned by his subordinates, he insists upon respect. All of which makes the doctor the "professional" worker and the nurse merely a "technical" one.

3

The Disruptive Medical System

A s they try to address the nursing shortage, nursing organizations often talk about recruiting people who have had one career and are interested in making a switch. Faith Henson is one of those older, second-career nurses. She began her nursing career at the age of fifty-five. When she was working nights at the hospital, she occasionally had to call doctors at home to report changes in patient status. One might think that doctors would respond politely and expeditiously to the nurses' calls. Not so, Henson says. Each doctor has a different idea about when it is necessary or appropriate for a nurse to call.

Henson outlines the dilemma. "You have to know each doctor well enough to know when and for what reason to call. For example, Physician A wants you to call them for any change in vital signs. Physician B doesn't want you to call them unless a patient is dying. Physician C says you should call only if this or that is happening. So if you wake them up in the middle of the night and it's not in the ballpark of what they want to be woken up about, they can be very abusive."

If a physician is exhausted after a difficult day and does not want his sleep to be interrupted, he may pass the buck. Henson remembers one particular night when she had a patient who had come out of surgery to her intensive care unit and developed serious breathing problems. He had been stable for a few days before developing the problem. The patient was so frightened that he asked her to call his wife and daughter. Suspecting that the patient had developed a pulmonary embolism, a potentially fatal complication, Henson called the surgeon who had performed the patient's operation. He refused to come and told Henson to call the patient's cardiologist. The cardiologist, who may have been equally exhausted, told **77** Henson to call the patient's pulmonologist, or lung specialist. He also refused to come in and told her to call the covering pulmonologist. "By this time the patient was coding" (going into cardiac arrest), Henson says, "and I couldn't get anyone to come in."

The patient died. Since the hospital required Henson to call the various doctors to apprise them of this fact, Henson telephoned the patient's pulmonologist. The next morning, when he came into the hospital, the pulmonologist was furious, Henson reports. "He came right up to me and said, 'Faith, don't you ever call me to tell me a patient has died. I can find out when I get here in the morning.' I said, 'Okay, you put that in writing, because two weeks ago, you had a nurse written up for not calling you.' There's no consistency. It's very, very difficult to deal with."

While dealing with "superiors" who are rude or abusive is hardly unique to the medical workplace, nurse-doctor relationships have certain unique features that make them a serious public health issue. Poor nurse-doctor relationships drive nurses out of hospitals and sometimes even out of nursing, and they jeopardize the lives or recovery of patients.

Nurse-Physician Noncommunication

If people are responsible for the care of a sick, vulnerable human being whose condition can destabilize in a matter of minutes, it's essential that they remain in close, sometimes constant communication. When doctors are at the patient's bedside only a few minutes a day, if at all, nurse-doctor communication becomes imperative. "Whether it's information shared on rounds, noted in the chart, or discussed on the phone, the essence of patient care is communication between physician and nurse," says nurse Jean Chaisson. "Patient care is all about the exchange of valuable assessment and evaluation data, which are critical to making plans for maintaining or improving health and function of the patient."

Such communication is, however, even more critical in a system of structured inequality where the nurse's practice is, theoretically at least, subject to the doctor's order. Nurses simply can't do their jobs if they can't reach doctors in a timely manner. But communication about the changing status of the patient is one of the most complex aspects of dysfunctional doctor-nurse relationships. It's complicated by doctors who seemingly fail to understand why nurses are trying to reach them, by doctors who entangle nurses in their own internecine feuds and rivalries, by physicians who want to avoid uncomfortable issues, and by a system of care that has become increasingly fragmented. "I waste so much of my time every day trying to get a hold of doctors with concerns or questions about patient

78 treatment plans," says Susan Thomasy, a nurse at Newton Wellesley Hospital in Massachusetts. "I'm either worried about a patient, or trying to convey to the doc a concern the patient has, or can't read the orders clearly, or just don't understand what we're doing with their treatment. I need to find their numbers, speak with their secretaries to have them paged, wait for the page, and then if they don't call back, redo the above, and so on and so on."

In her years of experience as a nurse, Thomasy says there are a "handful of doctors who do it right." When they visit their patients, they look on the assignment board to ascertain who is caring for that patient and then seek out the nurse and ask relevant questions and answer any questions or address any concerns the nurse has. This, Thomasy says, shows "respect for nurses and for what we do."

And she adds, it is so rare. In most cases, nurses feel that they bear the burden of trying to facilitate communication with doctors who are so harried that they seem to flee from their approach.

"Most docs see the patient, scribble something in the orders of the patient's chart, and leave," Thomasy continues. "I try to keep a lookout for my patients' doctors and try to approach them each day, because it makes the patient's treatment so much safer and my day so much easier. But I'm often with someone else and they seem almost to sneak in and out and I miss them."

In most hospitals, physicians tend to make their rounds early in the morning. This is a time when nurses are making their initial evaluation of patients, when they are doing their own data collection, giving basic personal care, making sure patients are fed, or perhaps getting patients to the bathroom. Because what the nurse knows about the patient is crucial to the formation of a medical plan of care, it's critical for the nurse to provide her perspective on patient care issues during rounds. Similarly, information that the physician has is critical to the formation of the nursing plan for care. "But rounds are not conducted at a mutually convenient time," Thomasy points out. "Doing the work to create a real infrastructure for multidisciplinary teamwork has simply never been a priority in most places, and so rounds are conducted for the convenience of the physician."

The increasing fragmentation of care in the modern health care system makes nurse-physician communication even more of a nightmare. Many physicians, nurses say, continue to believe that the individual nurse is not working for the hospital and its patients but is working for them personally and that the nurse's sole priority is to care for the patients of that individual physician. But unless they are working for a physician or physician practice, nurses are employed by hospitals to take care of a group of patients who are admitted by a variety of physicians. This means that each nurse is juggling the demands of not one but many physicians.

Jean Chaisson offers a typical example. An elderly woman tells her primary care doctor that she feels weak, short of breath, and is having trouble sleeping because of a persistent cough. The primary care doctor admits her to a hospital unit with chronic lung disease plus heart failure. In this hospital this doctor will be known as her "attending" and "admitting" physician, but he will be only one of a larger medical cast of characters that may include a pulmonary doctor, a heart doctor, and a kidney doctor. If she is admitted to a teaching hospital, there will also be interns, residents, and fellows involved.

"One doctor will say she needs more fluids. Another thinks she should get less. One says she needs more diuretics. Another says she needs steroids. No wait, hold off on steroids, another chimes in. Consider antibiotics. No, maybe not." Chaisson offers a verbal pantomime of what often happens. Or, there's a patient who has just come out of surgery. "Surgeons are recommending fluids and postoperative treatments. There may be a cardiologist who recommends very different treatments, and an anesthesiologist who is coordinating the pain control. The nurse is trying to facilitate communication between disciplines who don't always have time to talk to each other."

To complicate further the already chaotic picture, there will be times when decisions about treatment will be made by a doctor who has never met—and who may never meet—the patient, as in the fatal case Henson described. This is the physician who happens to be "on call," that is, covering for another physician who is off duty, asleep, on vacation, out for the weekend, or performing surgery. So it's critical for the nurse to know the patient, be aware of all the suggestions, and be able to reach the various doctors in a timely fashion.

In today's environment, nurses are taking care of eight, ten, twelve, or even more patients—all of whom are sicker than ever and are in the hospital for briefer stays. Multiply those eight to twelve patients by the many physicians involved in their care and by the urgency of their needs and you begin to get a picture of the workload nurses now routinely juggle.

In April 2003, I met with ten nurses from the Massachusetts Nurses Association. The group of nine women and one man included nurses who'd been in the profession for twenty or thirty years and younger nurses with five or ten years of service. The nurses worked in Boston teaching hospitals, as well as hospitals and visiting nurse agencies in rural areas. These nurses recognized that physicians were under increasing pressure to see more patients and were relentlessly hassled by insurers. Instead of recognizing the mutual problems all clinicians encountered under managed care and cost cutting, and joining together to find ways to deal with them, nurses felt that physicians, wittingly or not, entrapped nurses in their own professional tensions, adding to the frustrations of an already difficult work environment.

One nurse spoke of the difficulties of simply getting telephone orders for a patient who'd just come out of surgery. The surgeon who performed the operation insisted that what the patient was experiencing was not a "surgical" but a "medical" problem. When the nurse responded that he was the doctor on the chart, he insisted that she find a "medical" doctor to deal with the patient's "medical problems." This goose chase, she said, took a great deal of time out of a far too busy schedule.

"You never know which doctor is dealing with which aspect of patient care," another nurse explained. This nurse had recently asked one of the doctors, an orthopedic surgeon, to order an incentive sperimeter, a device that encourages patients to cough after surgery. Although he could easily have written the order, he refused, arguing that the nurse should seek an order from someone in medicine not surgery. Although this surgeon may not have been ducking out just to catch an extra round of golf, the need to chase down a medical doctor complicated the nurse's workday.

Nurses also report that they have trouble doing their jobs, because physicians often have difficulty dealing with thorny issues like giving patients bad news and helping them make decisions about the termination of futile treatment.

Tomes have been written analyzing why physicians have difficulty navigating end-of-life decisions. Physicians may feel that the patient's death is a personal failure or they may not be well tutored in delivering bad news. Also, physicians are not reimbursed for spending time working through complex issues with patients. Many physicians thus retreat from end-of-life decision making, and nurses must often deal with the fallout of this avoidance.

Marion Phipps recounts a typical incident. As a clinical nurse specialist, Phipps has worked with bedside nurses to deal with the problems involved in caring for complex patients or groups of patients. After a decades-long career at Boston's Beth Israel Hospital, Phipps moved to the neurological unit at the Massachusetts General Hospital. There she recently worked with a young nurse who was caring for a ninety-six-year-old patient who had just had a severe stroke and whose family wanted the patient to have a full code (full-court rescue in the case of a cardiac arrest) rather than Do Not Resuscitate status (which would give the patient comfort measures only). On a Thursday night during the patient's stay, the man developed congestive heart failure, and medication was used to help him breathe more comfortably. The next morning, the nurse who took

over his care was concerned because his breathing pattern was abnormal. **81**
Sometimes he would even stop breathing. Phipps and the nurse suggested
that the entire medical team reassess the situation and try to talk to the
family about end-of-life care.

Given the patient's condition, neither nurse felt there was any clinical
justification to break the patient's ribs or burn the patient's flesh with electrical paddles while they did cardiac resuscitation. Even if his heart was
restarted, he would barely survive and have no quality of life. Yet, the staff
nurse knew that if the patient "coded" on her watch, she would be the one
to initiate CPR on the frail, dying man.

She thus called the neurological team to discuss the issues with them.
The doctors failed to respond. She then called the medical team that had
been called in to consult on his condition. When a young intern came by,
he refused to get involved. As the hours passed, with no plan in place,
Phipps said, the young nurse was left with a man who could go into cardiac arrest at any minute and she would have to act. Phipps said the nurse
wondered whether the same thing would have happened had it been a
doctor who called the team. She suspected they would have responded
differently to her serious and urgent concerns. The young nurse felt like
the doctors simply blew her off.

Patty Healey, an ICU nurse at a Boston teaching hospital, says that
some doctors will simply ignore her when they feel she challenges them.
"I may say that the patient's symptoms are such and such, and her blood
pressure isn't stable. I tell them I don't agree that we should give her a
medicine they have prescribed at this point, because we don't have adequate knowledge about, for example, her fluid status." Doctors, she says,
often misinterpret what are collegial, clinical concerns as a challenge to
their authority. "When doctors feel challenged," Healey continues, "what
they very often do is turn around and walk away without responding to
me at all."

Other physicians may not be as passive in their resistance. In some
rounds, instead of responding respectfully and collegially when she raises
a concern, Healey says that "in the past year I have been physically
bumped out of the rounds. Doctors will physically back into me so that I
am not part of the group. It's happened to me—even with women physicians."

Verbal Abuse

Doctors today may be exhausted. They may be frustrated by the burdens
of having to take care of more and more patients. They may be irritated at
managed care interference. Many may not understand that nurses are not

82 making random calls to physicians in the middle of the night but are legitimately concerned about patients and cannot do their job without a doctor's orders. Whatever the rationale for physician behavior, as the study by the VHA on doctor-nurse relationships concluded, when nurses pick up a phone to make a routine call to a doctor, or take their posts at the bedside, they face the distinct possibility that a doctor will not only blow them off but blow up at them.

Tim Sweeney* began his nursing career six years ago working in a for-profit hospital in Texas. "I never like to set up a morality play between doctors and nurses," he says, "but the culture in the South was just incredible. Physicians would come in and just start screaming at you. As a nurse you have multiple patients, but most doctors I worked with in Texas didn't seem to get that. In Texas, if a physician came in and you weren't right in there, because you were working with another patient or talking with another physician, they would get right up next to you and be physically threatening with their stance. I'm a guy and I found it offensive and unreasonable. You can imagine what a woman would feel like."

Sweeney cited a conflict that occurred when he was taking care of a young patient who arrived in the ER with a major heart problem. The cardiologist who examined the patient wanted to perform surgery immediately, but to do that he needed permission from the boy's legal guardian, which meant someone had to find the guardian. When Sweeney took more time than the cardiologist felt was appropriate, Sweeney says, "He wouldn't let me finish trying to find who we needed. He got right in my face and started screaming, 'Can you get on the phone! Can you get somebody right now!' It was right in front of the patient, other RNs, and ER physicians. No one stood up for me. It was standard, acceptable practice. I told him to get out of my face, to step away, because he was too close."

What Sweeney found so interesting was that doctors who were abusive to nurses seemed to be Jekyll-and-Hyde characters. "There was a gastroenterologist in town who was actually my gastroenterologist. I went to see him as a patient. He was so nice. I was really impressed at how he treated me as a patient. Three days later, he came in while I was working in the ER to work on a gastroenterology case. As soon as he walked into the room, it was like he was a different person. He started screaming at the nurses. I was starting an IV on another patient who was in critical condition, and he said, 'Well, I guess nobody's going to move too fast around here,' implying I was lazy. His expectation was that I would be there to serve him and only him, as though the ER wasn't full of other patients and other physicians."

While many nurses say that they have excellent relationships with physicians, most of the nurses I interviewed have had some experience with a physician who throws a temper tantrum, screams, and humiliates the nurse in front of patients, family members, physicians, and other clinicians. "You call because you've identified a problem," said a nurse from western Massachusetts, "and what you often get is a very demeaning attitude." A nurse at the Royal Victoria Hospital in Montreal recently asked a female surgeon to clarify an order. "I don't need to repeat the orders for you," the surgeon snapped. "You're only here because we need you. I wish that one day we won't need you."

Nurses say they are particularly at risk for this kind of abusive behavior if they try to teach patients how to cope with their illnesses or if they question physicians about an order, a potential mistake, or a chosen treatment plan.

A major part of nurses' role is to educate patients about their treatments, their procedures, changes in lifestyle, diet, exercise, how to cope with an illness, and how to deal with medications and other treatments when they are discharged home. Many physicians understand and value this function. "The nurses' role in educating patients," says Dr. Glenn Bubley, an oncologist and prostate cancer researcher at the Beth Israel Deaconess Medical Center, "is of paramount importance. Patient education cannot be done by doctors alone. Nurses and doctors both try to reinforce what the side effects of the drugs are. So if I tell a patient a drug could cause thrombocytopenia (low platelets) and therefore may lead to bleeding, I usually rely on the nurse to reinforce this message. This is a potentially dire effect, and patients absolutely need to hear this from more than the physician."

"Patients often pretend that they understand things when talking to their doctor," Bubley explains, "yet they sometimes get greater comprehension when talking to the nurse. Very many patients, especially older patients, feel more at ease asking a nurse questions than they do asking their doctor, particularly regarding those side effects that are potentially life threatening."

Bubley states the case eloquently. Some doctors, however, seem to interpret this kind of teaching as an unwanted interference, as meddling in "medical" issues or trespassing on "medical" turf.

In Florida, Connie Barden described a recent experience. Barden has been a critical care nurse for years. She was the president of the American Association of Critical Care Nurses and is a cardiovascular clinical specialist at a hospital in Florida. Her job is to help nurses and doctors deal with complex cases. One of these patients was an eighty-three-year-old

84 man who was on a ventilator in the ICU because of problems with his heart, lung, and kidneys. The old man could no longer communicate, and his family members, who served as his health care proxy, were confused about the meaning of a Do Not Resuscitate order. Because the nurses caring for the patient were unclear about what the family wanted, they asked for Barden's help.

Barden met with the man's two daughters. As often happens in crisis situations, the family didn't understand what was happening with their father and seemed not to understand what the physician had explained to them. "This is one of the reasons we have nurses," Barden explained. "Sometimes physicians explain things to patients, and they just don't understand. Families vary in their ability to hear things in the middle of a crisis, and physicians don't have a lot of time to spend at the bedside, so nurses serve as interpreters."

In this case, the daughters had reams of questions. Barden explained the patient's status. The family asked Barden questions about the man's prognosis, but, Barden says, "I never go there. I don't give families percentages" or "likelihood of survival." When they asked Barden if she'd ever seen anyone in their father's condition get off a ventilator, she said that, yes, she had. She also went on to explain the meaning of a DNR order. In the end, after a forty-five-minute conversation, the family decided to make their father "DNR."

When Barden came to work the next morning, she found a frantic phone message from one of the patient's daughters. "I hope we didn't get you into trouble," the daughter blurted out when Barden returned the call. The daughter explained that when the physician came in at night to talk with the family, someone had referred to the meeting they had with Barden and to the comments she had made. "What are you doing listening to a nurse?" the physician exclaimed. "You should know better than to listen to the nurses in the hospital. Who you need to be talking to are the doctors."

Barden went in search of the doctor and asked him what had happened. He explained that he felt the patient was doing very badly and would never make it out of the hospital. Since Barden had accomplished what he had apparently been unable to do—get the family to request a DNR order—the issue seemed not to be the outcome of the discussion but the very fact that it had taken place at all. According to the family, he insisted, Barden had contradicted him, and he feared that this would create problems. Barden clarified what she had, in fact, told the family and the conversation ended.

In her view, the conversation did not, however, resolve the dilemma. Barden felt that the doctor should have talked to her about his concerns rather than tell the family not to listen to a nurse. "Can you imagine what he would have done had I told patients and families they should never listen to their doctor?" she asked. "It would never occur to me to do such a thing. Not because I'm afraid of doctors or want patients to defer to them, but because all of us have to cooperate if patients are to get through the process of illness."

In this particular case, Barden felt increasingly wary of doing her job with this patient and family, because she feared further flack from the physician. "Over the next couple of days," Barden says, "I went and visited the family to make sure they were okay, but I was skittish with them. I noticed I was very reluctant to get in the middle and try to interpret any more information for them for fear it could put us in an awkward spot. This deprived them of a resource or lessened the resource. To be honest, I was much more reserved than I would have been, absolutely."

Physical Abuse

In the case of some doctors, verbal abuse of the kind Barden describes may be a warning sign of such poor impulse control, and such poor attitudes toward nursing, that the doctor may end up physically assaulting a nurse. On September 26, 2001, Anne Dolan* reported to work as usual. Dolan, an operating room nurse at Montreal General Hospital who'd been a nurse for twelve years, had spent most of her time working in the intensive care unit. Earlier in the year, she had taken a two-month training to be an operating room nurse, and since March she had been scrubbing in the operating theater. On that particular Wednesday, she was scheduled to do a rotation in orthopedic surgery. She had been assigned to work in one operating theater when suddenly she was asked to work in a different theater. It turned out that the surgeon whom she would now be assisting was known to be sometimes physically abusive to "underlings." This morning he'd come into the OR and, true to form, he'd begun berating the staff. The nurse assigned to work with him refused her assignment and Dolan, a relatively new nurse, was asked to replace her.

Although Dolan understood that the physician had a bad reputation, she took the assignment. "To me," she said, when recounting the incident two years later, "you have to be professional. I had worked with this surgeon on night, doing trauma." She thought, therefore, she could handle him.

What she didn't understand was that, at least for this particular surgeon, the level of stress on nights is often lower than on days. At night, the surgeon might have only one or two surgeries, or maybe none at all. On days, surgeons book multiple cases back to back. Since health care

86 cost cutting has limited surgeons' incomes in Canada as well as in the United States, money considerations mean even more surgeries are booked. If anything goes wrong to delay the assembly line of cases, surgeons—already working in an anxiety-provoking field—may become more anxious and irritable. They may thus take their frustrations out on those who have a lower rank in the hospital hierarchy.

Although Dolan thought she could manage the surgeon, she was, she said, nonetheless worried enough about his reputation to ask a more experienced nurse to scrub with her. Because she was relatively new at the job, she didn't want to be distracted by any of his antics and felt that moral—and, if necessary, clinical—support might steady her in case he "started acting up, or going crazy."

Both nurses scrubbed and worked with the physician on a femoral nailing. In this operation, a titanium rod or "nail" is placed into a femur that has been damaged by either a fracture or cancer. In the operating room, the surgeon creates a canal inside the femur, inserts a titanium rod to stabilize the bone, and fixes it in place with one screw at the head of the femur and two at the base. Although the surgeon seemed a bit unsettled by a new spiral blade they were using in the hospital, the operation was going well. The more experienced nurse stood on the opposite side of the operating table and didn't lift a finger throughout the procedure.

Near the end of the operation, the surgeon asked a circulating nurse to release the traction on one leg of the operating table. The table moved away too quickly and the motion upset the already tense surgeon, who screamed at the nurse. The quick release of the table also jarred a basin that held the drill the doctor would use to drill the hole in which the last screw would be inserted. When Dolan reached out to remove the drill to maintain its sterility, the surgeon misinterpreted the gesture. He thought she was contaminating it as well as other objects in the sterile field. Without hesitating, he reached out and grabbed her hand and shook it "nonstop," Dolan said.

Because the patient was under epidural anesthetic—an anesthesia that leaves the bottom half of the body without sensation while the patient remains conscious—Dolan tried to stay calm and keep her voice low. Quietly, so as not to frighten the patient, she told the surgeon he was hurting her and asked him to let go of her hand. The experienced nurse watching from across the table also asked the surgeon to release Dolan's hand. He finally did, but the harm had already been done.

The surgeon put in his screw and left the operating room. Dolan, her hand painful, stayed while the resident sutured the patient. After she cleaned the table she left the OR, shaken and hurt. Her hand was blue and swollen, the marks of the surgeon's fingers imprinted on the flesh. When the head nurse of the operating room saw the distraught nurse, she came **87** up to her. When she saw the hand, she immediately took a photograph and also called the director of nursing, the manager of the operating room, and a member of the human resources department. Then Dolan went down to the emergency room, where X rays were taken. After that, Dolan was examined by a physician she knew and with whom she felt comfortable. He brought Dolan to a hand surgeon, one of the most respected in the hospital, who diagnosed tendon damage and advised putting her arm in a cast. This hand surgeon also approached the surgeon who had hurt Dolan, and the surgeon came up to speak to her.

"He told me that the operation had gone well and that he hadn't wanted this to happen," Dolan recounts. "And then he said, 'But you know it was your fault.' "

Susan Mullan, who is in her early fifties and has been an operating room nurse for over twenty years, is the president of the nurses' union at the hospital. She told me that once news of what happened to Dolan circulated among OR nurses at Montreal General, the response was both unequivocal and unusual. Although everybody had known about this surgeon's behavior for years, the consensus was that "this surgeon had crossed a line."

"We all knew this wasn't the first thing this particular surgeon had done," Mullan told me as we sat late one spring afternoon in a café near the McGill hospitals. "The surgeon had thrown a mallet. He had wrenched one of the resident's arms so badly he dislocated the elbow. He threw the X-ray machine out of the way and in doing so hit the X-ray tech." She paused, catching her breath to catalogue his conduct, "And that's just the physical stuff. The verbal stuff is worse because it's constant. A constant stream of yelling, cursing, swearing, slamming instruments around on the table, just saying that nothing is right, nothing is any good."

The problem, Mullan said, is that while this particular surgeon acted out physically and verbally, he was not alone. "There are about three or four who are really verbally aggressive with nurses. The others are a little more subtle but it's still there. They're degrading of your work efforts. They make snide remarks like 'How come we never have the right equipment in the room? How come we're always running late? Why is the set never right? Why can't you read the book and do it properly?' What it creates for nurses and others is a very threatening, hostile work environment," Mullan concluded.

Until Dolan's arm was hurt, according to Mullan, nurses responded like victims of battered woman syndrome. Even strong feminists took the abuse, she explained, because most of the time it occurred during the sur-

88 gery itself, and nurses who protest feel they are putting a patient at risk. "Are you going to distract the surgeon? Are you going to do something that's going to make him lose his concentration? Then by the time the surgery is over, people are too tired or busy to deal with it. And when the issue is verbal abuse, there is no visual evidence, nothing to rally around."

This time, however, the nurses had a visual reminder, a nurse with a cast on her hand. The evening of the incident, Mullan and her colleagues called all the OR nurses in the hospital and asked them to come in the next day, whether they were scheduled to work or not. She asked them what they wanted to do. Did they want to go back to work, and back to business/abuse as usual, or did they want to do something about it? Mullan went around the room and asked each nurse, as well as the orderlies, who were also involved, what she or he felt comfortable doing. "I told the nurses we had to decide what we wanted to do and do it together."

All of them said they did not want to go back to work under such conditions. All of them agreed to a day off work in protest. They also demanded a meeting with the board of directors of the hospital. Coincidentally, the board was meeting the next day and the nurses, accompanied by their injured colleague, made a presentation to the board.

"We said that there had to be something done with his behavior," Mullan continued. "The surgeon had crossed the line. We told the board it had to take a stand on this. It could no longer go on. Every doctor in the hospital knew about it. We pointed out that the board was our employer. Under health and safety laws, it has to provide us with a safe working environment. If it wasn't prepared to do something, nurses would refuse to work. We asked that the surgeon not be allowed to work until he had learned how to control his anger and that he properly apologize to Dolan and her colleagues."

The board was surprised by this show of cohesion. Members of the board, she added, were well aware that other nurses in the hospital would support the OR nurses. Judging from articles that had appeared in Montreal newspapers, the public too would be supportive.

"The chairperson of the board was the president of Alcan," Mullan recounted. "He was a very distinguished-looking man, and after hearing our presentation he told us that if that type of behavior had happened at Alcan, he would have dealt with it right away and it would never ever happen again. There was zero tolerance."

Mullan said that the thing that distressed her the most was what happened after the meeting was over. "The nursing representative on the board came up to me afterward and said thank you for doing what they were never able to do. Isn't it a sad state of affairs that our nursing leadership has to wait for the union to do something? It says a lot about the state of nursing. You have these people who theoretically can talk the talk, but **89** they haven't walked the walk for us."

Because of the nurses' action, the doctor was suspended. Eight months later, he returned to work. Mullan and other OR nurses believe he attended some kind of therapy or anger management seminar, because his behavior notably improved. But they were never informed of any treatment, nor were they informed that he would be coming back to work. One day he simply reappeared in the OR. Although the nurses demanded that he formally apologize to Anne Dolan and the other nurses, he never did.

Since few nurses report assaults by doctors to the police or even to unions and professional organizations, it's difficult to determine how large a problem this is. What we do know about violence against nurses comes from general workplace statistics and some studies conducted by nursing organizations.

According to the United States Bureau of Justice, nurses rank high on the list of workers who are subject to nonfatal physical assaults. Between 1992 and 1996, nurses were the victims of an average of 69,500 incidents of nonfatal workplace violence a year.[1] According to nurses, most violence occurs at the hands of patients and the majority of acts of violence take place in the emergency room or on psychiatric wards.

Nurses who responded to the FIIQ survey questionnaire said that most violence was perpetrated by patients and families. But the union had an interesting section on violence perpetrated by doctors. "Fifteen percent of respondents reported that doctors had thrown an object at them; 7% say they were grabbed, shoved, or pushed back, and 5% report they were hit with an object. The final toll is heavy," the report continued. "If we add the threats of assaults, the picture is even gloomier; 28% of respondents faced verbal intimidation at least once, and these threats were accompanied by a cutting object in 7% of cases." And after listing a variety of other abusive behavior, the FIIQ commented, "We must also add assaults of a sexual nature: intimate questions, light touching and fondling, lifting clothes."[2]

The International Labor Organization says that nurses are three times more likely to be exposed to violence than any other professional group who work in health care.[3] Nurses are likely victims of violence because they spend more time with patients and families and are thus the ones likeliest to be close at hand when a frustrated or mentally ill patient or family member explodes. Because women are often targets of violence, patients and family members may consider nurses to be less threatening, or to be safer targets of their anger and frustration. The sense of entitlement of some male physicians, who may consider themselves to be supe-

90 rior to female nurses, may also result in acts of violence or bullying. The problem, however, is that few analyses of violence against nurses discuss physician involvement or quantify whether incidents reported are physician related. Because of this, one is forced to rely on anecdotal evidence that should be the impetus for further investigation and research.

Nurse Susan Schultheis was working at the VA hospital in Portland, Oregon, when she got into an argument with a doctor about patient care. The physician lashed out in anger, pushed her up against a wall and then dragged her down the hall by the arm. Schultheis was so traumatized by the incident that she had to go for counseling.[4] Several years ago, when I visited the University of Massachusetts Memorial Hospital for Nurses Day, I met a group of demoralized, exhausted nurses. They seemed to have absolutely nothing to celebrate and could only ventilate their distress about working conditions and workloads. Kate Maker, president of the Massachusetts Nurses Association union local in the hospital, told me about a nurse who had a startling experience. While working in the OR, a surgeon had thrown a small bowl of blood at her at the end of an operation. She did not report it to the police or even to the union. I tried to track down the nurse, but I could only find another nurse who had witnessed the incident. Another nurse explained that the nurse in question was in the OR with a surgeon who was doing a Triple A (abdominal aortic aneurysm). When he saw how the nurse was spattered with blood he had thrown, he laughed.

I was stunned to hear this, but she was not. Why should she be? she said. It had happened before. Not to her but to another nurse when the same surgeon was doing a vascular operation. To make sure the vessel being operated on worked, he aimed it at a nurse and covered her with blood. She had to leave the case. She apparently reported the incident to the hospital, but nothing ever came of it. She did not go to her union or her professional association.

Hospital Management and Nurse-Doctor Relationships

If poor nurse-physician relationships have a serious impact on nurse retention, why don't hospital administrators, many of them nursing managers, intervene to improve relationships? One major reason seems to be that hospital administrators consider doctors to be revenue generators—the proverbial geese who lay the golden eggs of patient admissions to the hospital. They may thus subordinate issues of staff morale to their perception of how to assure institutional survival.

Over and over again, administrators have told me that if doctors are too frequently or aggressively chastised, they may threaten to bring their patients elsewhere. "The name of the game in hospitals these days is volume," as one vice president of nursing at a major teaching hospital candidly expressed it. "If there's going to be any positive margin, you've just got to keep bringing the patients in. The physicians are seen as the key driver of volume. You don't want to mess with them."

So bad conduct may be rationalized away. In a community hospital the doctor may be viewed as just having a bad day, as "not really meaning it," or "being under a great deal of stress." In a teaching hospital, where, as one administrator explained, "faculty and chiefs are like kings, popes, rabbis, and priests," people tend to rationalize physician conduct with "Oh, he's just eccentric. But he's a brilliant scientist, you just have to let it go."

Nurses thus find there is never a good time to act. When things are going well, one doesn't want to jeopardize patient flow. When times are tough, hospitals may try even harder to cater to physicians. "We're in terrible financial shape," another vice president of nursing in a teaching hospital explained. "For us it's all about improving volume, so we're always meeting with physicians to find out what we need to do to enable them to increase volume."

The conversation, the administrator said, goes like this. "If each physician brought in only one more admission, that's 2,000 discharges, and that would mean blah blah blah blah in revenue. We're asked to figure out what gets in the way or what makes doctors dissatisfied. They'll tell us, 'I have trouble scheduling my cases. Patients tell me the floors aren't staffed well enough. The place is too dirty.'"

In this environment, hospital managers may be loath to ask doctors— the perceived institutional drivers—to recognize that nurses are in fact the engine that makes the hospital run. Pointing out the simple fact that no driver can win the race if his engine is poorly maintained—or has been entirely removed—does not seem to get on the agenda. Doctors who have been the victims of abuse or bullying also tell me that when the bully is a high-performing doctor, CEOs won't do anything to curb the behavior for the same reason. A number of nurse executives assured me that with or without formal policies, egregious cases of disruptive physician behavior are always addressed. "A physician recently humiliated a nurse in the middle of the recovery room in a very public way," a hospital administrator told me. "I really wasn't going to let that one go. That particular chairman (of a medical department) was very supportive. We had a meeting about this incident and there was a formal discussion with a member of the labor relations department, who is responsible for verbal abuse. The physician did apologize to the nurse and publicly came to a staff meeting to talk about it. There probably should have been a more formal kind of discipline. But I don't think anything was put in the guy's record.

92 Maybe that should be there. If a nurse had done it, I would have formally disciplined the nurse and it would have been put in her record."

Many hospitals have zero-tolerance policies that discipline or deal with any employee who is abusive. When it comes to nursing, these policies may not exist, or when they do, they may not be well advertised or effectively implemented. "Do we have a zero-tolerance policy on abuse?" the VP of nursing continues. "I don't think so." He pauses and then adds, "No, wait a minute, if it's about verbal abuse, I think so. But the fact that I don't know how to answer that question shows that it's not well known in the organization, and I don't think many people would come forward if they had a problem."

Nurse managers are supposed to be key in creating a safe work environment. But repeatedly nurses have told me that nurse managers either failed to support them when a conflict occurred between a staff nurse and doctor, supported the doctor instead of the nurse, or swept the problem under the rug.

"You write report after report," one nurse said, "and nothing happens. They are sent down to the risk management department or to human resources and, from the nurses' point of view, disappear into a drawer."

The perception that hospital administrators or medical chiefs never discipline doctors, says the psychologist Larry Harmon, may be due to confidentiality rules, which prevent hospitals from revealing any disciplinary action taken against an employee or staff member. Nonetheless, many nurses seem to be well aware that their colleagues were frequently "written up" or disciplined. They were not aware that the disciplining of physicians was also routine. Is that because of a concern for privacy or because it rarely happens? Whatever the answer, from the nurses' point of view, their concerns seem to have been rendered invisible and their complaints seem to disappear into a black hole. Many insist that doctors who are abusive or disruptive continue unfettered in their behavior.

Sometimes staff nurses feel that nurse managers side with the abusive physician. One nurse in New York State told me about a physician who had slapped her in the face in the emergency room. She slapped him right back. When her nurse manager heard about it, she was reprimanded but the doctor was not. Some nurses have told me that when they report a physician, a nurse manager will ask them whether they really want to persist in pursing a complaint that could, as one put it, ruin a physician's reputation.

Another way nurse managers may tacitly support abusive physicians is to allow nurses to engage in the individual boycott of disruptive doctors that Susan Mullan and Anne Dolan described. This seems to be a common strategy, particularly among operating room nurses, who have more

opportunity than floor nurses to influence decisions about which physi- **93**
cians they are assigned to work with.

Larry Harmon believes nurse managers tolerate this kind of behavior
because many simply don't know how to deal with physician behavior.
This is a problem worldwide. Tom Keighley, the former editor of the
journal *Nursing Management* in the United Kingdom, explains that managerial tolerance of the boycotting of difficult doctors reflects the learned
powerlessness of the manager, not just the learned powerlessness of the
nurse. "Behind it is the view that the doctor cannot be challenged,"
Keighley explains.

Nurse managers may have learned this from experience, he elaborates,
or because they were educated to believe that the doctor's power should
be maintained at all costs. "Often, the doctor has been talked to or disciplined. In the UK," he goes on to explain, "the doctor would often be
suspended for two years, on full pay, whilst there was some half-hearted
investigation. Then he would be brought back into the organization without having changed his behavior, and the manager feels absolutely disempowered. Sometimes complaints don't lead to any action. So the managers have learned not to do that and to simply say, 'Okay, we'll work
around them.'"

Given both real and perceived limits on their sphere of action, nurse
managers may thus endorse the kinds of strategies of resistance and adjustment that allow individual nurses to escape an abusive physician while
allowing the abuse to continue, albeit directed toward someone else.
They thus give nurses an unofficial safety valve, allowing some of them to
act on their disaffection while physician abuse continues.

The powerlessness reflected in this indirect way of dealing with problems may also reflect the fact that many nurse executives may themselves
be victims of abuse from medical chiefs. In the fall of 2002 I was asked to
speak to a group of nurse executives from small Southern and Southwest-
ern hospitals in the United States. When I raised the issue of doctor-
nurse relationships, some of them talked about their problems dealing
with physicians and administrators. One nurse executive described sitting
at meeting of hospital higher-ups who routinely ignored or dismissed her
comments and attempts to raise issues pertaining to the delivery of nursing care. She seemed as disarmed by these experiences as the nurses she
manages.

Another vice president of nursing described an encounter with a senior
physician. The doctor began shouting at her. When she told him not to
speak to her in that tone, he simply raised the pitch. She said that she held
her ground and reported the incident to her CEO. This provoked a visit
in which the CEO commiserated with her about the surgeon but

94 nonetheless warned her about creating too much conflict with physicians. Doctors bring money into the hospital, she was told. We can't afford to alienate them. You just have to take it, he said. She did not make the counterargument that if doctors alienate too many nurses, they will quit and doctors won't be able to admit the patients upon which volumes and margin depend.

During the break, I went into the ladies room, where I overheard a revealing conversation between the vice president of nursing who had spoken up and a colleague from another hospital. The colleague congratulated her on standing her ground and raising the issue with her CEO. The nurse executive replied, "Yes, but you have to be careful about how many issues you raise. After all, it's our job to protect the CEO."

If nurses at the highest level of management worry about protecting the powers that be, imagine the worries of lower-level managers and staff nurses.

It is thus understandable that in his report on nurse-physician relationships, Alan Rosenstein explained that 51.5 percent of nurses did not view the policy for handling disruptive behavior as effective (compared to 69.5 percent of physicians who thought their institutions had effective policies).[5]

The net result is that many doctors are allowed or, to use popular jargon, "enabled" in their bad behavior. This bad behavior, in fact, becomes a self-reinforcing cycle. Too often there is no "time out" for the doctor who screams, humiliates others, throws tantrums—or objects—or physically assaults a nurse. The doctor who gets away with what he (or she) can get away with passes on a not-so-subtle lesson to doctors-in-training. When hospitals don't step in or nurses don't object, abuse of some form is considered acceptable behavior. Indeed, patients would be shocked to learn that the managers of health care systems in most countries tolerate patterns of behavior so counterproductive that they contribute to dangerously poor, even life-threatening levels of communication about critical patient issues.

4

Fatal Synergy

In May 2001 the Provincial Court of Manitoba released its *Report of the Manitoba Pediatric Cardiac Surgery Inquest: An Inquiry into Twelve Deaths at the Winnipeg Health Sciences Centre in 1994.* The inquest had lasted three and a half years, included 278 days of testimony from eighty-six witnesses, and comprised fifty thousand pages of evidence. The report, running nearly six hundred pages, reads like a murder mystery. Among the victims were Gary Caribou, born August 22, 1993, who had surgery on March 14, 1994, and died on March 15; Jessica Ulimaumi, born August 18, 1993, who had surgery on March 24, 1994, and died on March 27; Vinay Goyal, born March 2, 1990, who had surgery on March 17 and April 18, 1994, and died on April 18; and nine other victims. The oldest was three and lived for one day after his operation. The youngest was two days old and died the same day of his surgery.

Who was the culprit? Was it murder? What did these children die of? Was it their disease? Or prematurity? No, they died from a surgeon's incompetence and because physicians and hospital administrators systematically ignored the warnings and concerns of expert nurses and doctors. The cases led to the longest-running medical inquest in Canada's history. The inquest report documented that these babies and toddlers were the victims of a fatal synergy—a collision of poor doctor-nurse relationships, poor doctor-nurse communication, cost cutting, and a refusal of hospital higher-ups to attend to nurses' concerns, heed their warnings, and thus allow them to rescue patients in dire need.[1]

Failure to Rescue

According to recent studies, in the United States alone an estimated 44,000 to 98,000 patients die every year from medical errors, more than from motor vehicle accidents, breast cancer, or AIDS.[2] Although the term "medical errors and injuries" conjures up the image of physicians or surgeons prescribing the wrong dose of a medication or cutting off the wrong leg, many of these errors and injuries have to do with nursing care. A medication error kills you only when someone administers the medication. In the hospital, that's almost always a nurse. In the Manitoba case, nurses were involved, witnesses to an unheeded Cassandra's warning about a surgeon's incompetence.

Those who are concerned about hospital errors and injuries have argued that every patient death or incident of patient harm is the result of a process, not a single event. It's a result of small "system failures" that jeopardize patients and that finally result in some fatal error—or many. Those system failures involve multiple players, not just physicians. "All hazardous technologies, including medical care, possess layers of barriers and safeguards. These defences take a variety of forms: technological, administrative, educational. Most important is culture—the cluster of attitudes, beliefs and values held by the individuals of the organization," write D. C. Aron and L. A. Headrick in an article on medical errors and injuries and their relation to physician education. "Ideally, in combination, the defensive layers are impermeable," the authors explain. "In reality there are always weaknesses in the defences. The layers are more like slices of Swiss cheese containing many holes that are continually opening, shutting, and altering their positions. . . . For a mishap to occur, the holes in many layers have to line up, at least momentarily, to permit a trajectory of accident opportunity–bringing hazards. When an adverse event occurs, the important issue is not who blundered but how and why the defences failed."[3]

One of the major roles a nurse plays in the health care system is to make sure those defenses don't fail and that treatments, medications, and procedures don't kill or harm patients. Nurses are part of an elaborate fail-safe system that is supposed to catch errors before they happen. When a nurse gives a medication, for example, she first asks whether it is the "right dose" of the "right drug," given at the "right time" through the "right route" (i.e., orally, intravenously, intramuscularly), to—and this of course is paramount—the "right person." The fail-safe function of the nurse also includes the administration and monitoring of treatments or surgeries. If, for example, a physician "orders" that a patient be given intravenous fluids, the nurse's job isn't simply to hang an IV. She makes sure the patient is able to tolerate the fluid load. If a doctor says a patient is

ready to be discharged home, a nurse should share what she knows about
the patient's home environment with the physician. She must always be
able to relate critical information to the physician, and part of the physician's job is to take that information into account.

Nurses' monitoring, judgment, and skill have always been key to patient survival, and it is certainly so today in our intricately complex, increasingly fragmented, high-tech medical system. That is precisely the
conclusion of an important study done at the University of Pennsylvania
School of Medicine where physicians Jeffrey A. Silber and his colleagues
identified a problem they called "failure to rescue."[4] These researchers
explored incidents when patients died or came to harm after surgery.
Some of these patients would have died no matter what doctors and
nurses did to save them, but some of the deaths were preventable. When
a preventable death occurred, it happened because hospital staff didn't
"rescue" the patient. When the researchers compared hospitals with the
same adjusted case mix, they found that some were indeed better at "rescuing" patients than others. Working with researchers Linda Aiken and
Julie Sochalski, and their colleagues at the University of Pennsylvania
School of Nursing, the investigators have identified critical factors in patient rescue. Hospitals have to have enough educated staff to recognize a
problem when they see it. That staff must be with patients enough of the
time to know the patient and observe and detect problems before or as
they happen.

Nurses, the researchers explain, are the educated, eyes-on, hands-on,
twenty-four-hour-surveillance, early-warning and early-intervention system in hospitals. These researchers add a critical caveat: Identifying a
problem isn't sufficient to implement "rescue." Staff must have enough
status and authority in the institution to mobilize resources, be it the ability to change a medication, to consult expeditiously with a physician, or to
be attended to when they alert doctors or administrators to problems.

A system, however, that deems nurses to be subordinate and defines
them as medical tools, or as hysterical/emotional women who should not
have "theories of their own," will not give them the authority to rescue
patients. Similarly, if nurses are supposed to limit their contributions to
"nursing" and are never to venture into the terrain of "medical issues,"
their fail-safe function will be severely limited. We have seen this in major
cases that have reached public attention in the United States, England,
and Canada. Although these health systems are very different, in each
case the powerful players (physicians and hospital administrators and
CEOs) view the role of the nurse similarly. I want to begin this discussion
with the Manitoba case because it is amply documented and because the
discussions I held with one of its major participants, the senior operating

98   room nurse in cardiac surgery, Carol Youngson, illustrate so many of the problems nurses encounter.

Failure to Rescue in Winnipeg

In the case of the Winnipeg Health Sciences Centre (HSC) pediatric cardiac surgery program, the holes in the system lined up perfectly and remained that way for months. This allowed twelve children to die and others to suffer potentially preventable complications. The stage for this particular tragedy was set in June 1993, when the pediatric cardiac surgery program at the HSC Children's Hospital lost its cardiac surgeon. Because of numerous problems, Dr. Kim Duncan left the program for a job in the United States. Duncan felt that the hospital administration and the larger university failed to support what was, in fact, a relatively small pediatric cardiac surgery program. He also worried that such a small surgical program did not furnish surgeons with enough patients to maintain their surgical skills.[5]

After Duncan's departure, these problems were not remedied. Physicians and hospital executives were loath to close the program because sending children out of the province to have heart surgery would be more costly. They were determined to find a replacement for Duncan. Given the ongoing problems, size of the program, and lack of resources, the HSC could not hope to recruit a surgeon at the height of his or her career. So they chose to seek someone who was just starting out, even though this young doctor would be entering a program with serious drawbacks. To complicate matters, in 1994 the hospital was undergoing cost cutting and restructuring conducted by an American firm called American Practice Management. Connie Curran (whom we'll hear about more in a later chapter), a nurse turned management consultant, was the APM consultant hired by the Conservative government of Manitoba to save money. Over the next year, Curran and her colleagues arrived in Manitoba and began to slash nursing jobs and change the administrative structure of the hospital. Reporting patterns were disrupted, heads of departments changed and shifted, and lines of authority and responsibility in clinical care became ambiguous (79–92).

The Manitoba doctors working in this highly charged atmosphere finally found someone they considered to be a prime candidate for the job. He was an American-trained surgeon, Jonah Odim. A graduate of Yale University and the University of Chicago Medical School, he had trained at the renowned Boston's Children's Hospital. Odim, the staff was told, had excellent recommendations. He was supposed to be brilliant. That's what the surgeons and cardiologists who ran the hospital thought and what the anesthetists, intensivists, and surgical and ICU nurses were led **99** to believe.

As the inquest later revealed, no one in charge of the program probed his record. Because lines of authority had been disrupted in the hospital restructuring, contacting real people at Boston Children's Hospital fell through a very large crack. Doctors, who reviewed Odim's recommendations, read letters that told them little about his competence. No one talked with anyone in Boston who had actually worked with and supervised Odim. The doctors responsible for hiring Odim, the inquest revealed, thought the pediatric cardiac surgery program at Boston Children's was brilliant and assumed Odim must be too. He wasn't. If they'd bothered to call Boston Children's Hospital, they would have been told that Odim was not considered a brilliant young hotshot. In fact, he was viewed as mediocre (115–125).

When Odim arrived in Winnipeg in February 1994, Carol Youngson had been a nurse for twenty-five years and was chief operating room nurse at the pediatric cardiac surgery program. She was looking forward to working with Odim. So were her colleagues who worked on the neonatal and pediatric intensive care units, where the babies Odim operated on would be sent to recover. Because he was a young surgeon, and newly out of training, Youngson said she and her colleagues had expected that Odim would restart the program gradually, taking on lower-risk cases and working up to more complex ones. Odim, however, immediately scheduled the most complex cases.

Because teamwork involves practice and trust, Youngson suggested that the team of operating room nurses, anesthetists, perfusionists (the people who operate the complicated bypass machine), and the surgeon do some mock run-throughs. When presented several times with this suggestion, Odim refused. Cardiologist Niels Giddins was the chief of the Variety Children's Heart Centre. Children would first be seen by Giddins, who would diagnose their problems and refer them to the surgeon. Giddins never made sure that such run-throughs were standard operating procedure (127–131).

Odim did meet with the heads of each nursing department—the pediatric intensive care unit (PICU) nursing and the nurse neonatal intensive care unit (NICU) nursing—as well as with the director of nursing, Isabel Boyle. Donna Feser, the PICU manager, asked Odim how he wanted to approach the postoperative care of his patients. In response, he gave her an article that she did not find to be helpful. NICU nurses who asked the same questions were also given a journal article, which, according to a NICU nurse, "didn't tell us what Dr. Odim's approach would be" (132, 133).

100   Odim's resistance to the nurses' suggestions and questions was symptomatic of his difficulty communicating his needs and approaches with both nurses and other doctors. "Before an operation, it's very important for a surgeon to explain what he is going to be doing so that nurses can get the proper instruments ready and the anesthesiologist can have the blood, fluid and medications the patient will need," Youngson explained in one of our interviews. "It's also important for the doctor to communicate what he's doing during the operation."

The process of securing the proper equipment for an operation is very complex. A cardiac operation, Youngson explains, can require forty different kinds of sutures and many different kinds of needles: half-circles, quarter circles, needles of different circumferences. Each operation—say, an atrial septal repair or a ventricular septal repair—involves a different kind of suture. Similarly, there will be a different suture for sewing up a hole in the heart or putting in a canula, or tube. As chief operating room nurse, it was Youngson's job to make sure that equipment was on hand for each particular operation. To do this, however, she needed to know what devices Odim wanted. She thus provided the surgeon with the different catalogues from medical equipment companies so that she could order equipment well in advance from suppliers in say Germany or the United States. When Youngson asked Odim what he wanted to order, he would tell her that "what you used in the past will be fine," adding that he didn't have time to look over the catalogues she'd given him.

"I would approach him beforehand and he couldn't tell me. At first I thought it was because he was just ignoring me," Youngson speculated. "But I came to realize it was because he didn't know himself what he wanted, because he was so junior and inexperienced" (137–140).

Youngson recalls one particular case which required a specialized measuring device for determining the diameter of the blood vessels. Odim didn't request any of these devices for the upcoming surgery, but Youngson thought, "Well, I'd better order them anyway." She did and, of course, he needed them. "If I hadn't done that, I would have been in deep, deep trouble. We would have had to send someone off to the adult side of the center, which would have taken more than ten minutes. Then we might have had to sterilize the equipment, which would have taken more time. So the whole thing could have taken more than a half an hour. All the time the kid's on the bypass."

Over the course of her career in the OR, Youngson had worked with over 150 surgeons and assisted at thousands of surgeries. An experienced operating room nurse like Youngson may not know how to perform the surgery she's assisting on, but she certainly knows what each surgery involves, step by laborious step. Without this detailed knowledge, she can't assist and order the proper equipment. She also knows good surgical technique when she sees it and is alert to any warning signs of inexperience or incompetence. Almost as soon as Odim started operating, inexperience is what she and her colleagues observed.

When Odim did his first open heart case on March 7, problems occurred with "Odim's lack of familiarity with the OR setup," his "problems with cannulation," and "his treatment of nurses" (137). Over the course of the next few weeks more problems occurred. Surgical repairs were failing and had to be done over again. "Cases that were routine were turning into nightmares and marathons," Youngson recounted.

"We were doing bypass surgery that involved putting tubes, or canulas, into the vessels so that blood bypasses the heart and is put through a machine that oxygenates and heparinizes (or thins) it," she told me. "There are techniques for putting in canulas that are pretty basic for cardiac surgery. These are things residents are allowed to do. But Odim had trouble putting in the canulas. They would fall out. There would be tears in major vessels coming out of the heart, which would require a lot of suturing and blood loss. The bypasses would take longer."

Over and over again, Carol Youngson stood by as the inexperienced surgeon took twelve or fourteen hours to do a surgery that an experienced surgeon would finish in three or four. Patients started to die, others suffered preventable complications.

Gary Caribou, an aboriginal child, died just a month after Odim began to perform surgery. The inquest concluded that the death was "possibly preventable" (159). Then one after another, Jessica Ulimaumi, an Inuit child, and Vinay Goyal died. Jessica Ulimaumi died when Odim had serious problems in the OR, sent her to the ICU, and tried to deal with them there without any other OR staff present. Although appropriate nursing staff was available had he called, he didn't (169–177).

Other babies were sent to the PICU and NICU in an unstable condition, and more surgical procedures were done on these units without appropriately trained surgical nurses (168). Within a month, three young patients—whose surgeries were considered low to medium risk—bled to death because of failed repairs. Others suffered complications.

The surgeon's attitude toward the nurses appeared to be ambivalent, if not hostile. He did not seem to tolerate differences of opinion on what he considered to be "medical issues," and he made sexist comments about the nurses (140). When Jessica Ulimaumi was operated on on March 24, Youngson told the inquest, Odim blamed the patient's extensive time on the bypass machine (eight hours and forty-three minutes) and his need to redo the heart repair on Youngson's alleged failure to provide him with the "right kind of suture material" (174).

102   Youngson and her nursing colleagues in the OR, PICU, and NICU were so concerned they felt they had to take action. They went through the proper channels, talking first to the head nurse and then to Isabel Boyle (204). On April 20, Daniel Terziski was operated on. NICU nurses testified that Odim "failed to assist the NICU in planning for Daniel's postoperative care" (217). When problems developed in the NICU, Odim asked neonatal ICU nurses to assist at a surgical procedure for which they had no training. When the patient died, they again met with Boyle and catalogued the problems that occurred in the operating theater and in the NICU. Odim seemed to believe that a nurse is a nurse is a nurse and that any nurse can do any nursing activity.

The nurses were alarmed not only because of the number of deaths but also because of what kinds of patients were dying. It soon became clear that families of immigrant and First Nation children were being steered toward the program while those who were white, Canadian, and better connected were being told to take their kids out of the province.

The nurses also approached their medical colleagues about the quality of Odim's surgical technique. In the spring of 1994, Youngson and other nurses spoke to Dr. Nathan Wiseman, head of the Division of Pediatric Surgery at the HSC. They implored him to "scrub" for one of Odim's operations. Rather than interpreting this as a collegial request that stemmed from both their clinical expertise and deep concern about patient care, Wiseman told Youngson he did not take orders from nurses. When Irene Hinam made a similar request, he similarly declined to take her concerns seriously.

The nurses were hardly the only ones concerned. Perfusionists were alarmed at Odim's lack of competence, as were anesthetists. Ann McNeill, an anesthetist who'd delivered anesthesia at many of Odim's failed operations, also hoped that Wiseman would intervene. In the absence of action to protect these fragile patients, Youngson and the nurses continued to try to stave off problems. Over this period, the nurses were so concerned about the situation that they wanted to quit. Well aware that only a few RNs had the specialized knowledge and skill they had acquired over years in the program, they felt that their departure would put patients in further jeopardy.

So they continued to raise their concerns. "Doctors would tell us if we didn't like it, we should just quit. Or they'd blame us. They'd say that I couldn't adapt to a new surgeon, because I'd become so used to working with the surgeon who'd worked here before," Youngson recalls.

Youngson doesn't deny that she and the previous head of the team had, after a few years of working together, developed an excellent partnership. Nor does she deny that she and Odim didn't like each other very much.

She does, however, point out that the teamwork she and the former sur- **103** geon had achieved was the result of years of work—work she was pre-pared to put in with Odim. As for their mutual dislike? "Hell," she says, "I've worked with a lot of surgeons I haven't liked."

In May, with the death of the fifth patient, Alyssa Still, the program's mortality rate reached 50 percent, with other infants experiencing serious and preventable complications. Although it had been unwilling to act on the earlier alerts from experienced nurses, the hospital abruptly sus-pended the surgical program when the anesthetists threatened to with-draw their services unless the pediatric cardiac surgery program was eval-uated (257).

Nathan Wiseman, the surgeon who had refused his nursing colleagues' pleas to observe Odim in action, was asked to form and chair a committee to look into the program's ongoing problems. Although OR nurses were not the only ones who had serious concerns and who played a role in the program, Carol Youngson was the only nurse who was appointed to the Wiseman committee. NICU and PICU nurses were excluded from par-ticipation (273).

As Youngson described it to me and to the inquest, she felt intimidated and outnumbered on the committee. "I felt that my role was to support Ann McNeill," she told me, referring to the spokesperson for the anes-thetists who had withdrawn their services. "I didn't open my mouth until she spoke and then I jumped in and supported her."

Every time she tried to intervene, Youngson said, she felt she was "practically laughed out of the room" because she was "just a nurse." In-terestingly, Youngson notes, none of the concerns of nurses that she voiced at the meetings were mentioned in chairman Nathan Wiseman's minutes.

When the committee met, according to witness testimony at the in-quest, major issues about Odim's competence and communication prob-lems with the entire team were left unaddressed. Nevertheless, the com-mittee (many of whose members seem to have felt pressured to go along with the decision) determined that, at least temporarily, Odim should only perform low- and medium-risk surgeries. The program was restarted. Within a short time, however, he was again performing a full range of pediatric open-heart procedures. Again, nursing's concerns were ignored and unrecorded. And, again, babies started dying (320–324).

By this time, Youngson found she could no longer tolerate taking the tiny patients from their parents and bringing them to the operating room. "When I take a patient from a parent, if the patient is old enough to un-derstand, I usually tell the child, 'You'll be seeing mommy and daddy soon,' or I tell the parents, 'You'll see your baby in the ICU in six or ten

104 hours.' After a while, I felt like a liar. I couldn't look them in the eye and tell them they were going to see their child, because half the time I didn't think the child was going to come out alive."

"In December," Youngson continues, "we lost three neonates, bang, bang, bang. One bled to death. Another had a canula in and Odim knocked it out and destroyed the repair. The repair on this three-day-old baby's heart was complete and things were looking pretty hopeful. As I briefly looked away, I heard a gasp. I looked at the heart and saw that the aortic canula, the tube that returns oxygenated blood from the bypass machine, had been knocked out. In his efforts to restore it, Odim destroyed his repair. The baby died on the table."

This thirteen-hour case finished on a Sunday night. The next day Youngson went directly to the medical director and to the director of nursing. Finally responding to the concerns of Youngson, other nurses, and doctors, the hospital required Odim to have another cardiac surgeon present when operating on complicated cases. But several times Odim operated without him.

By this time nurses were distraught. Babies were sent to them in the PICU with an open chest, with excessive bleeding, with clots, or with a need for a pacemaker. Several nurses had already requested not to work with the program. Carol Youngson decided that if things continued as they were, after February, she would no longer be involved in pediatric cases (355).

Youngson still did not tell parents to take their children and run. No one did. Nurses did, however, continue to talk about their concerns to hospital and medical higher-ups like the clinical head of surgery, Dr. Robert Blanchard, and the president of the HSC, Rod Thorfinnson. But these physicians and administrators transformed clinical into medical or emotional concerns. Thorfinnson insisted that the problems that occurred should only be aired in front of the Medical Advisory Committee not the Nursing Council.

In December 1994, Odim did another complex open-heart surgery on a neonate without requesting help from an assistant surgeon. The baby bled to death in the OR. This twelfth death was Odim's last case. ICU physicians said they would no longer refer patients to him and the program was stopped.

After the program was suspended, two physicians from Toronto's Hospital for Sick Children were called in to conduct an external review. On January 9, 1995, doctors were informed of the appointment of these two physicians and were asked to prepare written submissions to them. Nurses were not informed of the appointment or asked to provide written comment. This was "sadly in keeping with the way that nurses had been **105** treated through the process," Judge Sinclair wrote (449).

On January 13, Blanchard sent out a memo to the sixteen doctors involved in the program telling them that the two physicians would be at the hospital on January 25 and "urging them to make themselves available on that day," but "again the nurses were left out of the loop" (452).

These reviews (and the subsequent inquest) documented the same serious problems delineated by the nurses and decried the program's mortality rate. As a result of the review, however, Winnipeg Children's Hospital sent out a news release announcing the program's suspension. Parents whose children had died under Odim's care were stunned when they read the news. They soon discovered that this was Odim's first job as surgeon, that he had no experience with complicated surgery, and that the anesthetists had threatened to withdraw their services. "They went wild," Youngson said. They brought their complaints to the provincial and territorial government, which demanded an inquest that delved into the functioning of the program since its founding in 1981.

Youngson was soon notified that she and other nurses would be represented by the hospital's attorney during the proceedings. She and Irene Hinam, Carol Bower, and the unit manager Karin Dixon met with the hospital's lawyer, director of nursing, and a senior administrator. At this meeting Youngson revealed that she had made copious notes about those operations that had gone wrong. So did nurse Carol Bower. The nurses presented their notes and opinions to the hospital. "Here," Youngson said, "you should take a look at this."

Several days later, the hospital told Youngson and her fellow RNs that the hospital's attorney could not represent the nurses because of a conflict of interest. The hospital had cut them loose and the nurses were told to seek their own legal representation. With the help of the Manitoba Association of Registered Nurses, the nurses got legal representation.[6] During the inquest, Canada's longest running, Youngson and the nurses testified about their experiences. Youngson herself testified for thirteen days, five of which were under cross-examination by the physician's attorney. Lawyers for the anesthetists, the Health Sciences Center, and the victims' families also questioned her.

The inquest report reads like a riveting whodunit, except you know who "done it" right from the beginning. Physicians and administrators consistently made invidious distinctions between "nursing" and "medical" issues and declared nurses' concerns off limits, because nurses did not have medical expertise. For example, hospital president Rod Thorfinnson, insisted that it wouldn't be appropriate to bring up nursing concerns

106 to various hospital bodies, including the Nursing Council, because "while nurses were involved in the program, it was in his opinion a medical and surgical issue, not a nursing issue" (455).

When Judge Murray Sinclair delivered the report and recommendations of his inquest, he succinctly stated the relationship between the hospital and the medical view of nurses helped create this tragedy. In his conclusion, Judge Sinclair's ire is contained but clear, and his comments are worth quoting in their entirety:

"The evidence suggests that because nursing occupied a subservient position within the HSC structure, issues raised by nurses were not always treated appropriately.

"Throughout 1994, the experience and observations of the nursing staff involved in the program led them to voice serious and legitimate concerns. The nurses, however, were never treated as full and equal members of the surgical program, despite the fact that this was the stated intent of the administrative changes that the program underwent in June 1994. Intensive care unit nurses, for example, were never properly involved in the review team that assessed the program during 1994, and nurses were not properly involved in the Williams and Roy Review [reviews that took place after the program was shut down]. The concerns expressed by some of the cardiac surgical nurses were dismissed as stemming from an inability to deal emotionally with the deaths of some of the patients. As well, any concerns over medical issues that the nurses expressed were rejected as not having any proper basis, clearly stemming from the view that the nurses did not have the proper training and experience to hold or express such a view. In addition, while HSC doctors had a representative on the hospital's board of directors, nurses did not.

"Historically, the role of nurses has been subordinate to that of doctors in our health-care system. While they are no longer explicitly told to see and be silent, it is clear that legitimate warnings and concerns raised by nurses were not always treated with the same respect or seriousness as those raised by doctors. There are many reasons for this, but the attempted silencing of members of the nursing profession, and the failure to accept the legitimacy of their concerns meant that serious problems in the pediatric cardiac surgery program were not recognized or addressed in a timely manner. As a result, patient care was compromised" (477–478).

Failure to Rescue in Bristol

In what has been called an "eerie parallel" to the Winnipeg case at the turn of the twenty-first century, nurses at a pediatric cardiac surgery program in Bristol, England, also watched patients die unnecessarily.[7] Led by

Professor Ian Kennedy, an inquiry began in 1998 to look into the deaths of between thirty and thirty-five children who were operated on by surgeons at the Bristol Royal Infirmary and the Bristol Royal Hospital for Sick Children. The inquiry, with its 900,000 pages of documents, testimony by 577 witnesses including 238 parents, and examination of over 1,800 children's charts, provides another window onto how medical tragedies happen.

As in Winnipeg, the program—one of nine designated cardiac surgery centers in England—didn't have enough patients to allow surgeons to maintain their skills. Cost cutting and restructuring was also a factor. The hospital had been restructured and departmental authority and lines of communication between units were fragmented. In this case, a different element was added into the mix. Children were operated on and attended to by adult cardiac surgeons and, due to short staffing, sometimes by adult cardiac nurses. Sue Burr, an expert in pediatric cardiac surgery and Royal College of Nursing adviser in pediatric care, told me that these nurses, as they themselves testified, didn't have enough familiarity with the population they cared for to understand that the death rates they were witnessing were unacceptably high.[8]

In this case, however, nurses did not act to alert authorities to the problems. Instead, a consultant anesthetist, Stephen Bolsin, alerted the public and authorities to problems with two surgeons, James Wisheart and Janardan Dhasmana. What is particularly interesting is that although the nurses in these institutions had knowledge of the problems well before Boislin made them public, they felt too disempowered and intimidated to speak out.

In her written statement to the inquiry, nurse Patricia Dorothy Fields explained that the hospital was "very much medically dominated" and that nurses "had a lot of work to do in order to overcome the medical dominance in existence at the time, to be allowed the opportunity to give a balanced, progressive view on nursing issues." But, according to her testimony, the division between nursing and medical issues was strictly maintained. Although Fields was supposed to be a nursing leader and a nursing officer (i.e., manager), she stated that she could not comment on key issues in the program. She testified that she "did not recall that there were significant problems with the cardiac surgery during this time," nor did she see "any surgical results," since these were considered a medical issue involving only the consultant medical staff.[9]

Sister Sheena Elizabeth Disley reported that managers could not "guarantee that paediatric nurses would only look after children, and not occasionally adults if we had no children on the unit at the time."[10] Although she felt that a dedicated pediatric unit would have helped with their difficulties in recruiting nurses, nurses apparently did little to lobby for such a unit.

Nurse Kay Armstrong's written statement and her response to intensive questioning present the most disturbing picture of the effects of the nurses' intimidation and subordination. In her written testimony, Armstrong said unit nursing managers had no control over their staffing and budget and no control over the number of nurses in the unit (these decisions were apparently made by senior nursing administration). She described the effects of hospital restructuring: the loss of a special nurse counselor, whose job it was to support patients, and the elimination of the position of director of nursing services. She added that nurses were afraid to raise the alarm about what they considered to be serious patient safety issues. In principle, "any member of the staff was at liberty to discuss any issues which were causing them concern with the theatre sisters, directly to management, or with their union representative, should they feel that necessary," she wrote. But in actuality "the majority of staff were unwilling to make formal complaints because of their concern about job security."[11]

In her oral testimony, Armstrong's responses painted an even more alarming picture. Under intense questioning, Armstrong said that she and her fellow nurses noted problems with the two surgeons but were afraid to raise them.

"Why?" Chairman Kennedy asked.

"Because he would seem to disapprove of what was being said to him, but he would not answer you or give you a satisfactory answer; he would be more likely to walk away."[12] Armstrong said that other members of the surgical nursing staff were similarly fearful of raising their concerns with the physician. Armstrong also testified that she felt similarly intimidated by a Mr. Dhasmana, whose "temper would deteriorate" when he was tired.

When physician Stephen Bolsin discussed his concerns with the nurses, they listened but did nothing to voice their concerns publicly.

"Why not?" the chairman queried.

"We were not in a position, I do not feel, that we would have been listened to or that there was anything we could do about it, but he [Bolsin] was, and he was doing that." Indeed, Armstrong added, the very fact that Bolsin discussed his concerns with the so-called team was a stunning departure from business as usual for these nurses. "His was an uncommon attitude among the consultants in that he would discuss what he was doing with nurses and with whoever happened to be in the coffee room at the time."

Because the nurses were not pediatric cardiac nurses, Armstrong said, she did not realize the operations the two surgeons performed were tak-

ing too long. When asked about another surgeon, whose operating time **109**
was much shorter, she agreed but would not speculate about why that
might be. "I am not really clinically trained to comment on that."

The nurses, Armstrong did say, found it hard to scrub for problem
cases. "It was very hard to have to scrub for those cases when you realized
that it may well end with the child dying." Indeed, the nurses working in
the OR found it so hard that in mid-1994 seven of the nine boycotted the
two surgeons. "We took that choice ourselves. That we did not wish to
scrub for those complex cases anymore. . . . We did not actually approach
the surgeons or take a stand against the surgeons and tell them we were
not willing to scrub. Those two people (the other two nurses) were willing to do those cases, so it did not affect the throughput of the children at
the time."

When Chairman Kennedy asked Armstrong if the nurses took their
concerns to management, she said they did not. When he asked if they
were willing to pursue their concerns by making a formal complaint, she
stated that they were not. When he asked why, Armstrong gave a sobering
view of the results of nurses' socialization. "I think the problem is that
nurses probably undervalue themselves, and you always feel that you will
maybe not be listened to should you make a complaint about something,
so it very rarely gets any further than possibly the Sister of your first line
manager level. I think there is always the fear, as well as, that you could
end up being suspended or—"

Kennedy interrupted, "Was anyone ever suspended for raising a concern, so far as you are aware?"

"No," Armstrong replied.

"So what was the basis for this concern that a nurse might lose his or
her job?"

"I think it is based on the fact that nurses have always felt in awe of senior management and hospital consultants. That is changing slowly now,
but that has been the case."

"I was not brave enough," Armstrong concluded during her examination.

The American Experience of Failure to Rescue

In the United States nurses are often viewed as ahead of the pack in having a voice and winning advances in their institutions, but many nurses
have the same problems. Nurse researchers Patricia Benner, Christine A.
Tanner, and Catherine A. Chesla have for years studied nurses on ICUs.[13]
They paint a picture of nurses who are knowledgeable and effective and
document the many instances of nurses working well with doctors. They
also dissect, in vivid detail, what happens when nurses aren't able to res-

110   cue patients, not because the nurses' educated eyes don't identify danger, but because the traditional medical hierarchy makes it impossible for the nurses to mobilize the necessary resources.

In one incident the authors describe, a nurse is trying to alert physicians to a major complication following surgery for an abdominal aortic aneurysm.[14] The nurse recognizes the patient has developed a "dead bowel" after the surgery. Because of a complication of the surgery, blood supply to part of the patient's intestine was compromised and part of the bowel died. In such cases, if the necrotic tissue isn't quickly removed, the millions of bacteria contained in the bowel can leak into the peritoneum, from whence it can penetrate the blood supply and gain access to the entire body. This can lead to rampant infection (sepsis), shock, and death. Like a burst appendix, a dead bowel is a surgical emergency. Speedy remedial action is essential.

The experienced nurse immediately recognized the problem and did what nurses are supposed to do, report all the signs and symptoms (distended abdomen, mottled knees, unstable blood pressure, acid accumulation in the body, irregular heart rhythm, and falling temperature) to the doctors in attendance, who were in this case surgical residents. Unfortunately, the residents insisted the patient didn't have a dead bowel.

The nurse paged the senior resident, but he was unavailable. So was the surgical attending. Another surgeon came into the room, agreed with the nurse, and told the residents to operate on the patient immediately. Nonetheless, the perhaps insecure residents wanted to wait for the attending, but the nurse insisted, "You don't have the time to wait for this attending." She told them, "Someone's just going to have to make a decision and do it. The senior resident has the ability to operate. This woman is going to die."[15] They still didn't operate.

The patient coded. But it was too late to save her. On autopsy, the nurse's clinical assessment was confirmed. The patient had a dead bowel. Summarizing the experience, the nurse said, "They [the residents] had the ability to look at the same things that I saw, I mean maybe in their eyes I'm just a nurse, but they had someone even telling them what the problem was." But they didn't listen.[16]

The Failure to Rescue Bobbi-Jo Rivard

In 2002 Bobbi-Jo Rivard and her husband were awarded $21.4 million in a medical malpractice suit against three physicians at the University of Massachusetts Medical Center in Worcester (which consists of three hospitals: University, Memorial, and Hahnemann). Details in the case, which produced one of the largest malpractice awards in the state's history, re-

veal an interesting behind-the-scenes story of hospital efforts to cut Caesarean section rates and physician failure to attend to nurses' clinical judgments.[17]

The problem began at Memorial Hospital on December 26, 1996,
when Rivard was transferred there after her family physician had tried unsuccessfully for three days to induce labor, because she was two weeks
overdue. The doctor had administered Pitocin, a medication that stimu-
lates contractions, but Rivard did not go into active labor. She was transferred to the care of obstetricians, because she had now become a high-
risk case that required specialist attention.

On December 29, the second day of Pitocin at Memorial—the fifth day
of attempted induction—Mrs. Rivard felt ill and again asked for a C-
section. Again physicians said it was unnecessary. Soon after, obstetrician
Jane Hitti became involved in her case. Hitti proceeded with the Pitocin
administration. Despite rupturing her membranes to induce labor and additional Pitocin, no progress was made for several hours.

As the labor arrested, the nurses monitoring her and her baby's status
began to notice that her uterus did not relax between contractions as it
should in a normal labor. Soon after the fetal heart rate began to show abnormal decelerations and other signs of fetal distress. The patient again
asked for a Caesarean, and the nurses refused to continue the Pitocin administration. One nurse told a resident that she would have to get someone higher up to give her the order, because she wouldn't do it.

A first-year resident, Gabrielle Reine, and a fourth-year resident,
Melissa Mead, were involved in the case. They ordered continued Pitocin
despite the signs of fetal distress and arrested labor. The nurses insisted
that the attending physician should be brought in and advised that a C-
section should be performed. At 3:30 the next morning, Jane Hitti again
arrived on the scene, examined Rivard, and found minimal change in the
cervix, which had become swollen and filled with fluid edemitis—usually
a sign that it will not be able to stretch further to accommodate the de-
scending baby. Hitti again refused the patient's request for a Caesarean
and ordered more Pitocin. Over the next few hours, in front of the patient, her husband and mother-in-law, the nurses and physicians struggled
over whether to continue the Pitocin, with the nurses refusing to give it.
The nurses went up their chain of nursing command, bringing in the
nursing supervisor and resource nurse. The latter tried gently to suggest
that the OR was ready anytime for a C-section.

At 6 a.m., as the nurses and residents were arguing, there was a prolonged deep deceleration in the baby's heart rate and the patient was
taken to the OR for an emergency C-section. In a situation like this, the
baby needs to be pulled out as quickly as possible, because it is essentially

112 without oxygen until it is delivered. To facilitate the process, Mrs. Rivard received general anesthesia to relax her uterus. However, the baby's head was so tightly wedged in the pelvis—attorneys argued because of the strength of the Pitocin-induced contractions—that there was great difficulty releasing him. In fact, one nurse, braced by another, pushed her hand up the vagina to dislodge the baby's head. The doctors needed to extend the uterine incision in a T shape to deliver the baby—fifteen minutes after the initial incision was made. During these fifteen minutes, the baby continued to be severely distressed.

When Michael Rivard was born, he was limp, pale, and without a heartbeat for eighteen minutes. The child remains profoundly handicapped. He can't walk or talk and is fed through a gastric tube surgically implanted in his stomach. To breathe, he is dependent on a tube that is permanently inserted into his trachea. He has cerebral palsy, cortical blindness, and needs twenty-four-hour care, which is delivered in a nursing institution.

According to Rivard's attorney, the doctors were so resistant to performing a C-section because the hospital was putting enormous pressure on obstetricians to reduce their C-section rate. In the mid-nineties, clinicians and hospitals were pushing to lower the national Caesarean birth rate. Given that the United States has the highest Caesarean rate in the industrialized world, this was a laudable aim, but in this case it went tragically wrong. What is also striking about this case is that the doctors—even younger, less experienced ones—were adamant in refusing to listen to experienced nurses. This in spite of the fact that they were all women. The combination proved tragic for Michael Rivard.

Building Failure into the System

As they recount the details of their conversations and conflicts with physicians and physicians-in-training, nurses followed the established rules of deference and went through all the appropriate channels in all of these cases. Some played the nurse-doctor game according to its intricate rules. Clinical diagnoses were masked as "reports" of signs and symptoms, and it was sometimes left to inexperienced doctors to make the "diagnosis." Treatment recommendations were disguised as suggestions or hints: "Do you want to turn up the dopamine?" "What size gloves do you need so you can do it right?" "The OR is ready when you need it." Some nurses went through all the channels and begged and pleaded, "Please just come and observe the surgeon's technique." "Please do the surgery now." Some vented to each other but not to senior management. Some withdrew their services, perhaps even their concern, and certainly their advocacy.

In these cases of bad outcomes, doctors and administrators didn't listen, patients suffered, and senior nurses were forced to stand by and watch as junior doctors—who could really not be expected to know more—exercised authority with poor judgment. Senior doctors, unaccountably in some cases, couldn't be reached, and there was no mechanism in place to allow a veteran nurse's judgment to supersede a novice physician's.

Recall the concerns of nineteenth-century physicians, that the private duty nurse with a front-row seat—and possessing the knowledge to understand the real meaning of the acts being performed on the patient—would steer patients away from physicians she considered to be unsafe or incompetent. Nurses occupy a front-row seat today. By dint of their own knowledge and experience, they have valuable opinions about medical decision making but may be reluctant to present them.

Nurses' comments on their experiences are very illuminating. Carol Youngson told me several times what she said at the inquest: as more babies died, and more were delivered into her arms for what she feared would be certain death or terrible complications at the hands of an inexperienced surgeon, she wanted to tell the parents to take their babies and run. Nurses claim that one of their major roles is to act as their patient's advocate; when asked why she didn't warn parents about Odim, she answered, "Well, first of all, when I see these parents, we are literally at the door of the operating room. They have gone through all of the pre-op teaching sessions. They have gone through all of the stress of preparing themselves for this particular event. And I can't imagine anything could be more stressful for a parent than something like this. I could sort of paint a picture of what it would be like if I had gone out to this parent and said, 'Stop, you can't do this, take your baby and run, or whatever.'"

"What would have happened then would have been that all hell would have broke loose. They would have called Dr. Odim. They would have called Dr. Wiseman probably, called the director of nursing up. There would have been this big group of people come to this, wherever we were, waiting room, wherever. I would have been very upset by then, probably crying. There would have been Dr. Odim and Dr. Giddins and whomever, calm, cool, collected. I would have looked like an overemotional, almost crazy person. . . . Would the parents have listened?" No, she said, they wouldn't. They would have thought she was "overreacting" or "overemotional," and she would have been fired and "there would have been more kids come in, the next day or the next week."[18]

This episode exposes the limits of nursing advocacy and illuminates the terrible bind in which nurses find (or put) themselves in our health care system.

114   Advocacy, after all, doesn't merely involve making suggestions that a patient can easily follow, or engaging in conversations in which there is no risk of conflict. The term comes from the Latin for "counselor" and "voice." It often refers to a legal advocate and implies a willingness to take risks for one's client or patient. An advocate, says *Webster's* dictionary, is "one who pleads the cause of another in a court of law," or who "defends, vindicates or espouses a cause by argument." The very term suggests a willingness to go up against others, to go to the limits of one's powers to defend another.

In this case and so many others, we see the structural and historical impediments to both advocacy and rescue. Carol Youngson and her colleagues and many of the other nurses we have mentioned had the right education, and they certainly had the right experience. But they had the wrong institutional socialization and lacked the institutional authority and respect to act on their knowledge and experience. Because advocacy in nursing is so often viewed as an individual rather than a collective responsibility, they also lacked—and sometimes did not solicit—external support from nursing groups when they finally asked for it.

In their hospital, they lacked institutional respect and regard for their work and knowledge. They were told they occupied a limited space, and in some instances they seemed to have stayed in that space. In the tradition of their socialization, neither Youngson nor any of the other nurses made an issue of Odim's refusal to do a run-through of upcoming surgeries. While disappointed in his reaction, Youngson testified that "it was not her place to insist that the surgeon participate in a dry run."[19]

Before the Wiseman committee was formed, Youngson and other nurses, like the anesthetists, debated whether or not to withdraw their services from the program. The nurses felt that their withdrawal would not have had sufficient impact, unlike that of anesthetists, and that the program would have continued without them. Their withdrawal would, they felt, have deprived patients of expert OR, PICU, and NICU nurses that were even more necessary given the inexperience of the surgeons. So they stayed. But what if their calculation was wrong? What if their withdrawal of services would have forced the hospital to listen? Why didn't they join the anesthetists in their protest? Wouldn't that joint protest have had even more of an impact? Again, nursing socialization in medical institutions makes it extremely hard for nurses to take that risk. Their training teaches them that they must sacrifice for the patient. But does it teach them when that act of sacrifice itself compromises the patient's health?

As Judge Sinclair concluded in his inquest report, because of the "historically subordinate role of that the nursing profession has played in our health care system," Youngson's actions were not unprofessional.[20] In-

stead, one could argue that, proclamations from professional nursing organizations about patient advocacy notwithstanding, they reflect precisely
the level of "professionalism" and "advocacy" that is possible under such
severe constraints.

Failing to Rescue Nurses

The nurse-doctor synergy I've described in this chapter is a complex interaction between people who appear to be victims and their apparent vic-
timizers, in which the former adapt and acquiesce and then end up per-
petuating their victimization (which is precisely the internal dynamic that
makes oppression so insidious). Some nurses obviously rebel against this
dynamic, some negotiate a partial rebellion, and some submit. Whichever
course they take, it affects their commitment to their profession.

Although there don't seem to be any studies judging the psychological
impact of physician abuse on nurses, many of the nurses I talked to about
their relationships with physicians seemed to exhibit an almost chronic,
low-level sense of despair and depression about the situation. Limited in
the kind of external action they feel they can take to protect themselves
against "superiors" with higher status, and poorly educated in effective direct communication with doctors and direct strategies to confront bullying in the workplace, nurses can turn the anger and resentment they feel
against themselves. Some may become depressed. All of this, the psychologist Larry Harmon says, is likely to have a negative impact on job performance.

Some of the nurses I talked with often referred to themselves as battered women who keep on taking it and feel more and more demoralized,
isolated, and powerless. They felt beaten down by physician disregard and
abuse.

Faith Henson, whom we met in chapter 3, presents an interesting example of this dynamic. Unlike many nurses, who come from a working-
class background, Henson is an upper-middle-class woman. Her husband
is a math professor at the University of Illinois at Champaign/Urbana.
She worked as a potter before she became a nurse in mid-life. Yet, her
sense of self was, like the clay she molded, reshaped by her experiences in
the hospital. Nurse-doctor relationships at Provena/Covenant, she said,
were just awful. For the entire time she practiced, nurses seemed to be
barely visible to physicians—except as objects of derision and disrespect.

"In all the time I worked at Provena," Henson says, "I never had a doctor call me by my name. I didn't think that was unusual. They wouldn't
call you anything. I'd never had any doctor say anything pleasant to me,
like 'Isn't it a beautiful day?' or 'thank you.'"

After years of fighting the hospital for better staffing and working conditions, Henson was fired, she believes, for trying to organize a union. She pulled up stakes and moved to San Francisco, where she now works in the intensive care unit at UCSF Medical Center. The hospital is in a more liberal city in a more liberal state. It's a teaching hospital associated with a highly respected nursing school, and nurses in the institution are members of a nurses' union, the California Nurses Association, and thus have greater protection when they exercise voice.

Her first day on the job, Henson recounts, she had a transformative experience. "A resident came up, put his hand on my shoulder, and said, 'Thank you for helping me.' I had never had that happen. Never. Doctors here call you by your name. I had an attending come back and thank me for taking care of our patient." When he did, Henson said, she was so stunned that she had to turn away so he wouldn't see the tears in her eyes.

When nurses feel powerless to protect their patients, they may end up blaming themselves for the problems they or their patients endure. The nurses whom Benner, Tanner, and Chesla interviewed blamed themselves for not fighting hard enough for their patients, not being assertive enough, or not manipulating enough.[21] Often nurses may blame themselves or each other much more than the abusive physicians and the larger system that has enabled the abuse.

One of the things that I have found most impressive about nursing is how easily nurses bad-mouth one another and nursing culture in general. Get nurses together and you will begin to hear familiar mantras. "Nurses are their own worst enemies" is perhaps the most popular. Then there's "Nurses eat their young."

Nurse-physician relationships are one of the exacerbating factors in this culture of negativity. Larry Harmon, for example, says that he finds that abusive physicians can have a deleterious effect on how nurses relate to one another. Abusive behavior creates a general level of tension on the unit. When a doctor is disruptive, nurses may also disagree about how to deal with it. Some nurses want to act to confront the physician, take the issue to management, and push as hard as is necessary to correct the problem. Others insist that to act will be too dangerous. "You have to pick your battles," they tell another nurse, "and this isn't one of them." Others deny the extent of the problem, insisting that "boys will be boys" or that physicians are having a hard time and nurses need to sympathize with their dilemmas. Whatever the response—or excuse for inaction—it can provoke dissension among people who could otherwise act together in a cohesive and perhaps effective manner.

Anne Dolan is a case in point. When I talked to her about her hand injury (see chapter 3), I was struck not by how traumatized she was by her experience but by the sense that she was ashamed of—rather than outraged about—what had happened. She had refused to talk to the media about the event at the time and did not want to revisit it now. Reluctant to discuss the issue, she was adamant that her name not be revealed. She just wanted to forget about it. "No one knows this has happened to me," she said, almost as if she were at fault.

She told me that she no longer works in nursing. I assumed that she blamed the physician who hurt her, but that was not the case. Dolan said she left nursing because of the nurses and residents who wanted her to act more assertively than she was prepared to act. Since a number of them had been abused by the surgeon, they wanted Dolan to make his attack a police matter. But Dolan refused. As she depicted him, the doctor seemed almost to be another patient for whom she was obliged to care. The nurses and residents who supported her and urged her to take even stronger action were reconfigured as the aggressors.

Another nurse, a graduate of the University of Pennsylvania School of Nursing, also expressed great disaffection with the nurses she encountered when she moved into the workplace. Her first job was at the New York Hospital during the heyday of cost cutting. Veteran nurses, the young woman said with some disdain, were overworked yet afraid to complain or fight for themselves. She then went to work for a traveling nurse company that provides nurses on a temporary basis to hospitals across the nation. The conditions in the hospitals she worked in were even worse. "When I challenged physicians, a lot of them were older, and they simply would not answer my questions or give me a reason for their actions. I had a patient who was dying. He was an end-stage cancer patient who had two seizures. He had one seizure, and the physician wouldn't let me give him anything to stop it. It stopped on its own. When it happened again, he would not let us give him medication. The patient's wife was there and it was very upsetting to her."

"It was a very hostile environment," the woman continued. "It appeared that all the hospital cared about was the bottom line and that was it. All the incident reports I filled out should have been very alarming to the quality assurance people. I have no idea if they were ever followed up. No one ever contacted me. The hospital treated the nurses badly. They treated me like scut labor."

Many of the nurses who have encountered the most serious difficulties with physicians no longer work in nursing. Carol Youngson has quit nursing altogether. She works as a forensic investigator for the government of Manitoba. She has not even kept up her nursing license. "The whole experience just took the joy out of it for me," she said recently.

Hundreds of nurses I have interviewed have cited physician-nurse relationships and a culture of acquiescence to abuse as one of the reasons they want to leave the bedside and become advanced practice nurses. Many

118 nursing students have also told me that after watching nurse-doctor relationships and seeing how working nurses have adapted to low-level battering, they have seriously questioned their choice of career. Several years ago, I taught some classes to students at the McGill University School of Nursing in Montreal. Few of the students seemed unaffected by Western society's focus on medicine and its poor image of nursing. Many of the students told me they received little support from family or friends when they announced that they wanted to go into nursing. The attitude was "If you're bright and ambitious, why don't you go to medical school?"

Students said that this attitude even contaminated social gatherings with friends and other university students. If they went out to dinner with friends who were in other fields and a medical student was at the table, everyone's attention would be trained on him—or her. What are you learning? What will you be specializing in? were questions addressed to the med student. The nursing student was an object of curiosity because she hadn't decided to become a doctor—of medicine, that is. One student said, almost in tears, "After so many people ask you why you're not becoming a doctor, you begin to wonder if you've made the right choice." She eventually decided she'd made the wrong one and went to medical school.

Already set up to question their choice of profession, the experiences these students had once they entered the hospital for their clinical apprenticeships didn't help. One of my classes took place just as the students had gone onto the floors at the McGill University Health Centre. I asked the students what they noticed when they went into the various hospitals in the system. I didn't mention the word doctor. Nor did I ask them about negative experiences.

But they recounted negative experiences—with doctors. A number of students said they were shocked at how little doctors and nurses communicated with one another about patient care. They were surprised that doctors, or doctors-in-training, did not routinely round with nurses or consult them about their mutual patients. They were also shocked at how doctors talked to nurses. One student was teamed up with a veteran nurse. She and the nurse had a question about a patient and, because they couldn't reach the resident, they discussed it with the attending physician. Furious that the nurse had gone over her head, the resident assailed the nurse and nursing student, "reaming out" as the nursing student put it, a nurse who was her senior. The senior nurse said nothing while the junior resident fulminated in the hallway, where everyone could hear her tirade.

Another student told the class that she had been teamed up with a veteran nurse who was working in labor and delivery. One of the obstetricians was rude and abrupt with his patients. The student was surprised that the nurse who was "mentoring her" did nothing to curb the physi- **119** cian's behavior. When the student later asked the nurse about the physician's behavior, she found the nurse's response to be even more alarming than her silence. "That's not our concern," she told the student.

The students' distress about the gap between what they had been told in nursing school about nurses' power and autonomy and the reality of their daily subordination—and their tacit acceptance of that subordination—seemed almost palpable. What were they doing here? some wondered. Is this the kind of treatment they could expect when they became real nurses? Why didn't veteran nurses respond to physician abuse or challenge physicians' decisions?

American nursing students express the same questions and concerns. Many of the women and men I talked to had been raised in a period where women's expectations had dramatically shifted and where women had won significant advances in the workplace. Numerous strategies—legal attempts to transform "hostile" workplaces, media campaigns, high-level reports—have been mobilized to make gender inequalities a public issue and to combat and transform patterns of abuse in the workplace. As a result, while status hierarchies are still alive and well in almost every workplace, many professional women no longer tolerate the kinds of behavior to which nurses are routinely subject.

Nurses, on the other hand, seem to be socialized to adapt to pernicious working conditions and physician behavior. This creates a disconnect between nurses who have been in the work force for several decades and those entering nursing today. Of course, it's true that the white caps and white hose have been replaced with the stethoscope and that nurses are now, they proudly point out, part of the "multidisciplinary team." In some hospitals doctors round with nurses. Some doctors and nurses have excellent working relationships.

The problem is that younger women and men aspiring to assume what they consider to be their rightful place in the professions don't view this as an advance, they view it as a given. Why are nurses proudly trumpeting their membership on the health care team? they may wonder. Aren't they supposed to be full members of the health care team? It's great that some nurses diagnose and prescribe, but why are doctors still dissing bedside nurses, throwing scalpels at them in the OR, and excluding them from the highest decision-making bodies in the hospital? And why are nurses taking it and so few using the many mechanisms of protest and complaint that women and minorities have used to such good effect in other settings? Why didn't Anne Dolan, hand in cast, walk out of the hospital and to the police station? And why do nursing schools, nursing organizations, and even some unions seem so silent on the subject?

120   This was not what promotional campaigns to enhance nursing's public image have led new recruits to expect. The disjunction between what students have been taught to believe a nurse deserves and how nurses are treated and respond to that treatment fuels an invisible exodus from the bedside. It explains, in part, why many nursing students and new nurses are so quick to question the profession, leave it entirely, or seek out areas which they feel have higher status and in which they will be treated with more respect.

It's hard to blame them. Ideally, nurses shouldn't have to conduct a mass walkout of an operating room or engage in heroic whistle-blowing to be heard. Society should recognize the obvious: a dysfunctional system of nurse-doctor interaction can lead to near misses, to delays in providing needed care and attention, and to an environment where clinicians' energies are consumed by frustration and demoralization instead of used in empathic communication with patients.

"To not have a system set up to make sure this communication doesn't happen is just astonishing," Jean Chaisson comments. "You wouldn't have a situation where you are building a new office building and the architects aren't going to talk to the structural engineers. You'd be out of business in six months."

5

Making Matters Worse

The week before Christmas 2003, a friend who's an oncologist invited me to attend the Kenneth B. Schwartz Center Rounds at the Massachusetts General Hospital (MGH) in Boston. The Schwartz Rounds are sponsored by the Kenneth B. Schwartz Center, which was founded when Kenneth Schwartz, a cancer patient, left money to promote more compassionate care and better interactions between patients and their caregivers. Held in a variety of different hospitals in Massachusetts and around the country, they are supposed to be a "multidisciplinary forum where caregivers discuss important emotional and social issues that arise in caring for seriously ill patients."[1]

That particular day, close to a hundred men and women gathered in a large glassed-in room in the Wang Ambulatory Care Center. At the front of the room a physician dressed in a short white lab coat with the name "Dr. Thomas Lynch" embroidered on it in blue script sat next to a woman in a red knit sweater and skirt. When Lynch opened the discussion, he explained that rather than addressing heavier issues, today's rounds would be devoted to reading and discussing letters patients had sent to their caregivers. These letters, with the names of patients and caregivers deleted to protect privacy, had been copied and handed out so that members of the audience could read them aloud.

Lynch proceeded to call on different people to read the letters. As he called on physicians, Lynch always identified them, whether male or female, by title, first name, and last name—for example, "Doctor John Smith, would you please read your letter?" Whenever he called on someone who was not a physician, he used only their first name and omit-

122 ted any identifying title. The woman sitting next to him, for example, was never introduced and was referred to only by her first name. Since this was a public meeting, many people in the room, including me and a friend who came with me, were unfamiliar with the participants. The only people we could readily identify were physicians. As for the others, we discovered they were nurses or social workers only when Lynch specifically asked them to comment on an issue from a nursing or social work perspective. (That's how I learned that the woman sitting next to Lynch was in fact a social worker.)

With the exception of two letters, all were written to doctors, praising doctors. One of the letters was written to the hospital president. One was written to a nurse. Without exception the letters were extraordinarily adulatory. "Thank you so much, doctor. You affect so many lives in so many ways everyday." "Thank you for your warmth, humor, honesty, and caring," and "please extend my appreciation to your office staff and to the ambulatory staff on the oncology unit." (The writer evidently did not send a letter to the staff.) "Your nurses and your receptionists were as kind as could be, even by the guy who parked our car, kindness and thoughtfulness was shown."

In most of these letters doctors were given credit for all the knowledge and skill that went into the patients' care. When nurses were mentioned, it was exclusively for their compassion. The letter written to the nurse, which was the shortest, thanked her for being cheerful and running around the hospital to get compression stockings. What was even more interesting was the fact that doctors were generally given credit for nurses' training, for nurses' kindness and empathy, and for nurses' attentiveness. The nurse in these letters was the *doctor's* nurse, not the patient's nurse or even the hospital's nurse.

As I sat listening to this session, given by what was supposed to be a fairly progressive group, I marveled at the endurance of the reigning paradigm. Palliative care is supposed to be about teamwork. But the rendition given in these letters and endorsed by this meeting is that, to paraphrase Join the Army ads, the doctor is a "team of one." If I were a nursing or social work administrator listening to this, I would wonder what was wrong with nursing and social work at the MGH. Why, I would ask myself, do nurses and social workers make such a limited impression on their patients? But no one asked those questions. Nurses and social workers, it seemed, were supposed to sit and bear witness to patients' adulation of their physicians and accept the patients' understandable but erroneous impression that doctors employ and train nurses and social workers and are responsible for their every deed. No one suggested that Lynch might identify non-physicians by name and tell the audience what func-

tion they play on the team. When the meeting ended, apparently everyone was supposed to feel rewarded and refreshed.

Leaving the meeting, I turned to my friend, a molecular biologist who
doesn't work in health care, and I asked him what he thought. Did he
think the format reflected a really multidisciplinary team at work? "Multidisciplinary?" he asked. "Everyone was basically accepting the public
fiction that the patients also share, that the doctor knows everything and
knows it best. Everybody in the room was always deferring to the doctor,
to daddy, and all the other people who took care of them—whom they
may like and who provide them support—they seem to think are all helping daddy. Nobody challenged that. It would have been interesting to see
how they would have reacted if that were brought up," my friend continued. "You can have a conversation about this today, a conversation you
couldn't have had thirty years ago. People could say, let's stop and look at
this. Nurses could initiate that kind of conversation. But it seemed to me
that they didn't even seem too troubled about it. They didn't get after
them for selecting those letters, letters that only talked about doctors.
Why not? Is it always like this?"

That, of course, is a most relevant question.

In her book *Gender and Discourse*, the linguist Deborah Tannen reminds us that "human interaction is a 'joint production': everything that
occurs results from the interaction of all participants."[2] While doctors
have been socialized to ignore and disregard nurses, and sometimes even
abuse them, nurses have, in turn, been socialized to adapt to, enable, or
perpetuate the problems that make their work much less satisfying. Like
medical socialization, this nursing socialization has a long and complicated history.

Back to the Future

Although Florence Nightingale is often said to have founded nursing in
the mid-nineteenth century, women—and men—have been giving nursing care for centuries. While individual nurses probably practiced in almost every civilization and era, the development of Christianity transformed nursing by making compassion and good works a religious
imperative, by giving nursing an organized structure and home, and by attaching to it a very specific sets of images and moral metaphors and thus a
series of rigid moral scripts.

Building on the Egyptian and Jewish traditions of providing social welfare to the sick and poor, early Christians made acts of charity and of self-
sacrifice—particularly to the poor, sick, and vulnerable—central to the
believer's duty to serve God. Easy access to nursing care was one of the

124 most tangible benefits of membership in the early Christian community.[3] The early Christian's obligation to help and show compassion to others was an avenue not only to salvation but to atonement and redemption through self-mortification, which immersion in the stench and suffering of illness could also provide.

To follow this particular path to redemption and salvation, one did not originally have to be a woman. In the early Christian community both men and women provided nursing care. Orders varied in the types of vows or promises men and women made, the degree of their isolation from the world, their commitment to prayer and contemplation, and their class background. These religious communities built some of the great hospitals that exist to this day like the Hotel Dieu in Paris and Santo Spirito in Rome. In all these settings, monks provided care for men and nuns for women.

The Protestant Reformation, however, transformed both nursing and hospitals throughout Europe. In Protestant countries, authorities closed monasteries and convents and the hospitals and hospices they ran. All church property and funds were confiscated. Skilled nuns and monks were expelled from hospitals they'd run, often for centuries. Hospitals that had once been financed by the church became dependent on individual charitable donations. Additionally, a lay manager and his wife generally replaced a religious superintendent.

When Catholic clerical authorities launched the Counter-Reformation, they encouraged believers to proclaim the greater glory of God by performing acts of service. The religious zeal thus unleashed produced hundreds of nursing orders, whose impact we still see today. One of the most influential of these was the Daughters of Charity, founded in 1617 by the French priest Vincent de Paul, who was later canonized. De Paul wanted to bring greater organization to the charitable care provided to the sick in their own homes. The uncloistered lower-class women he recruited took vows that could be renewed annually. They received payment for their work through contracts that were negotiated with local authorities.[4] Working with the well-born St. Louise de Marillac, de Paul created the Dames de Charité, a society of unvowed, uncloistered upper-class women who functioned as would a charitable association today.[5]

The Daughters of Charity established an enduring social bargain. Lower-class women chosen for their devotion and moral probity received "a steady wage, free accommodation, clothing, security, a modicum of comfort in illness and old age, a decent burial and also the sense of social promotion that membership of such an esteemed community entailed."[6]

In England the quality of the institutional care of the sick declined and did not recover until the mid-nineteenth century. Nonetheless, hospitals were established during this period and nurses sometimes founded them. According to Deidre Wicks, in the seventeenth century hospital nurses were "poorly paid and highly regulated."[7] During the reign of George III many wealthy English people traveled to Europe and returned with stories of the excellent nursing care available in European hospitals. This produced a series of reforms that altered hospital nursing in Britain.

In England during the seventeenth and eighteenth centuries, nurses also provided care in the community. Independent nurses worked in the homes of both the rich and poor, took care of sick children, and delivered babies. The work of the nurse is difficult to define during this era. Did a nurse do the same work as a doctor? Was a midwife a nurse? Was she paid only to deliver babies or was she also paid to tend the sick? Was a nurse also viewed as a healer? wise woman? old woman? The answer seems to be that there was no clear difference between these categories of healing. "Women irregulars moved across the different health care categories," acting sometimes as midwives, healers, nurses, and layers-out of the dead, Wicks explains.[8]

The same blurring of distinctions held true in the American colonies. In *A Midwife's Tale*, Laurel Thatcher Ulrich provides a detailed picture of a late-eighteenth- and early-nineteenth-century midwife who not only delivered babies but functioned as a nurse, healer, and physician.[9]

The historical record indicates that there was no clear differentiation between the work of religious men and women and the work of physicians. Nurses diagnosed conditions and prescribed remedies. Some of them grew the herbs and mixed the remedies their patients drank, performed procedures like bloodletting, and prepared and applied poultices—mixtures of bran, mustard, flax, or other substances that were put on wounds and inflamed areas. They also fed and bathed patients and created calm, orderly environments where patients benefited from a modicum of cleanliness, ate nutritiously, and got much-needed rest.

As a routine part of her training, for example, a Daughter of Charity was taught how to perform minor surgery as well as to apply leeches. On completion of her preparation, Nelson explains, she set off from her motherhouse in Paris to work for a provincial hospital that had contracted her services, equipped with "three boxes of lancets and ligatures plus a case of surgical instruments."

In England, nurses took a "cautious and conservative approach to therapeutics, and one which relied on regimen, herbs and basic physical care, where this was necessary." Typically, doctors were summoned only by the rich and only for the most serious cases. Nurses in this period also delivered what would now be termed, in the fashionable nursing jargon, "holistic care."[10]

126   Although religious nurses would undoubtedly have attributed their success to divine intervention, their knowledge of herbs, minor surgery, proper diet, and hospital organization played a more significant role.

The Angel's Arithmetic

For many men and women, nursing represented an excellent social bargain. In periods of economic and social chaos, belonging to religious orders promised an escape, or at least a respite, from the insecurities, tumult, wars, famine, disease, and pestilence that were so pervasive for so many centuries. Living and working in monastic or tertiary orders gave people permission to abstain from the responsibilities and dangers of family life in the Middle Ages. Religious orders offered a vocation and a home to aristocratic or well-born men who were unable to inherit property. They offered widows and unmarried women shelter and a useful occupation. Families could unburden themselves of the lifelong responsibility of providing food and shelter to an unmarried daughter by sending her to a convent. These nurses were promised salvation as well as the benefit of a community of like-minded women engaged in purposeful work outside of the home.

To perform this work, nurses, whether male or female, had to gain knowledge that few possessed. Monks and nuns and those in secular orders had easy access to the caregiving services delivered by other members of their community. They also had certain freedoms that would otherwise have been unavailable. As Nelson writes of the Daughters of Charity, "The combination of obedience to their rule and utter faith that they were the instruments of God's will was capable, on occasion, of empowering these women to use their initiative and exercise their judgment" in ways that would have been otherwise unthinkable.[11] Well-to-do women who directed convents controlled huge budgets and were sometimes more successful in attracting patrons and their funds than were male orders. Similarly, ministering to the needs of others conferred higher social status on women, which was particularly important for those of humbler origins.

As in all bargains, however, nurses paid a price. Whatever accomplishments religious nurses achieved, whatever freedoms they enjoyed, whatever respite they had from the dangers of life, whatever respect they accrued, "occurred wholly within a framework of submission, obedience, and indifference."[12] Religious orders demanded that nurses not only cultivate knowledge but also anonymity and that they sacrifice every shred of their individual identity. They gave up their given names and adopted new ones assigned by the community, and they lived and worked where the community dictated. Not only were they required to be obedient to

God, they had to give unwavering obedience to their mother or father su- **127** perior and to their order.

In these communities, nursing was considered a calling. Nurses were called by God to do His work and were guided in the performance of that work by His will. Indeed, the eternal salvation nurses sought was dependent on the belief that it was God, not the individual nurse, who was responsible for whatever successes nurses managed to produce when caring for patients. In Christian theology, "good works" were certainly supposed to bring tangible benefits to others. But to attain the goal of eternal salvation, good deeds had to be conducted with the appropriate spirit of deference—which meant they could never be attributed to the individual, but rather only to Divine agency. "Nurses," Nelson remarks, "thought of themselves as God's instruments who did not deserve credit for themselves." Although humility served the goal of institutional survival as well as spiritual salvation, nurses cloaked their work—and any acknowledgment of the technical and scientific mastery it demanded—with the same hush of awesome mystery.

Another key element of that script was the shunning of conflict. For religious orders, the rewards that came from the care of the sick were possible only because nuns functioned in a hierarchical, male-dominated structure. They had freedom within their cloister, hospital, or lay order. Nonetheless, no matter how powerful they were, nuns were subject to the will of male clerics. One of the strategies for the success of all the religious orders, particularly religious sisterhoods, was the avoidance of open conflict with either ecclesiastical or municipal authorities. When the church had almost totalitarian statelike powers, no one, after all, wanted to invite the close scrutiny of ecclesiastical authorities. "Religious orders maintained their independence," Nelson explains, "in large part, because they were so adept at flying under the ecclesiastical radar. In other words, they tried to avoid attracting the attention of the bishop whose opposition could be disastrous to the future of a community which could be taken over by another religious order or entirely suppressed."

Nurses and their communities had to receive some remuneration and acknowledgment to survive. But since virtue is its own reward, pay could be minimal. What nurses could accept were compliments for their deferential behavior and angelic virtues. These habits of mind, heart, and soul became for nursing what the feminist legal scholar Isabel Marcus calls a "moral script."[13] Nurses' lives were governed by a series of scripts that prescribed the behaviors and attitudes that were considered appropriate for their sex, their class, and their religion.

For religious nurses, the carefully cultivated habits of self-sacrifice, devotion, obedience, silence, humility, and avoidance of conflict, unlike the

128   annually renewable vows taken by the Daughters of Charity, could not be abandoned at will. They were instead integrated into the self-definition of the nurse and of nursing. Religious affiliation tethered women to unpaid work, self-effacement, and the image of the angelic, saintly, and mystical. Being part of a religious community offered nurses learning, protection, and lifetime security, but it also submerged an individual's identity (even a medieval nurse's identity) into an anonymous mass. Nursing was so firmly attached to the divine that it seemed, Nelson says, almost "outside of the realm of the ordinary or the individual." Nurses, as Nelson's book title so aptly argues, were to "say little and do much"—not only because their spiritual beliefs demanded self-sacrifice but because the link between their work and the divine seemed to render its content beyond description. Any deviation from the script meant not only punishment by the community but, far more frightening, the loss of their eternal soul.

Nineteenth-Century Professionalization

The fusion of nursing and moral virtues would become one of the building blocks of the nineteenth-century secularization and professionalization of nursing. Indeed, it is one of the elements that make the story of modern nursing both so intriguing and so frustrating.

In England and other Protestant countries, the revival of nursing began early in the nineteenth century, several decades before Nightingale set foot in the Crimea and there, according to historical myth, founded modern nursing. One of the first manifestations of this renewal took place in the late 1830s in the German Rhineland. In a town called Kaiserswerth, the Lutheran pastor Theodur Fliedner and his wife Friederike Munster established a hospital, a penitentiary, and an orphanage. Like other nineteenth-century reformers, Fliedner was motivated by religious concerns. Simultaneously inspired by the success of the Daughters of Charity in France and concerned about growing interest in Catholicism and liberal and socialist thought, Fliedner wanted to deliver care to the sick and poor while simultaneously inoculating his flock against dangerous ideas and trends. His cunning solution was to incorporate both Catholic and socialist forms and ideals in an institution that trained a new cadre of Lutheran nurses. Borrowing the early Christian term *diakonia*, used to describe the rooms in a house set aside for the provision of hospitality or the care of the sick, he and his wife called these nurses "deaconesses." Specially trained to care for the sick, these deaconesses were attached to a Lutheranized motherhouse modeled on the Catholic convent.

Similar religious and social ferment in other countries produced more nurses. In 1813, well-to-do women set up the first home care agency, the

Ladies Benevolent Society, in Charleston, South Carolina. Quakers cared **129** for the sick poor in their own homes and tended victims of the 1831 cholera epidemic. To provide trained nurses for the sick poor, the Quaker Elizabeth Fry established the Society of the Protestant Sisters of Charity in London in 1840. Anglican sisterhoods, notably St. John's House and All Saints in London, were also formed. St. John's House, an order that was modeled along Catholic lines, contracted its nursing services to London hospitals like King's College and Guy's.

In 1838 an even more interesting development occurred. For the first time since the Reformation, Catholics established a convent in England. With the passage of the Catholic Emancipation Bill in 1829, Catholics were formally emancipated in England and were allowed to enter public life, attend university, pursue careers in the military, and practice their religion publicly. Taking advantage of this opening, Bishop Griffiths, apostolic vicar of the London District, asked the Catholic Sisters of Mercy in Dublin to come to England to care for the sick. In 1839 six Irish nurses founded the Sisters of Mercy at Bermondsey, where they took care of both the rich and poor in their own homes. The Bermondsey sisters also answered the British Army's desperate plea for nurses during the Crimean War. Indeed, Florence Nightingale's relationship with the founding superior of the order, Mary Clare Moore, had a significant influence on her work (as did her studies at Kaiserswerth).[14] After the Crimean War the Bermondsey sisters established a hospital for sick children, the first Catholic hospital to function in England since the Reformation.

Religious nurses also played a critical role in the establishment of the American health care system. Most popular accounts of American nursing focus on the development of nursing during the Civil War. Yet, as early as 1823 the American Sisters of Charity, who later joined the French Daughters of Charity, took over nursing at the Baltimore Infirmary, the first medical teaching hospital in the United States. Over the next century, literally hundreds of Catholic women—Sisters of Charity, of the Incarnate Word, of Providence, and of Mercy among others—and Protestant nuns, such as those of St. John's House, traveled across the American and Canadian frontier to set up the only hospitals and health services available. By the 1880s, there were sixty Lutheran motherhouses in Germany and six thousand deaconesses. These deaconesses, who had moved across Protestant Europe and opened hospitals from Scandinavia to Eastern Europe, also established hospitals, like Boston's New England Deaconess Hospital, across the United States. Religious reformers also established hospitals, schools, public health clinics, and home care nursing in Australia and New Zealand.[15]

"These women," Sioban Nelson explains, "convinced local business and

130 community leaders to finance the construction of hospitals, persuaded physicians to contract with them for services, and ultimately worked with large railroad, mining, logging and other major companies to provide some of the first insurance plans that guaranteed medical care for sick and injured workers. These nuns also set up the first nursing schools in America, like the nursing program at Bellevue Hospital in New York."

Early-nineteenth-century nurses shaped the thinking of mid-nineteenth-century "secular" reformers like Florence Nightingale. Although often considered to be secular women in the modern sense of the term, mid-nineteenth-century nursing reformers were first and foremost religiously and socially motivated. Even when they were Protestants, most borrowed the forms of the Catholic religious order, secularizing them to fit into the modernizing hospital.

The nineteenth-century nursing reformers wanted to improve the care of the sick, enhance the health of the public, and provide socially useful work for respectable women who wanted (or needed) to work outside the home. This last goal was no less important than the others. With the advent of industrialization and urbanization, women's economic role in the home changed radically. In rural areas, people were pushed off small family farms. Whether in urban or rural settings, the production of many goods, like cotton, wool, and everyday clothing, was increasingly taking place in large factories. Women's manufacturing and farming labor was no longer as important as it had been in the past. But women still had to work to survive.[16] As Florence Nightingale wrote, "the majority of women in all European countries are, by God's providence, compelled to work for their bread."[17] Apart from dreadful jobs in crowded, polluted factories or servile labor for upper-class or aristocratic families, respectable lower-class women had little decent work available to them. Women in dire need could also become prostitutes. Those women who, as Nightingale put it, were forced to "live by their shame" could look to nursing as "an avenue of honest work."[18]

Lower-class women weren't the only ones looking for suitable employment. Upper-class women who wanted to do purposeful work had only one acceptable option—marriage. If women didn't want to depend on a man and become the "domestic angel" who brought spirit and light to the drawing and dining rooms—they could become governesses or teachers in someone else's family.[19]

In Protestant and even Catholic countries, reformers like Nightingale found the perfect occupational opening in an institution that cried out for reform—the hospital. Nursing reformers were genuinely appalled at the state of nursing care in hospitals. The hospital was linked to notorious "hospitalism," hospital-acquired infections that killed thousands of pregnant women following labor and delivery (40 to 50 percent of surgical patients), as well as patients hospitalized with other acute illnesses. In 1848, a professor of obstetrics in Edinburgh wrote that "the man laid on an operating table in one of our surgical hospitals is exposed to more chances than the English soldier on the field of Waterloo."[20] Inadequate nursing services certainly played a role in the high death rate in hospitals. Charles Dickens, in his famous portrait of the alcoholic nurse, Mrs. Sarah Gamp, in *Martin Chuzzlewit*, implied that nurses were all drunken thieves. This was a caricature, for there were certainly some competent nurses functioning in a variety of settings. Nonetheless, whether in Protestant or Catholic countries, it was clear that nurses needed more systematic training. Bursting with the spirit of evangelical zeal, reformers used the language and ideology of the day and tried to turn it to their own ends. Reformers insisted that women's sensitivities, natural proclivities, and "natural moral superiority" made them more suitable to the care of the sick than men. By harnessing women's superior moral energies to useful purposes, order could be wrung from the chaos of the mid-nineteenth-century hospital. Filthy, disorganized hospitals could be transformed into clean and well-ventilated places if nurses mobilized the correct demeanor, attributes, and skill. Their patients would be well fed, adequately clothed, and set on the road to health and moral probity. To do this, however, non-religious nursing had to be made respectable for respectable women.

This was no trivial feat. The nurses who came after Sarah Gamp were viewed not only as a danger to men in the hospital setting but as potentially endangered by them. Nuns were able to approach the naked male body because their habits—both what they wore and how they behaved—desexualized them. But what would happen to the new nurse, the respectable lower-class girl or upper-class woman who ventured into the modern hospital or into the homes of the well-to-do or the poor as private duty or visiting nurses? This woman was venturing into a public sphere that, Richard Sennett writes, was off limits to women. For women, the public domain was "where one risked losing virtue, dirtying oneself, being swept into 'a disorderly and heady swirl' (Thackery). The public and the idea of disgrace were closely allied," something that was not the case for men.[21] If a young woman was then to learn things no woman should be learning, "inappropriate behavior" could easily make a woman sexual prey to male doctors or male patients.

The training and outfitting of the newly minted nurse was designed to shield women behind a veil of religious or, later, civic virtue that protected them from unwanted sexual advances as well as from the stigma of

132 caring for the sick. According to Nelson, "Some of these young women were taught to visualize the dying Christ when they took care of male bodies. In order to suppress their maternal instincts, they were supposed to visualize the baby Jesus."

To educate them in their calling, respectable women of good moral character, but of the lower classes, were recruited first to hospitals and then home care and private duty nursing. They were then trained and supervised by women of superior social class and education. These upperclass lady nurses rarely had much experience in bedside practice. Their loyalties were divided between the needs and survival of the hospitals and profession they were reforming and those of the women they were supervising. Yet they became the leaders of the profession. Their sense of power over the nurses they supervised, exercised within the ambiguous power structure of hospital hierarchy, led to a lack of clarity about whose interests they in fact represented—one of the pervasive legacies of the nineteenth century. Reflecting traditional class and status hierarchies, upper-class reformers like Florence Nightingale looked down upon working-class women and wanted to refine them. In a typical exercise of upper-class arrogance, the reformers were convinced that, if left to their own devices, lower-class women newly recruited to nursing would quickly become another batch of Sarah Gamps. With upper-class tutelage, women of the lower orders would be taught to dress and behave appropriately.[22] They would, of course, also learn about diseases, suffering, death, anatomy, physiology, and chemistry. But Bible readings and prayer, which would help students cultivate the right moral character, supplemented this rudimentary curriculum. This supervision would be exercised in environments that closely mimicked the hierarchically organized monastic orders of the Middle Ages. The message was reinforced by the nurses' uniform, a modified version of the nun's headdress. In England, nurses were called "sister." Throughout Europe and the New World, they could not marry while they worked in hospitals. Moreover, they were underpaid for the arduous labor they performed, and their needs were subordinated to those of physicians and hospitals.[23] (Later in the nineteenth and early twentieth centuries, the military would also strongly influence nursing.)

While nursing reformers were careful not to tread on physician's toes, they held the common nineteenth-century concept of a woman's sphere and envisioned hospitals in which nurses inhabited their own female-controlled universe. Reformers wanted lower-class nurses to report directly to upper-class "sisters" (i.e., head nurses), matrons, or superintendents (directors of nursing). Nursing superintendents, reformers argued, should replace the lay manager and his wife. This nursing super-

intendent would report not to physicians but directly to hospital govern- **133**
ing boards.

This was a reform agenda with a revolutionary twist. It was one thing
for women to acquire knowledge and power and care for naked male bodies, when the nurses were God's agents, protected, as Nelson puts it, by
"vow and veil." It was quite another for them to go out into an unprotected workplace or community to be paid to care for the sick without either protection. It was one thing for women to seek education that would
place them firmly under the thumb of physicians and make them better
physicians' handmaids. It was quite another to seek power and control in
the hospital.

The great, and ultimately problematic, accomplishment of lady nurse
reformers was to build on traditional gender stereotypes as well as the
language of religious devotion to convince the public that respectable
women, and only women, should do nursing for pay. By defining nursing
as a vocation and a calling, the reformers made it possible for respectable
women to leave the confines of the family for paid work outside the home.
By portraying the nurse as subordinate to the physician, they neutralized
medical opposition to the few nurses who had received some training.
And by demanding little remuneration for nurses—and emphasizing the
moral, the practical, and the efficient—they rendered nurses' ambitions
palatable to both medicine and a broader public.

The template that was established in the nineteenth century is still operating in health care today. Following the pattern set by the pioneer
nursing reformers, nurses still tend to rely on what Charles Rosenberg
terms the "double-edged sword" of appeals to efficiency or moral uplift to
justify their existence.[24] Like the nurse who sought her place in the system by promising to bring order to the chaos of the nineteenth-century
hospital, the contemporary nurse promises to be a more efficient caregiver and simultaneously to humanize the impersonal health care system
of the twenty-first century.

Today, as we have seen, many doctors still treat nurses not as members
of a unique discipline but, as one nineteenth-century physician once pro-
claimed, "merely one of the means of cure, like the administration of
medicines or the performance of operations."[25] And many nurses still play
the part, albeit reluctantly. Although nurses have persistently fought to attain what the historian Margarete Sandelowski refers to as "a socially valued place and distinctive identity," the persistence of the nineteenth-
century template prevents nurses from taking advantage of cultural
openings and changes in women's position in society; nor can they enlist
public support to redress inequalities that ultimately hurt patients far
more than they hurt nurses.[26]

Overadapting in the Present

Nurses, unlike other women in the workplace, seem reluctant to make private knowledge public when it comes to problematic gender relationships. They have not made a social issue out of the kind of abusive behavior many other working women have brought to public attention and have somewhat successfully fought. Of course, nurses have on occasion successfully fought for and won better treatment. But as I observe nurses dealing with this issue, I note more resignation than open rebellion, more adaptation than activism, and more depression than outrage. Sometimes nurses even defend their abusers. As we have seen, many nurses also tend to embrace the gender stereotypes of angels, saints, and martyrs that are used to legitimize poor treatment. They often teach one another how to enable doctors to mistreat them or how to conceal the realities of their mistreatment. Similarly, they may resist efforts to improve relationships or even attack those who are trying to protect them from abuse.

Nurses challenge the power and prerogatives of doctors on a daily basis. Advanced practice nurses and nurse practitioners have made some notable incursions onto medical turf. But in an era when patients view themselves as consumers and are more supportive of challenges to medical paternalism and domination, both advanced practice nurses and ordinary staff nurses seem reluctant to raise public awareness about the negative consequences of their subordination for patients. Nor do they borrow the strategies that other women and oppressed groups have successfully adopted to fight against mistreatment. There are, for example, few hostile workplace suits against hospitals for allowing doctors to continue disrupting nurses' work.

When nurses protested, John Bell Thompson, a surgeon and former head of the Erie County Medical Center's cardiothoracic surgery program, was suspended in 1998 because of his bad behavior toward the nurses he worked with.[27] We have seen that nurses in Montreal, after years of abuse, finally rebelled against their surgeons. These cases, however, tend to be exceptions. Nurses in Winnipeg brought their concerns to their union but didn't pursue them. They didn't go to their professional association. Nor did nurses in Bristol, England. Nurses rarely, if ever, leave the operating room and walk to the police station when a surgeon attacks them with what is today a lethal weapon—blood products or a bloodied instrument. For nurses in the United States, organized protest is more difficult than it is in other countries since few nurses belong to any organization whatsoever and only 17 percent are members of unions.[28]

Protests mounted by these organizations do not always yield results. Although unions and professional associations will sometimes fight hard for nurses who have to deal with abusive doctors, they may not consider **135** nurse-doctor relationships a pressing issue or part of their organizational mandate. Doctor-nurse relationships are a "professional issue," one union activist told me. "The individual nurse has to deal with the individual doctor about it," this otherwise assertive woman said. I'm sure she would never tell a nurse that she ought to deal with hospital administrators as an individual rather than as part of a group of concerned trade unionists.

Some union activists I've spoken to tell me that they don't consider nurse-physician relationships to be a central issue. They say that nurses aren't as preoccupied by these problems as they are by staffing and mandatory overtime. That may be the case. But I find it interesting that when I talk to nurses in the very same union, they flood me with stories of bad physician behavior and the negative impact it has on nurses in the workplace.

One union staffer explained that she feels the gap between rhetoric and reality has to do with nurses' sense of powerlessness. "They just don't feel this can change, so why bother raising the issue."

Professional associations—groups of nurses organized around their specialties, like critical care or oncology—also seem to do little about the problem. Nor do academics deal with it head on. Many nursing academics seem to feel that the problem will be solved when more nurses get a better education and become "worthy of respect," as one dean of nursing put it when I talked with her about doctor-nurse relationships. Why should doctors consult with bedside nurses? she asked indignantly. They are poorly educated and haven't earned physician respect. When more nurses go into advanced practice or become nurse practitioners, then physicians will treat them collegially, for they will have earned physician respect. Such was the subtext of her comments.

Given this complicated socialization, nurses tend to respond in a variety of indirect ways to their subordination and to difficult doctors. Some, as we've seen, engage in an informal, individual boycott of physicians they find hard to deal with. Although this tactic may solve the problem for the nurse who successfully boycotts that particular physician, it simply shifts the problem to others.

Nurses may follow the rules of the doctor-nurse game and choose indirect means to deal with problems. When it comes to discussions of end-of-life care, many nurses try to deal with their fear of physician retaliation by waffling or hedging. "If a patient asks a nurse, 'How do you think I'm doing?' or 'Do you think I'm going to die?'" explains Cynda Rushton, an expert in palliative care nursing at the Johns Hopkins School of Nursing, "this puts the nurse in the difficult situation of having to struggle with what she knows factually from data about the patient, what she knows

136 from her experience with taking care of this patient, and what she knows from taking care of other patients. She has a pretty clear picture of what is happening, but she feels compelled to maintain the culture, to be subservient to the physician's overt or covert message that this is something you, as a nurse, have no authority to speak to the patient about."

So, Rushton says, instead of asking the patient a direct question like, "How do you think you're doing?" or "Do you think you're dying?" the nurse will hedge.

"The nurse may ask indirect questions," Rushton says. "Or he may divert it back to the doctor: 'You'll need to talk to the doctor about that.'" This frustrates both nurse and patient, explains Rushton. It also means that the nurse is put in the position of subverting himself. He makes a public statement that reinforces the nurse's subordination to physicians. And of course, it deprives the patient of the nurse's assistance in this very complex area, not to mention adding to the patient's suffering and to potentially higher health care costs.

Like battered women conforming to a conventionally accepted moral script, nurses are constantly told they don't know, don't have authority, and shouldn't talk about medical matters. Not surprisingly, some internalize the message and believe that physicians' disregard, disrespect, and abuse is the normal state of affairs. These nurses adapt to it by trying to placate the doctor.

Some RNs are reluctant to confront disruptive physicians, because they believe that doctors are better than nurses and deserve to use their power and authority as they see fit. When I've raised the issue of doctor-nurse relationships, a few nurses will jump to physician's defense, commiserating with the difficult burdens they bear, the stress of their work, and insisting that doctors just need to release steam. Some nurses tell me that I'm "doctor bashing." For example, some years ago my colleague Bernice Buresh and I talked about physician-nurse communication at a conference of the American Nurses Association. It was surprising to see how many nurses raced to the defense of physicians. Several nurses reminded us how difficult life had become for doctors under managed care. This was the wrong time to take them to task about their bad behavior.

In her book *Nurses and Doctors at Work*, the Australian sociologist Deidre Wicks talks about how nurses have seized "limited opportunities" and how their "non-compliance and resistance" has "allowed them not only to do their work, but to carve out significant areas of practice within the dominant power relationships."[29] While it's critical to consider how nurses have mobilized to maneuver around the obstacles they confront, it's also important to analyze how these very strategies can perpetuate the stereotypes and dominance they were intended to counter.

While applauding nurses for their ability to "carve out significant areas **137** of practice" and "do their work" in spite of medical interference and disregard, I want to consider why some of these strategies may become counterproductive. Because patients have such a high stake in effective communication between doctors and nurses, I don't believe the public can afford to sit out this issue or just hope it gets better. How nurses negotiate their relationships with doctors can have a significant impact on anyone who is sick and vulnerable and in need of medical and nursing attention. Whether nurses' ways of dealing with difficult doctors or medical biases and prejudices are effective is a public issue, not a private, internal matter for nursing or medicine.

The Moral versus the Political

One way that nurses negotiate battles with doctors is by reinterpreting problems and disputes between doctors and nurses as moral rather than clinical or political problems. An article by Adele Pike entitled "Moral Outrage and Moral Discourse in Nurse-Physician Collaboration" is an excellent example.[30] Pike, then a clinical nurse specialist at the former Beth Israel Hospital in Boston, describes a paradigm case. A frail seventy-two-year-old man is admitted to the hospital with a cascade of symptoms and problems—failure to thrive, possible pneumonia, severe urinary tract infection, irregular heartbeat, and unstable blood pressure. He has a fever whose cause can't be identified and is unresponsive to treatment. Over the course of his admission the old gentleman is poked and prodded. In spite of his continued decline and his family's concerns about the painful nature of the remedies prescribed, doctors seem intent on using increasingly invasive measures. The nurses disagree. They want to begin palliative measures. They are overruled and, when those measures are initiated, the nurses feel it is far too late. The patient dies and the nurses are left with what Pike calls "moral outrage."

"Moral outrage," she writes, "is disturbingly common among nurses working in acute care settings. An emotional response to the inability to carry out *moral choices* or decisions, *moral outrage* is characterized by energy-draining frustration, anger, disgust, and a sense of powerlessness." Pike then describes conflicts about what she terms "constraints of moral action" that take place on acute care wards of hospitals.[31] Then she uses another example to explore how nurses can use moral argument and reasoning to create collaboration and eliminate "moral outrage."

More than ten years after this article appeared, nurses continue to frame disputes with doctors in moral terms. When I broached the subject to a group of nurses at a Boston-area hospital, a professor of ethics from a

138 local nursing school insisted that doctor-nurse relationships did not make it on her priority list of ethical problems nurses faced.

This recasting of clinical concerns and disagreements in moral or philosophical terms is both cunning and potentially worrisome. Instead of denying the problems they encounter with doctors, reframing the issue in moral terms allows Pike and her colleagues to consider and write about these problems. In nursing practice, this moral reframing also seems to have allowed some nurses to use the language of morality to negotiate with physicians. But these positive results may also have unintended negative consequences. Pike, for example, never uses the terms "medical" or "clinical" when she discusses the disagreements nurses have with physicians. Instead she interprets power inequalities and clinical disagreements in entirely moral terms. Yet, the dilemmas these RNs identified centered on clinical judgments, knowledge, and action. Studies confirm that unmanaged pain retards healing and can lead to death and that patients who are in too much pain develop serious and costly complications. Studies also document the costs and suffering involved in delivering futile treatments that only prolong the patient's dying. Of course, these conflicts have moral and ethical—not to mention legal—ramifications, but they are fundamentally about the wisdom and efficacy of a particular course of medical treatment. Were these disagreements originally articulated in clinical rather than moral terms? If not, why not?

In considering the moral aspects of these problems, nurses follow the contemporary practice of focusing on the ethical dimensions of clinical practice and decision making. But recasting their conflicts with doctors in moral terms does much more. It addresses their long-standing lack of status as much as it calls attention to critical issues of patient care. Redefining clinical/medical disagreements as moral or ethical issues gives nurses the "moral" high ground and removes the disputes from the medical terrain on which nurses have been historically so disadvantaged. If the dispute is medical, then the nurse may believe she is on shaky ground. She may not have been socialized or schooled to refute the physician's claim that MDs have more experience, more insight, and more knowledge about clinical conditions and concerns than do RNs. Recasting clinical issues as moral ones levels the playing field for the nurse. In fact, according to some nursing theorists, on the moral terrain nurses have a distinct advantage. Theorists who increasingly frame nursing expertise as morally "good and just" contend that nurses "know themselves" better than physicians and are closer to the patient than doctors are.

To turn clinical disputes or inequalities in power into ethical issues offers another advantage. It allows nurses to bypass nurse managers or hospital administrators who, they often complain, don't support them, or

physicians who may oppose them, and seek help from ethical experts. A **139**
more empathic doctor who specializes in ethical issues, a nurse ethicist, or
an outside ethics consultant can be called in to adjudicate the dispute and
may be more prone to side with the nurse than the doctor.

Translating clinical disagreements into moral debates, however, risks
concealing nurses' clinical and medical knowledge and judgment. It rati-
fies the doctor's—and public's—view of the nurse as a woman of virtue
and high moral standing who won't tread on medical turf. As nurses teach
this moral formulation of conflict resolution to students, one must also
ask whether the new nurse who is tutored in the art of moral argument
will be skilled in the kind of clinical argument and communications
strategies necessary to create effective collaboration. Finally, focusing on
morals and ethics may actually sweep problematic nurse-physician relationships off the table and out of public sight.

Another way nurses try to circumvent or reconstruct their disputes
with doctors is by claiming a higher or more holistic status in the realm of
caring. Over the past few decades, what academics would call a caring discourse has permeated nursing. Nursing scholars and researchers like Patricia Benner have focused on how nurses "know" the patient. The nursing literature is filled with discussions of nursing as "the art of self," of
nurses who need to "know themselves," and of "the therapeutic use of
self." These concepts are used to capture the way nurses use their life experience, their behavior, and their emotional self-presentation to build
trusting relationships with patients. While some of these discussions contain sound critical analysis, such as that offered by the feminist sociologist
Arlie Hochschild in her book *The Managed Heart*, the caring discourse in
nursing may cleverly disguise nursing's perennial struggle with medicine.[32]

"If you read the caring discourse in nursing closely," Sioban Nelson argues, "you'll find that many theorists of caring actually put down the
technical and medical. It makes medical and scientific knowledge far less
important and actually devalues empirical and medical knowledge." She
continues, "The focus on holism and on the ethical and moral nature of
care considers it more important data than medical knowledge. The holistic nurse is totally in tune with the patient. On the other hand, as nurse
theorist Sally Gaddow writes, doctors 'only have statistics, laboratory reports, and the latest survey of commonsense.' In this formulation, the eth-
ically superior nurse can actually know what is required in a situation even
if it is contradicted by that data. Medical knowledge is instrumental and is
not the most important thing, most important is being in tune with the
situation and having intuition."

Nelson also points out an often-unnoticed irony in some of the caring

140 discourse. "It's all about the nurse not the patient. Under the guise of being humanistic and all about the patient, one of the ironies is that this kind of discussion is really about the nurse's interiority, how the nurse relates to the work." In spite of this, Nelson believes that "nurses are reluctant to let go of that moral reframing, because they contend it gives them superior clinical insight and allows them to try to overrule doctors in the rhetorical arena if not in the clinical one."

Although I have written a great deal about caring in nursing work, I too am often uncomfortable with the way discussions of caring skirt perilously close to traditional gender stereotypes. Rather than depicting caring as a skill—what Benner calls the "skill of involvement"—it almost seems as if some nurses trivialize their caregiving skills by adopting the very sexist self-definitions that have been consistently used to denigrate and sentimentalize their work. When I first went into the hospital to observe nurses, for example, I noticed how nurses would routinely repeat the phrase "Nurses care and doctors cure." Or they would recite a standard mantra, "Nurses are the patient's advocate." Or, equally popular, "Doctors take care of diseases and nurses take care of the people who have them." Some academics and nurses' organizations translated these thoughts into more official-sounding statements used in the definition of nursing diagnosis, which puts nurses in charge of the "human response to illness," while doctors are in charge of—what? The inhuman response?

One nurse related a fascinating story about her work with a patient who was supposedly dying of congestive heart failure. The nurse realized that the patient was on the wrong medication and was getting bad medical treatment from her physician. She told the woman to get a second opinion and that she needed a more effective medication. The patient, like many elderly people, had no idea she could challenge or change her physician, but she followed the nurse's advice. When the nurse saw the patient again, the "dying" woman had been resurrected. She'd seen a new doctor, was on new medication, had dropped pounds of water, and was doing well. When I commented that the nurse had a great deal of "medical knowledge," she and other participants in the room recoiled, almost in horror. I felt like I'd waved a string of garlic or a cross in front of a vampire. A number of professors insisted that this nurse was mobilizing not "medical" but nursing knowledge.

This same process of claiming and disclaiming is evident in the complex issue of nursing diagnosis and nursing notes. Although nursing diagnosis developed in the 1950s, it became much more popular in the 1970s when nursing was trying to find a home of its own in academia and to prove its professional bona fides. Since sociologists like Eliot Freidson and Amitai Etzioni and others insisted that a true profession must have its own "knowledge base" and language, one of the things nursing diagnosis did was give nursing its separate knowledge and language. This move was always controversial because it not only gave name and visibility to the unspoken and invisible nonmedical work of the nurse, but it also repackaged the medical work of the nurse in a new nursing vocabulary.

Because disease is the linguistic currency of modern medicine, nursing diagnosis has focused on "client-centered problems." This "placed more emphasis on the nurses' independent practice compared with the dependent practice driven by physicians' orders." If the off-limits act of physician diagnosis focuses on disease, then nursing diagnosis "is a clinical judgment about individual, family, or community responses to actual and potential health problems and life processes."[33]

"Nursing diagnosis will take a 'medical problem' like stress incontinence and turn it into 'an alteration in elimination due to stress incontinence,' instead of just telling you the patient has stress incontinence," says Jean Chaisson, a critic of what she considers to be a misuse of nursing diagnosis. "Or they'll say alteration in tissue perfusion due to pulmonary embolus." But this is a pulmonary embolus. "Why don't they just come out and say it?"

"This is a response to the fact that physicians said nurses can't diagnose, so nurses, particularly nurse academics, said, 'Yes, we can. We have nursing diagnosis.' What we should have said and should be saying is that medical language is our language," Chaisson argues. "We, doctors and nurses, work together. Language is something we share. If you think there's a nurse in America on a coronary care unit who can't read an EKG and recognize cardiac ischemia, then I hope you're wrong, because the patient will be dead. So why do you need to call it 'alteration in tissue perfusion due to cardiac ischemia?' Why not just say 'cardiac ischemia' and claim that these words belong to nursing, not just to doctors or a group of special nurses like NPs and APNs who've been given a special dispensation to use them?"

Chaisson and others argue that nurses should use language that describes the educational, preventive, and similar activities not adequately described by disease-focused words. But here again, she feels that speaking in English (or whatever the local language may be) rather than code would help both doctors, payers, and the public understand what nurses do. "If we're trying to help people understand what we do to educate the patient, or to prevent problems, then let's just say it instead of inventing terms like 'knowledge deficit' that turn off other team members," Chaisson continues. "We want them to read our notes, because we need them to understand not only what we're doing but also what the patient is experiencing and living through. If doctors don't read nursing notes then

142 maybe we have to ask ourselves why. Of course, they need to be taught about the value of nursing notes, but we have to make our notes comprehensible. We have to ask ourselves who we are writing notes to—each other or the team?"

As I have observed nurses taking care of patients, I am struck by how little nursing's self-definitions, language, and catchphrases reflect the complexity of what nurses really do. The reality is that nurses are often as disease focused as doctors. Their specialties are in cancer, critical care, diabetes, and rehabilitation. If their work, to cite only one example, is in oncology, then their work is all about cancer—the disease *and* the patients who have it. When the problem at hand is curing the patient or at least achieving remission, their work is as much about cure as it is about care. Nurses are the ones who administer chemotherapy. They are the ones who monitor the side effects of treatment. They often tell doctors when and what to prescribe to manage side effects like nausea and vomiting, pain, and anorexia. They have tremendous knowledge about disease as well as about the treatments, procedures, medications, and experimental protocols.

Of course, nurses talk about palliative care and when to stop aggressive treatment. In the time they spend with patients, they elicit crucial information about how patients are living and how their disease and treatment affect them. But why, I wonder, are nurses so quick to allow doctors to claim total control over—and thus to efface their participation in—the highly valued process of cure, when they are in fact crucial to so many curative activities? Why are they so willing to relinquish their knowledge of medicine and their participation in diagnosis and treatment when they are often central to both? For most patients, instrumental activities—like giving a good shot, knowing how to manage equipment like IVs and other medical devices, and giving medication and treatment on time—actually constitutes caring.[34]

I have come to understand that nurses' dismissal of their contributions may represent an attempt to gain status and legitimacy within the narrow space in the medical world they have been assigned. Indeed, the focus on care seems to set up a kind of competition with physicians that nurses may believe they can win. They may think they can't win the knowledge and status competition, but perhaps they believe they can win what I've come to think of as the intimacy competition. If nurses win this competition, doctors may whine a bit—"If nurses are the patient's advocate, then who am I?" a surgeon once exclaimed in frustration, "the patient's enemy?"— but like physicians in the nineteenth century, doctors in the twenty-first seem to be perfectly happy allowing nursing to lay claim to sentiment and moral virtue.

While it's critical to focus on the skills of caring and the impact of dealing with the whole human being, radically shifting the terrain from the clinical to the moral, or discussing nursing uniquely in terms of "caring," paints nurses into another kind corner. It conceals nurses' mastery of medical and technical skills and dismisses the importance of that mastery to patients. It also deprives nurses of a way of demonstrating the true nature of their holistic approach. If a nurse's approach is truly holistic, she not only knows about relationships but also has medical and technical expertise. A nurse's holism ensures that, in the Swiss cheese of errors, the holes don't line up perfectly.

The sociologist Daniel Chambliss contends that traditional ethics, now mirrored in nursing ethics, obfuscates the kinds of problems nurses encounter in their daily working lives. Because most of what nurses confront are issues of power, particularly with doctors, Chambliss believes that standard ethical accounts often miss issues that are critical to nurses. Medical ethics focus on the dilemmas "in which the lone individual must decide the right thing to do. Philosophical medical ethics largely assumes this freedom of the practitioner to choose; the ethical problem lies in deciding what choice is morally right. But in nursing, the problems are frequently those over which nurses have no control; they are not dilemmas, in the sense of an individual's quandary at all, and the language of 'ethical dilemmas' hardly works for a profession whose work is so determined by the choices of other, more powerful actors."[35]

These issues, Chambliss explains, should not be addressed in ethics rounds, because nurses often consider these problems practical or political rather than ethical. They belong in the political and public relations arena, where nurses must illuminate how the power politics that plays out at the bedside compromises patient care and hampers nurse retention and recruitment. Will the nurse, taught to argue morally, be able to argue politically? Will she be skilled enough in the art of power and politics to renegotiate the political arrangements inherited from the nineteenth century?

When I observe nurses in the workplace—hearing how they talk, seeing how they dress, noticing how they adapt to or subtly resist physician authority—I am sometimes reminded of the religious nurses of earlier periods. The religious nurse both was hampered by and cannily used difference and deference. Deference allowed the religious nurse to avoid notice and thus avoid sanction and insure survival. The behavior produced by deference also made the nurse different and thus valuable.

Today, the same strategies still help nurses navigate power and authority in the modern hospital. The problem is that strategies for eluding or defying physician power may also keep the nurse subject to it. Modes of

144   dress and address may make nurses seem more accessible, but they also make them more forgettable—indistinguishable members of an anonymous, semicloistered mass. In countries where nurses have adopted the pajama-like outfits with hearts and flowers, my colleague Bernice Buresh points out, this new uniform makes nurses look immature and silly. "The old nursing uniform made younger nurses look older," Buresh comments. "The new uniform makes older nurses look younger."

It also sends out another signal to doctors: we're not a really a threat to your power and authority. Similarly, in allowing or enabling doctors to continue their bad behavior, nurses not only avoid the worst but, as Larry Harmon has explained, perpetuate it. The doctor who faces no complaints for his bad behavior, Harmon explained, will feel that his strategy to control mistakes, and those who might make them, works. Nurses who accept abusive and bullying physician behavior also fail to take advantage of the public sympathy and support that they may elicit if they made these private acts of "disruption" public. In today's world, abuse and abusers receive little sympathy. Since nurses can connect their own suffering to that of patients, they have a powerful argument to mobilize in the service of change. In their reluctance to mobilize collectively to challenge physician prerogative on a global scale, they may inadvertently conspire with the medical system to perpetuate the nineteenth-century image of the nurse as one who is primarily involved in making the hospital "a place of joy."

Because of the potent cocktail of difference and deference, nurses may fight the very visibility they say they seek and limit their full integration into the health care team. On this subject, a vice president of nursing at a major teaching hospital recently told me a disturbing story. The chief of medicine in the hospital approached him and explained that he'd been discussing how residents navigated their six- to eight-week rotations on the units. The residents complained that it is always difficult for them to get to know the nursing staff and that this makes their work more difficult. The chief resident suggested what he thought was a great idea. The hospital should take a photograph of every member of the nursing staff, with his or her name underneath, and post these pictures on the units. Residents could thus scan the photographs and easily identify the nurses with whom they'd be working. "I thought, what a great idea," the nurse executive said. (Photographs are routinely used to help nurses and other staff identify interns and residents. In most teaching hospitals pictures of the newly arrived crop of interns are posted on each unit.) "I went out and talked to my leadership team and they also thought it was a great idea."

Little did he anticipate the reaction he would get when he took it to the wards. "The minute it got down to the managers and the staff nurses it was . . . ," he paused and sighed, "it was absolutely no way. They were **145** adamant. No way."

Why do they want to see our names with our pictures? the nurses had asked. What are they really trying to find out? What if we do something wrong? They jumped immediately to the conclusion that the only product of visibility would be negative.

"It created all kinds of issues connected to vulnerability and worry," he continued. "To be honest with you, I didn't really work through it with them and talk about what's really going on here. I should have explained that the intent is really genuine and that I think it would really be helpful to increase communication. I was so shocked and disappointed. It really surprised me—the fact that they wanted so badly to remain anonymous."

Given nurses limited experience with positive credit and accountability and their socialization in negative credit and accountability, the nurses' reluctance is, sadly, all too predictable and has significant implications for the presentation of nurses and nursing, not only in the hospital and other health care settings, but in the public and media presentation of health care.

Think about it, when was the last time you saw a nurse—an ordinary bedside nurse—appear as a major player or expert source in a media discussion of health care? I don't mean in what you've read about nursing shortages, nursing strikes, or killer nurses. I mean in the daily coverage of health care innovation and medical work.

PART TWO

THE MEDIA AND NURSING

I recently had an interesting conversation with my friend Laura, an architect who has two daughters aged twenty and twenty-five. Laura's elder daughter is in business school and her younger is about to enter medical school. Lately, Laura and her family have had a lot of contact with nurses. Laura's father was hospitalized because he had blood clot in one of his legs. When he went home, a home care nurse came every day to make sure he didn't develop further complications. Two years ago, Laura had also had a knee replacement operation.

Despite all her contact with nurses, Laura candidly admitted that neither of her girls has ever considered nursing. She has a friend, though, one of whose daughters is going to nursing school while the other is in medical school.

"I wonder why she chose nursing," Laura mused. "Maybe it's because she just didn't want to spend so long in school."

When I pointed out that this interpretation of nursing cast the profession in pretty poor light, Laura said, "Of course, nurses are wonderful, kind, trustworthy people. I'm sure they have to study to prepare themselves for their career, but you have to admit that no matter how smart a nurse is, she certainly isn't as smart as a doctor and doesn't know nearly as much. Doctors have to memorize so much. And they have to have an an-

148 alytical intelligence in order to synthesize all that material, analyze it, and come up with a diagnosis and treatment."

Nurses, I countered, also have to know a lot. Nurses may not know what doctors know, but they know things doctors don't know. They know how to handle people's emotional responses and needs, how to deal with patients' families, and how to help people cope and recover. And, I added, nurses also diagnose and treat.

"Think about when you were in the hospital," I suggested to Laura. "You may not have been aware of it, but nurses acted to prevent postsurgical infections. If you'd suddenly started to complain about shortness of breath or leg and chest pain, nurses would have instantly diagnosed a probable pulmonary embolism and acted to save your life," I explained.

All this was news to Laura. "Well, yes," she said, "I don't doubt that nurses may even diagnose some problems. But, Suzanne, you have to admit that no matter how smart they are and what they do, nurses are still operating on a field that has already been prepared for them by the doctor."

This conversation illustrates what many people believe: nurses are people, mainly women, who don't have the patience, stamina, ambition, curiosity, or intelligence to make it through medical school, and who work in a field wholly owned and operated by doctors.

Given this mind-set, it's not surprising that neither of Laura's daughters had considered nursing as a career option. Middle-class and especially upper-middle-class parents in many countries around the world would probably be loath to see their children become nurses, if they conceptualize nursing as way below medicine on the occupational ladder.

Sometimes, young people have told me, it's a student who puts a parent in his or her place if they suggest a career in nursing. At Regis College, a small Catholic women's college outside of Boston, I found dismissive attitudes toward nursing. The students in a class on health policy (not part of the nursing school at Regis) had been asked to read my book *Life Support: Three Nurses on the Front Lines.* When I asked them what they thought of the nurses I described, all of them were surprised that the nurses knew so much about diseases, treatments, medications, surgical procedures, and human psychology.

Had any of them considered a career in nursing? I asked. One young woman confessed that her parents had suggested she study nursing. "I was shocked that they expected so little of me," was her response.

These comments reflect the common view that nursing is not service work but servants' work. In 2003, the Swiss Nurses' Association initiated a suit to force the Swiss government to pay nurses as much as police officers. In Swiss society, nursing had been considered less important, demanding, or difficult than policing.

Too many people believe that care will be provided to the sick and de- **149**
pendent no matter how little attention is paid to the systemic supports
that underpin that care. This is reflected in media coverage of nursing,
which focuses on nurses' problems or failings but gives little ink to their
many accomplishments.

In a mass media culture, the way in which novels, plays, TV, movies,
children's books, and journalism portray nurses is critical to our ability to
retain and recruit nurses. Because the medical system so often conceals
nurses' judgments, diagnoses, and treatments, media exposure is essential
if people are to view nursing as more than an extension of the physician's
knowledge and judgment. Similarly, since people often think that nurses'
work consists of simple activities and pleasant relational interactions, the
media is central to helping us understand that nursing work is far more
than niceness.

I was reminded of this fact when I spoke with Irene Wielawski, a journalist. Although our interview focused on her professional experiences,
she also provided an interesting lens into how family members view the
nurses who take care of a loved one. At the time of our conversation,
Wielawski's eighty-three-year-old mother had just been hospitalized and
had emergency surgery. After her surgery and a short stay in the ICU, her
mother was transferred to a hospital ward. What Wielawski noticed was
how skilled nurses were in assessing her mother's physical and mental
condition. "The nurses were trying to determine how well oriented she
was, whether she was confused after surgery," she related. "So they chatted with her in a very cheerful manner asking her some mundane things
and then some very pointed questions about where she was. It was a very
elegantly choreographed conversation that checked whether she could
track information and remember conversations and information given
about her condition only an hour before."

While Wielawski clearly appreciated the significance of what appeared
to be little more than chitchat, her mother did not. "Oh, the nurses were
so nice," her mother commented. To her, they were just kind people engaging in not very important social give-and-take, not highly trained clinicians who knew exactly what they were doing, what kind of information
they needed to elicit, how to interpret it, and what role this would play in
her recovery. Some patients and family members can see past the "niceness" of nursing to its significance. If they cannot, their understanding
will probably not be enhanced when they pick up a book, open a newspaper, or turn on the TV.

From an analysis of children's books, television, movies, plays, novels,
hospital newsletters, press releases, and the journalistic media, one sees
that RNs are either largely invisible or depicted in ways that trivialize,

150 sentimentalize, or sometimes even demonize them. This is not because novelists and writers, producers, hospital public relations staff, or journalists are villains. It's because the system in which they work reflects, reinforces, and reproduces traditional assumptions about nurses' and women's work. As we'll see, these depictions of nurses are also a result of nurses' own action and inaction.

6

Dropped from the Picture

In Paris several years ago I visited an old friend who was dying of lung cancer. As I sat in his bedroom, my friend—still alert and full of his usual pithy observations and opinions—recounted the saga of his recent experiences in a major public hospital in Paris. What impressed him the most about his hospital stay, he said, was the nursing care. They were on top of every possible permutation in his treatment. In fact, he said he rarely saw a doctor. He gave the same high marks to the nurses who made it possible for him to be at home with his wife.

After leaving his house I strolled past a children's bookstore. As I glanced in the window, the cover of a bright red and blue book showing a cartoonish nurse bandaging a child's finger caught my eye. *Je sais qui nous soigne* (I know who takes care of us), the title announced. I couldn't resist a closer look and went into the store.

The book, I discovered, was part of a special series devoted to educating children between the ages of nine and thirteen about citizenship.

And what an education it provides. The text begins with a typical case. Julien comes down with a high fever and begins vomiting. He is then taken to the doctor. To help Julien understand the realities of health care, the book defines sickness and introduces children to the key players in the health care system. Physicians, always identified by their last name and title ("Dr. Chevalier"), are center stage. The book describes the training and knowledge of doctors in a variety of different medical specialties. Nurses, who are given only first names ("Gaston," "Lucile"), are defined by who they are not, instead of who they are.

"Who is a nurse?" the text asks. "The nurse," it answers, "is not a doc-

152 tor." The nurse is someone "whose studies give her or him just enough knowledge to follow and apply the decisions taken by the doctor or surgeon." Contrast this with the description of a physical therapist: "someone who has made long study and has a great deal of knowledge about the human body."[1]

My friend just described institutions in which nurses were central, not ancillary, players. But in this educational rendition of the health care universe, the nurse is barely connected to the patient whom she cares for. In all respects, the nurse-patient relationship is firmly mediated by the physician. In contrast, say, with the physical therapist, who helps the patient in a relationship unmediated by the doctor.

Some patients, like my friend, understand the critical nature of the nurse's role. Others have only a partial understanding of what nurses really do, focusing solely on their "caring" and kindness but not on their knowledge and lifesaving actions.

In a variety of polls, nurses consistently get high marks for their ethical and honest behavior and trustworthiness. The widely held view that nurses are honest and ethical but that their field is not dynamic, challenging, or intellectually demanding is the result of a complex set of factors that include media presentations of nursing.

The kind of fictional depictions of nurses I'm going to analyze in children's books, television, movies, plays, and novels may be dismissed as just entertainment. But as Philip and Beatrice Kalisch observe, "Entertainment fare does more than merely entertain: it communicates information about the social structure and shapes attitudes about ourselves, others, and the world at large."[2] Studies of the impact of entertainment media reach the same conclusion. In 1997 the Kaiser Family Foundation documented the impact of just one episode of the television show *ER* that dealt with the issue of emergency contraception following a date rape. "The entire 'date rape' vignette is no more than a couple of minutes long, and the mention of using birth control pills for emergency (postcoital) contraception is less than a minute." Yet, a week later, "the number of *ER* viewers who knew that a woman has options for preventing pregnancy even after unprotected sex increased by 17 percentage points."[3]

In 2002, another study by the foundation reported that "research has documented the role that entertainment TV plays as a source of personal health information. But beyond providing specific information about topics about topics such as cancer, heart disease, or HIV, the 'cultivation thery' of media studies suggest that entertainment media are also likely to play a role in shaping viewer's broader conceptions of the health care system." The viewer of a fictional account of the health care system may be even more influenced by TV than someone who reads a nonfiction account in a newspaper or magazine or watches a TV news report or docu- **153** mentary. He or she may believe they're being "taken behind the scenes to see the hidden forces affecting whether there's a happy ending or a sad one. There are good guys and bad guys, heroes and villains and innocent bystanders."[4] When they are not depicted as villains, nurses tend to be portrayed as innocent bystanders, spectators instead of central participants in the health care drama.

Beginning at the Beginning—Children's Books

This is certainly true of the books that present the health care universe to children and their adult readers—a parent, relative, friend, or perhaps a teenage baby-sitter. Since reading *Je sais qui me soigne*, I have searched out other children's books that illustrate how publishers and children's book writers view the health care system and pass these views on to children. In books published in Italy, Spain, England, Australia, Canada, Germany, Switzerland, and Japan a favored character is a child who is either sick or visits a sick friend or relative in the hospital.

To continue with the French example, in two other books, *Max va à l'hôpital*[5] and *L'hôpital*,[6] doctors have all the knowledge and make all the decisions. They read X rays, diagnose, deliver anesthesia, and perform operations. The nurse pushes wheelchairs or carts or takes someone's blood pressure. Sometimes the nurse is there to comfort a child when the child's parents go home by giving the child a teddy bear. In Germany, Switzerland, and Spain, books paint the same picture; in fact, *Max va à l'hôpital* has German, Spanish, and Italian versions.

A counterpart in the United Kingdom, Australia, and New Zealand is *Paddington Goes to the Hospital*. Busy nurses are seen hustling and bustling around Paddington bear, who has a dislocated shoulder. But while doctors take actions for clear clinical reasons, nurses just hang around or hang the odd IV, without explaining why they do what they do, or sweetly offer food and water.[7]

The Little Workmates books, published in England, includes *Nurse Nancy*, about a black nurse who still sports a nurse's cap. We learn, "This is Nurse Nancy. She is always very neat and tidy, and she works very hard looking after the patients at Story Town Hospital." We never get the slightest hint of what this "looking after" entails.[8]

Of the twelve books I examined from the United States and Canada, none made it clear why patients need nurses. *Jeanine the Nurse Paper Doll* is all help—helping doctors in the OR or the hospital, helping mothers in the maternity ward, and helping (it doesn't say whom) if patients are helicoptered to a hospital in an emergency. The only exciting and dynamic

154 thing in Jeanine's career is the red jumpsuit and helmet she wears for those excursions.[9] *Going to the Hospital*, in the Mister Rogers' Neighborhood series, shows us doctors who alone decide when a child is ready to leave the hospital and who are the only ones curious about the results gleaned from tests and other data. Nurses appear in photographs, but as extensions rather than users of medical equipment.[10]

One of the most detailed books I looked at is called *Ask Nurse Pfaff, She'll Help You*. The book features pictures of an actual nurse, who is also a captain in the U.S. Army. We see Nurse Pfaff taking care of patients young and old, from six to what looks like eighty-six. We don't know what kind of nurse she is or where she works—an interesting omission, since not many nurses work with such a daily grab bag of patients. What we do learn, however, is that she is "special," "kind and gentle with people," "dependable," "always there when patients need her," and "helps doctors." Although the text does tell us she teaches people how to get well, the words smart, intelligent, skilled, expert, curious, creative, or exciting never appear in print.[11] Mercifully, Nurse Pfaff doesn't wear a cap.

What's even more interesting is how the stereotypes about nurses remain constant even when the gender and race of the characters change. Thus, we get a black American version of the same moral script in *A Trip to the Hospital*, which is part of the Nick Jr. series created by Bill Cosby. Little Bill breaks his arm playing, and Grandma takes him to see Dr. Clinkscales, a tall black man in a white coat, blue shirt, and dark tie. The nurse, who is also African-American, is dressed in pink scrubs. (No matter what the race, religion, or ethnic background, boys still wear blue and girls pink). Her only activity is to lead the patient and his grandmother down the hall. Handsome Dr. Clinkscales does everything else—taking X rays, explaining fractures, applying the cast and reassuring the child.[12]

Books in Print

Things don't change much as we move from children's books to adult fiction. Although the script has changed for women in many other occupations in modern industrial societies, it remains pretty much the same for nurses and doctors. Nurses tend to be handmaids or horror shows.[13] Next to Nurse Ratched in Ken Kesey's *One Flew over the Cuckoo's Nest*, perhaps the most famous novelistic nurse is Charles Dickens's Mrs. Sarah Gamp, in his novel *Martin Chuzzlewit*. "She was," Dickens writes, "a fat old woman . . . and it was difficult to enjoy her society without becoming conscious of a smell of spirits. Indeed, she was so fond of her spirits that she separated from her husband long ago on the ground of incompatibility of temper in their drink."[14]

Mrs. Gamp, ever greedy for a shilling, is more concerned about how **155**
she will be paid and fed than how her patients fare. In one unforgettable
scene, she shares the care of a delirious young gentleman with a day
nurse, Mrs. Prig. When she arrives to take over from Mrs. Prig, her patient lies in an agitated state. At the sight of the young man, "a horrible
remembrance of one branch of her calling took possession of the woman;
and stooping down, she pinned his wandering arms against his sides to see
how he would look if laid out as a dead man. . . . 'Ah!' said Mrs. Gamp,
walking away from the bed, 'he'd make a lovely corpse.' "[15]

The nurse quickly became a symbol of all that the nurse reformers of
the nineteenth century opposed, and Dickens's essay "The Nurse in
Leading Strings" became part of the movement for nursing reform in England.[16]

From much twentieth-century fiction, one would never know nursing
had been reformed. Kesey's *One Flew over the Cuckoo's Nest* gives us one of
the most powerful nurse villains of all time.[17] Written at the beginning of
the 1960s, it became an artifact of the burgeoning rebellion against 1950s
conformity. In 1959 Kesey had taken part in experiments with hallucino-
genic drugs and then worked night shifts on a mental ward in the Oregon
Veterans Administration Hospital. Like R. D. Laing and others who were
influenced by radical critics of the psychiatric establishment, Kesey believed that inmates of mental institutions weren't really insane. Their behavior represented a higher level of consciousness and individual fulfill-
ment than a lockstep society was prepared to tolerate. As Laing famously
argued, society preferred to label "mad" those people it considered bad.

The book is narrated by Chief Bromden, part Native American and a
longtime asylum inmate. He relates the confrontation between Randle
Patrick McMurphy—Kesey's ultimate bad boy—and Nurse Ratched or
Big Nurse. McMurphy lands in the mental institution, because he refuses
to behave. He brawls and drinks and gets himself into so much trouble
that he's sent to the state work farm. At the work farm, however, he refuses to work, gets into more fights, and is shipped off to the state asylum
for observation. That's when he meets up with Nurse Ratched

Nurse Ratched is evil female power wielded mercilessly over men. She
has the doctors in the mental institution cowed and has total control over
them and the various male mental cripples in her charge. When McMurphy tries relentlessly to subvert her discipline and order, a struggle to the
death is engaged and Nurse Ratched takes no prisoners. She ends up driving one of the inmates to suicide. When, as a result, McMurphy attacks
her, she sends him off to be lobotomized, exulting at the vegetable who
returns to her ward.

Kesey's novelistic creature is devastatingly cruel. She has not a single

156   redeeming quality. Indeed, her villainy completely overshadows McMurphy's virulent racism and sexism. It's an extraordinarily powerful portrait of feminine evil. The book and the movie version (which I'll discuss below) made Nurse Ratched a nursing culture icon that continues to traumatize an entire profession. She may have faded in popular memory, but she lives on in the memory of nurses who teach nursing students about her in nursing schools.

And she isn't alone. There are the nurses in Joseph Heller's *Catch-22*, John Irving's *The World according to Garp*, and Samuel Shem's 1978 novel *The House of God*, about interns in a teaching hospital.[18] Shem portrays nurses as sex nymphs for whom the profession is merely the best route to marriage with a rich physician. Here, the patients are "gomers" and nurses little more than sluts. A typical passage: "I unbuttoned her dress and unhooked her bra and caught her little-girl breasts by their longing nipples. All over me, her dress was off her pantyhose were off her bikinis were off and she was going off." And so forth.[19]

In the 1990s the image of nursing changed with the times, but not necessarily for the better. For example, the heroine of Anna Quindlen's *Black and Blue* is a nurse and a battered wife.[20] Best-selling author Diane Johnson's *Health and Happiness* takes place in a San Francisco hospital where Head Nurse Carmel Hodgkiss's job is "to keep track of love and sex at Alta Buena." "Nurses were strategic about doctors, speculating on their hobbies and their wives," Johnson writes.[21]

Nurses are often villains in many popular medical thrillers. In Robin Cook's *Coma*, a promising young female physician discovers the dastardly plot to put patients into a coma in order to harvest their organs and sell them to the highest bidder. The evil woman who tends the comatose patients and runs the organ auction is a nurse. Cook's physician was one of the first in a long line of female physician thriller heroines who, like the affirmative-action queens on TV and in the movies, solve every problem to arise—whether medical or criminal—on the health care stage. In *Fatal Cure*, Cook's prescient 1993 send-up of managed care, a physician husband-and-wife team unearth the collusion between hospital administrators and insurance company executives.[22] In 1993 real-life nurses were beginning to organize mass protests against cost cutting by managed care, but in Cook's fictional universe they are noticeably absent and unconcerned about either the fate of individual patients or the larger system.

Nonfiction has been no kinder to the nursing profession. Since the second wave of the feminist movement in the twentieth century, women writers have scoured history to unearth any female subject neglected by patriarchal culture. They have revisited the professional and personal lives of famous figures such as Eleanor Roosevelt, Simone de Beauvoir,

and Marie Curie. But outside nursing scholarship, there has been little in- **157**
terest in overlooked pioneering nurses like Lavinia Dock, Lillian Wald,
Adelaide Nutting, Isabel Hampton, or Virginia Herderson, who established educational programs, launched community health campaigns,
and advanced nursing practice.

Most remarkable is that until fall of 2004 there has been no significant
modern feminist biography written for a nonnursing audience of the most
fascinating figure of them all, Florence Nightingale. When women's studies professors compile their catalogue of feminist "greats," Nightingale—
who unarguably viewed the fight to make nursing a respectable profession
as a fight for women's economic and social rights—rarely makes it into
the feminist pantheon. Perhaps because contemporary nursing has been
so closely associated with traditional femininity, no feminist biographer
has taken on the historical challenge of examining how patriarchal
iconography tamed Nightingale, transforming a tough, acerbic and complicated woman into a Victorian angel of mercy.[23]

TV Nurses

Fiction and children's books tend to reinforce social stereotypes about
nursing, but television is far more influential in shaping how we view
health care. Ever since TV was invented, doctor shows have been a dramatic staple. Acute care medicine fulfills all the dramatic requirements of
the television producer or writer. Like cop shows, acute care medicine
places characters in extreme conditions where the good guys can usually
win. Most of the time, death is vanquished, and heroic actions advance
scientific progress.

In his survey of the relationship between television and medicine,
Joseph Turow, a professor of communications at the University of Pennsylvania, traces the evolution of the TV doctor and analyzes the relationship between TV and organized medicine. This relationship turned from
flirtation to enduring romance with the first prime-time hit about a doctor in the 1954 series *Medic.* When the Los Angeles County Medical Association became intimately involved in the show, Turow argues, *Medic*
inaugurated what was to be "a symbiotic relationship between doctor-
show producers and powerful medical organizations that was to shape the
boundaries of medical portrayals on prime time for decades."[24]

With doctors and medical organizations providing sets, plot lines, and
technical advice, medicine "had leverage over the entire range of *Medic*'s
portrayal of medicine." The combination of television's desire to appeal
to a mass audience by avoiding controversy and medicine's desire to appear heroic at all costs meant that TV doctors would be the white knights

158 who controlled the health care stage and TV would help to maintain "medicine's cultural authority."[25]

Organized medicine's determination to keep nurses as handmaids on real hospital wards extended into television land. Turow explains that the unwritten rule was that nurses could not be portrayed in an accurate light if doctors were to be central characters in the medical drama. Thus, shows like *Doctor Kildare, Ben Casey, The Eleventh Hour, Breaking Point*, and *Marcus Welby, MD* established an enduring model in which doctors would often do work that nurses really performed. Turow explains that "packing all the elements necessary for a good doctor show into an hour while worrying about the nurses' role would have been impossible, they [the producers] contended."[26]

Nurses rarely moved beyond the virtuous, cheerful, or colorful presence in any of these shows. In fact, if there were any guardian angels around, they were doctors. They lingered lovingly at the bedside twenty-four hours a day. They followed their patients—even out of the hospital—appearing on a patient's doorstep to coax them to follow treatment plans or to help them deal with emotional and family problems. As Turow points out, TV doctors like Dr. Welby and his sidekick Dr. Kiley seemed to run one- or two-man ICUs. They not only did all the curing but also most of the caring.

In television's fifty-plus years, only a few shows have had nurses as their main characters. The first was the 1954 *Janet Dean* with Ella Raines playing a private duty nurse. Between 1962 and 1965 Shirl Conway and Zina Bethune starred in *The Nurses*, playing a veteran nurse and a student nurse. Nurses were not to appear as prominent characters for another fifteen years. In 1980, Peggy Anderson's book *Nurse* was adapted for television. The show portrayed an RN who was in charge of more than doctors' charts and love lives, but it only lasted a year. Another show that was centered on nurses rather than doctors was the ill-fated *Nightingales*, an Aaron Spelling production, about student nurses. It aired its pilot episode in June 1988 and ran from January 1989 until April 1989, when it was canceled. Portraying nurses as sexpots who spent more time in exercise class or dating than cracking books or in school, it generated a rare national campaign of nurses who protested the show's bimboesque depiction of both nurses and nursing students. Irate nurses first tried to coax Spelling to change his portrayal of nurses. When that failed, an outpouring of letters and calls resulted in the cancellation of the show.

Two TV shows have had more complex portrayals of nurses, the wildly successful *M*A*S*H* (1972–83), in which Loretta Swit played Major Margaret Houlihan, and *China Beach*. While some of the nurses on the show are depicted as silly, Swit's character, the Kalisches argue, became more nuanced over the years and certainly more professionally competent.[27]

Perhaps the best TV portrayal of nurses was *China Beach*, ABC's prime- **159**
time series about a group of nurses working in a surgical hospital close to
the action in Vietnam. The show, which aired from April 1988 to July
1991, starred Dana Delaney as Lieutenant Colleen McMurphy. Delaney
received two Emmys for *China Beach* and was much lauded by nursing
groups for her portrayal of a tough-minded, competent, skilled, and intelligent Army nurse.

Since 1991, however, nurses have not fared particularly well on TV.
Major series like *Chicago Hope, ER, Providence, City of Angels,* and *Strong
Medicine,* as well as duds like *Presidio Med* and *MDs,* all feature physicians.
Nurses have gone back to their roles as ancillary characters who add color
and authenticity to the scene but whose work remains largely invisible.
One of the most pathetic nurse characters on TV was the chief OR nurse
on the now defunct *Chicago Hope* (or "Chicago Hopeless," as I liked to
think of it). When the series began in 1994, its main characters were a cardiothoracic surgeon, a neurosurgeon, and the latter's soon-to-be-divorced
wife, who was also a chief OR nurse. While the doctors are involved in
the life-and-death struggle with disease, the nurse spends much of her
time fretting over her failing marriage.

There is, however, no better illustration of the paradoxical role nurses
play on television than *ER,* one of the most popular medical shows of all.
ER's first episodes premiered in 1994, and it is still going strong, particularly when it comes to stereotypical definitions of nurses. While *ER* does
occasionally give nurses more than a handmaid's role, it follows the same
tried and true formula. The doctors, both female and male, are in their
white lab coats or blue surgical scrubs. To distinguish the nurses, producers make sure to dress them—even the male nurses—in pastels. When
they refer to one another in conversation or approach each other in front
of patients, doctors (of course) say, "Dr. Green," "Dr. Ross," and so forth
while calling nurses by their first names. Doctors' lives are certainly not
picture-perfect Marcus Welby–like affairs. Many of them have personal
difficulties, serious character flaws, and leave behind them a string of
failed relationships, and sometimes even make mistakes that are fatal to
patients. Nonetheless, if patients survive on TV shows like *ER,* they generally do so because of a doctor, not because of a doctor and a nurse.

On almost any episode of *ER,* nurses—with the exception of whoever is
playing the head nurse at the time—are part of an ill-distinguished mass
of busy hands. Doctors, on the other hand, are both busy heads and busy
hearts. While they are using their brains to figure out the appropriate diagnosis and treatment, they also exhibit the most compassion and caring.

Today's TV docs have usurped even the narrow roles—of caring patient advocates and educators—that nurses have tried to claim as their
own. On one memorable *ER* episode, for example, a dying patient comes

160 on to the unit accompanied by a hospice nurse. The hospice nurse stands by helplessly, unable to figure out how to manage the patient's pain or cope with the patient's anguish. The patient begs for an end to the misery, but the nurse does nothing. Finally, Dr. Green comes to the rescue.

In another episode, Dr. Peter Benton is guilt ridden because he was unable to be with his mother during her final moments. In the next episode, he sits at the bedside of a patient who is dying of AIDS. In the hush of a now quiet emergency unit, Benton holds the patient's hand as he tries to ease his own and the dying man's suffering. In the same episode, after a child with cancer tells doctor-in-training John Carter he's bored to tears, Carter brings him video games and counsels him to be nicer to his sister.

Seven years later, we find Carter again taking the time to attend to children's every need, this time in the Congo, where he has joined a group similar to Médecins sans Frontières in which nurses still do a lot of the work, but the group is called Alliance des Médecins (Alliance of Doctors).

I do not want to suggest that doctors should *not* appear in a human, or humane, light on TV. The problem is that TV writers and producers are so fixated on physicians that they allow little space for nurses' work, caring or otherwise. When they are present, nurses furnish doctors with the instruments of cure and then obligingly get out of the way so that doctors can educate patients or engage in the emotional work of helping patients cope with their illnesses. These efforts are not, as they are in reality, shared by a team.

Doctors on *ER* and other TV shows are also at the center of most discussions of controversial health policy issues. In their 2002 Kaiser Family Foundation study, Joseph Turow and Rachel Gans analyzed the medical shows *ER*, *City of Angels*, *Giddeon's Crossing*, and *Strong Medicine* to see if these shows dealt with health policy issues and to determine who were the major actors in TV's fictionalized debate about health policy.[28]

The authors reported that health policy issues were, in fact, a staple of these shows. Doctors, the study goes on to say, "far outnumbered all other participants (in discussions of health policy issues). Physicians made up 64% of all characters. . . . Nurses comprised 4%." "The numerical dominance of physicians in health policy interactions meant that a large percentage of the arguments took place among doctors," the researchers concluded. Their further comments highlight the significance of these findings. "When creators of hospital TV programs choose which characters will argue about health policy, their decisions may be quietly asking and answering a question for viewers. The question: Who should legitimately be engaged in debates about non-clinical health policy within a hospital environment? The answer that we found: mostly doctors."[29]

Occasionally nurses get attention on *ER* when the show's writers and producers take on the problems that nurses experience in the workplace, such as the floating of nurses to unfamiliar units as a cost-cutting measure, the failure to provide enough nursing staff, or the refusal to pay nurses what they're worth. We do see nurses complaining about the job or nurses walking off the job. But while these are critical issues that must be raised, they are not balanced by an accurate portrayal of what nurses actually do in ERs. A realistic portrayal would help us understand why the cost-cutting measures highlighted by the show are so dangerous to patients.

In fact, in emergency rooms, the first person a patient sees is usually a nurse. Whether patients come walking through the door or are carried in via ambulance, a triage nurse or nurses will ascertain the level of seriousness of their problem and then make sure they are taken care of with the necessary speed by the necessary clinicians. "The triage nurse is using his or her knowledge and experience to decide how quickly the patient needs to be seen, where, and by whom," says Mary Ellen Wilson, president of the Emergency Nurses Association. "The nurse may order X rays or start blood work. Nurses will take vital signs and a history, assess the patient, and look at any records the patient has to find out what's going on. They'll be able to distinguish between indigestion and a heart attack. The nurse will say, 'This guy's having an MI (heart attack,) we've got to get him right back to the cardiac room,' or 'He's got a fractured left ankle, he'll go to the orthopedic room.'"

Although the law says nurses don't diagnose, in the ER as elsewhere, of course they do. When they think a patient is having a heart attack, not bad gas, they are making a presumptive diagnosis. The physician will, of course, determine what the final diagnosis is, but the nurse's assessment has been the first step in that diagnostic process.

TV's *ER* is also part of a teaching hospital. On the TV show, with rare exceptions, only doctors teach doctors-in-training. In a real teaching hospital, ER nurses also teach doctors. When Bernice Buresh and I went to visit Boston City Hospital's ER, it was clear how much power nurses had. At one point, a mother frantically arrived with a three-year-old boy who had swallowed half a bottle of Tylenol. The nurse in charge of the case had to deal with the anxious mother, sick child, and an equally terrified intern, whom she was teaching a procedure called lavage—pumping charcoal into the stomach to wash out dangerous chemicals. When, in spite of her lessons, the intern proved too inept to do the job himself, the nurse took over.

The Silver Screen—Sexpots and Sadists

For nurses, things aren't much better at the multiplex. After the 1930s and 1940s, when nurses played brave heroines, good, skilled nurses seem to be

162 few and far between. Good nurses appear in films like *Girl Interrupted* and *The English Patient*, but negative portrayals far outweigh the positive.

In two of the most popular movies of the 1970s, *M*A*S*H* and the film version of *One Flew over the Cuckoo's Nest*, nurses are either the dramatic or comedic fulcrum of the action. Robert Altman's 1970 hit movie about the life of a Mobile Army Surgical Hospital (MASH) unit appeared at the height of the protests against the Vietnam War. The film's antiwar commentary overshadowed its blatant sexism. The doctors portrayed in the movie numb themselves against the insanity of war with heavy doses of cynicism, alcoholism, sex, and black humor. No matter how many martinis the doctors down, how many nurses they bed, and how little attention they pay to army discipline, they are so competent that they operate without the slightest tremor or making the tiniest mistake. The nurses on the other hand, demonstrate no skill at all and are only sex objects.

Whenever a nurse is mentioned, it's because a doctor is commenting on the intricacies of her anatomy, not a patient's. "It's a good thing you have a good body, nurse, otherwise I'd get rid of you quick," one of the surgeons says during an operation. The chief target of the physicians' spleen is Major Margaret Houlihan, played by Sally Kellerman. A stunning blond, the major arrives as the base's chief nurse and is shocked by the blatant subversion of army discipline. She gets the nickname "Hot Lips" when she's caught having an affair with one of the doctors.

Because no recent movies or TV shows remind us of the lifesaving function that nursing routine actually brought to the hospital, we risk interpreting any nursing effort to instill order and discipline as the officious ravings of a straight-laced obsessive-compulsive. Similarly, this send-up of military nurses obscures the fact that, as Sioban Nelson has argued, military nurses were the ones who paved the way for a future generation of women to enter the military in combat roles.

Nurses are also porn film favorites. Go to the web and search for "nurses" and "images" and you'll get an astonishing array of Naughty Nurses, Naked Naughty Nurses (with salacious invitations to look under the uniform), Naughty Night Nurses, and a huge assortment of fantasy galleries. In the fall of 2004, in the middle of a severe nursing shortage, a British Columbia radio station, Z95.3, ran a series of TV ads featuring nurses wearing short skirts and skimpy tops, dancing Britney Spears–like to pop music. In the ad, an elderly patient banged his cane and demanded to know when he would get his sponge bath. Nurses in the British Columbia Nurses Union protested, and the station, as if stunned that the ads could create such a furor, sent an apology to the RNs and said it would withdraw them.[30]

To show just how enduring this Madonna and whore stereotyping is, ABC TV has just announced that it will be producing an American re-

make of the controversial British TV show about naughty nurses *No An-* **163**
gels. Although the British Royal College of Nursing has condemned the
show, which follows nurses who sleep with doctors in hospital linen clos-
ets and take drugs, that hasn't stopped American producers from launch-
ing this new effort.[31]

Since female doctors do not invite the same male fantasies, Philip Dar-
byshire and I have proposed one possible explanation for the enduring
popularity of the nurse as a figure of sexual fantasy. For men who feel
powerless because they are sick and vulnerable, sexual fantasy may relieve
a sense of anxiety. In mentally reimagining the nurse as an object of pene-
tration, the man reasserts his emotional dominion. He is no longer at her
mercy; she is at his.

Perhaps the most enduring portrait of the power of the nurse over her
male charges was in the 1975 movie *One Flew over the Cuckoo's Nest*. As
played by Louise Fletcher, Nurse Ratched seems to be the same perverted
caregiver she was in the book. Above her forehead, her pageboy haircut is
swept up in two teased coils that perch below her pristine white nurse's
cap. Starched to her core, she wears a white uniform that has never seen a
crease, white hose, and white, matronly shoes. We're meant to sympathize with McMurphy, the quintessential man's man, who detests all hierarchical authority. Looking at the movie with thirty years' distance, however, it's interesting to note McMurphy's rampant sexism. To him women
are "beavers," "cunts," and pussies.

Although Nurse Ratched remains a fixture of the culture, she's bested
in the evil department by Kathy Bates in her performance as Annie
Wilkes in the movie version of Stephen King's *Misery*.[32] Here we have not
only an evil nurse but also a genuinely psychopathic one.

Kind but Dumb

When nurses aren't busy killing patients or taking their clothes off, they
are often depicted as kind but dumb. In the 1999 movie *Nurse Betty*, Renee
Zellweger stars as the frustrated would-be nurse Betty Sizemore, a wait-
ress in a restaurant in a small town in Kansas, who is obsessed with a TV
soap opera and its handsome lead Dr. David Ravell. We learn that she
wanted to take nursing classes but her husband Del Sizemore, a used car
salesman who moonlights as a drug dealer, put an end to that. When one
of Del's deals goes wrong, two drug dealers come to their house and scalp
Del and then shoot him. Betty witnesses the murder and dissociates from
reality: she believes that she is actually a nurse in the soap opera she was
watching while Del died.

Betty runs off to Los Angeles to find her cinematic hero with the drug

164 dealers in hot pursuit. She purchases a nurse's uniform—yes, complete with the white cap—and finds a hospital complex that looks like the one shown on TV. In she goes to the office of the chief nurse to try to find her heartthrob and get a job. Rejected—thankfully—because she has no references, she exits the hospital via the emergency room exit. A car plows into an ambulance, a gunman starts shooting up the ER entrance, and a hysterical Hispanic woman begs the doctors to attend to the ambulance patient. Others are too afraid to help. But not Nurse Betty. Heedless of danger, she goes into the ambulance, and performs a critical procedure. How did she know how to perform this lifesaving feat? She saw it on TV.

Betty is instantly hired to be a pharmaceutical assistant until, the chief nurse tells her, her nursing credentials arrive at the hospital. She ends up finding her soap opera doctor, or at least the actor who plays him, comes out of her dissociative state, and her husband's killers are themselves killed. As the movie ends, she's playing a nurse on the same soap and plans to use her earnings to pay for nursing school.

The take-home message? Only losers want to be nurses, and any loser can function as a nurse if she watches enough daytime TV.

This is pretty much the same message given in the 2000 movie *Meet the Parents*, only this time it's directed at men. Ben Stiller plays emergency room nurse Greg Focker. Greg falls in love with Pam and goes to meet the parents. During their first, awkward get-acquainted meeting, Greg explains that he's just been transferred to triage. "Oh, is that better than a nurse?" Pam's mother asks hopefully.

In another scene, Greg is introduced to Pam's sister's fiancé, "Dr. Bob," and his father the plastic surgeon "Dr. Larry." Pam's father tells the two doctors that Greg is also in medicine. "Oh, which field?" Dr. Larry asks. "Nursing," says Greg. They all laugh uproariously.

"No, really, what field?" they repeat the question. To which Greg again responds, "Nursing."

There is a long, uncomfortable pause. Then Dr. Larry says, "so you didn't want to go for the M.D.?"

Greg explains that he thought about medicine and decided against it. "Just as well," Dr. Larry says, "the boards are a killer."

Worried lest the doctors think Greg is just a dumb nurse, Pam tries to prove that he's a smart one. In fact, tells them, Greg took the medical boards and aced them. Later in the movie, Pam's hostile father gets his CIA chums to look into Greg's background. Part of the background check reveals that Greg did indeed ace the medical boards. While Pam is infuriated that her father has invaded Greg's privacy, she nonetheless, proudly exhibits his MCAT scores.

It seems that the only way a nurse can prove that he—or she—is intelligent is to demonstrate he has what it takes to get into medical school.

In the 2003 film *Something's Gotta Give*, nurses are also used for comic relief. Jack Nicholson plays a multimillionaire businessman who is dating a young woman half his age. The couple find themselves staying with Mom, a millionaire playwright played by Diane Keaton, at the mother's elegant beach house in the Hamptons. Under the influence of Viagra, the Nicholson character has a heart attack. It's off to the hospital where he quickly exits without being pestered by any of those pesky nurses. It's the doctor, played by Keanu Reeves as a sensitive New Age guy, who treats the heart attack, monitors the patient, and educates Nicholson about how to deal with everything from his medication to questions about sexual function. We never see a nurse caring for a patient. When Nicholson is twice rushed to a New York hospital for panic attacks, nurses are only glimpsed pushing his gurney down the hall. It's a female doctor who advises him to relax.

A potentially useful nurse does appear early in the film, after Nicholson has his heart attack and has returned to Keaton's beach house. And what a nurse she is. As Keaton comes home after running an errand, she crosses paths with an ugly, obese middle-aged woman bursting out of her white uniform. The only unattractive woman in a movie populated by slim, long-legged beauties, she was hired as Nicholson's home care nurse. But Nicholson will have no more big nurses, so he fires her. Which means that Keaton will just have to play home care nurse, thus providing her with the opportunity to learn to love Jack.

The nurse's weight and looks could not send a more powerful message. Try as it might to portray itself as a movie about true love vanquishing the seductions of youth, this movie is all about surfaces. Diane Keaton, for all her charm and vulnerability, is only an aging version of one of the younger women who parade through the film. In terrific shape, wearing terrific clothes, living in a terrific house with a terrific career and a terrific daughter (who also has a terrific career), she is the icon of the dressed-for-success female who has it all, except for the right guy. Our brief glimpse of a nurse, on the other hand, is of somebody no one in this universe would want to be.

The PC Woman on TV and in the Movies

Something's Gotta Give illustrates one of the most profound and important contemporary shifts in the TV and cinematic depiction of the world of health care and the hospital: the industry's embrace of political correctness, particularly when it comes to women and minorities.

166   Since the advent of the women's movement in the 1970s, women have made significant inroads in American society. More women have fought for and won the freedom to move into traditionally male occupations and have become doctors, lawyers, bankers, stockbrokers, politicians, and journalists. Women in the professions may still be struggling with traditional patriarchal structures, but they are struggling on the lowest rungs of what are considered to be the highest occupational ladders. The problem is that the public in most industrial societies has not changed its view of women who remain in traditionally "female," caregiving professions, nor has it altered its view of the complexity of the work they do. Similarly, men have not entered these professions in numbers comparable to those of women in fields like medicine, the law, journalism, and business.

In my book *Prisoners of Men's Dreams*, I analyzed something I called dress-for-success feminism.[33] The dress-for-success feminist, I wrote, was the woman who moved into traditionally male fields of endeavor and advanced because she became as individualistic, competitive, autonomous, and materialistic as any man. Socialized in a "masculine world," these women often joined men in looking down on women who remained in traditionally female fields like nursing, teaching, and social work. While women climbing the ladder may have hit a glass ceiling, women still doing women's work were crashing against a shatterproof roof of class and gender prejudice in jobs that were poorly paid, and in which they were poorly treated. Moreover, they now had to deal with the scorn of those liberated women who looked down on the work they performed. Since women now have greater professional freedom, I argued, women's work will now be viewed as a second-class choice. In the nineteenth century, the woman to worry about was the woman who was not content to be a nurse and wanted to be a doctor. In the late twentieth and twenty-first, the one we wonder about, as I said earlier, is the woman who wants to remain a nurse and who has no desire to become a doctor.

One could write an entire book on the complex relationship between nursing and feminism. Just as many feminists have disdained nurses, many nurses have disdained feminism. New definitions of women's liberation have done little to advance the recruitment and retention of nurses in workplaces.[34]

While it is, of course, important to show the world that women have what it takes to work in jobs that were traditionally reserved for white men, TV has moved to a PC attitude that does not reflect the reality of health care work. On TV and in the movies the new, modern, successful, ambitious woman cannot be a nurse. She must be a physician, a medical student, or someone who at least aspires to be a physician. And so we have a string of female and minority doctors and med students on a variety of

TV shows and in movies: Dr. Kate Austin on *Chicago Hope*, Dr. Sydney **167** Hansen on *Providence*, the many female doctors on *Presidio Med*, Dr. Dana Delaney of *China Beach* (just promoted from nurse to doctor), and two female doctor leads on *Strong Medicine*. In the last we see a nice bit of gender bending: the most prominent nurse on the team is a guy, a nurse midwife.

Guided by their new PC formula, TV writers have no qualms even about dressing nineteenth-century women for twentieth-century success. In *Dr. Quinn Medicine Woman*, Jane Seymour played an intrepid frontier doctor, Michaela Quinn, who in the 1860s moved from Boston to a Colorado frontier town, where (from February 1993 to May 1998) she delivered the town's only health services. In fact, the idea of women providing health care services on the frontier is not at all far-fetched. But the person delivering those services would probably not have been a female doctor. Health care on the frontier in the 1860s and 1870s would likely have been delivered by a stocky woman clad in a flowing black habit, toting a six-gun and a medical satchel, not by a lithe, elegantly outfitted patrician doctor.[35]

Once again, when it comes to Hollywood PC, *ER* is the winner. *ER*'s first season began with one smart, ambitious female doctor, Sherry Lewis, who left the show after several seasons. Over the course of the last decade, *ER* has added even more smart, ambitious females—as doctors, of course. We've met the handicapped Dr. Kerry Weaver, chief of emergency medicine, and Dr. Hicks, an African-American chief of surgery. Then in rapid succession: Dr. Elizabeth Corday, an associate chief of surgery, and Dr. Jing-Mei Chen, a Chinese-American medical resident, among others. Interestingly, the only strong nursing character is the nurse manager, who unlike most nurse managers is never too busy with budgets or staffing problems to pitch in and care for patients.

What is more interesting is that even the most assertive nursing characters are turned into doctor wanna-bes. In *ER*'s third season, for example, Chief Nurse Carol Hathaway has an inferiority complex, begins taking pre-med courses, and finally sits for the medical school admissions test. Like Greg in *Meet the Parents*, she passes with flying colors. Only then does she realize that she loves nursing and doesn't want to be doctor. Seven years later, *ER*'s producers and writers revisited this contemporary moral script with a new head nurse character, Abby Lockhart. After an over-the-top doctor fires nurses who've taken job action to protest working conditions, Lockhart becomes so frustrated with nursing that she quits to go to medical school. This series of episodes produced a firestorm of complaints from nurses. Led by Sandy Summers of the Center for Nursing Advocacy, nurses protested the show's depiction of nurses and accused *ER* of aggravating the nursing shortage.

Living Out Loud is one of the only recent movies with a nurse as its main character. It stars Holly Hunter as a home care nurse whose doctor-husband has divorced her and married another physician, an Asian-American pediatrician. The abandoned nurse is lonely, so she hires a male prostitute and befriends the elevator man in her building. Finally, she gets her act together. How do we know this? She decides to go to medical school and become a pediatrician.

Is There a Nurse in the House?

In searching for a realistic or positive portrayal of a nurse in the entertainment or literary media, a few notable exceptions to the predominant stereotype turn up.

In the 1998 Pulitzer prize-winning play *Wit*, playwright Margaret Edson dramatized the last days of a terminally ill English professor, Vivian Bearing. The play follows Bearing from diagnosis to her stay on a hospital ward where she receives an experimental treatment for ovarian cancer. From beginning to end, the doctors who treat Bearing are oblivious to their patient's state of shock and feelings of terror. Bearing's nurse, Susie Monahan, is the only character who gets it, emotionally and medically. Monahan recognizes that the side effects of the high-dose chemotherapy may be too toxic for her patient. She intervenes when she realizes that the patient's doctors haven't addressed vital issues like pain control and helps the patient determine when to end futile aggressive treatment. Yet, the doctors consistently view her as their handmaid and resist her insights and suggestions. In the play's dramatic finale, Monahan forces the physicians to respect their patient's last wishes. Edson told me that the hero of the play is the nurse, the only real caregiver.[36]

Given the competition, Edson's Susie Monahan is a striking deviation from the norm, but she is ultimately overshadowed by the strongest portrayal of nurses to appear on either stage or screen, two AIDS nurses in Tony Kushner's magnificent play *Angels in America*. Kushner's six-hour-long production follows nurse practitioner Emily and bedside hospital nurse Belize. Belize, the central character throughout the play, struts his nursing stuff when he's assigned to care for the odious anticommunist lawyer Roy Cohn, who has terminal AIDS. In these scenes, Belize has several priceless confrontations with doctor and patient.

In the middle of the night, Cohn's doctor arrives on the unit and marches testily up to the nurses' station. Glancing suspiciously at Belize—who conforms to none of his notions of who a nurse should be or how a nurse should look—he barks, "Are you the duty nurse?" "Yo," Belize says defiantly. "Why are you dressed like that?" "You don't like it?" "Nurses

are supposed to wear white," the doctor insists. Without batting an eye, **169**
Belize retorts, "Doctors are supposed to be home in Westchester,
asleep."[37]

Belize is equally uncowed when he deals with Cohn, a closet homosexual who treats nurses—particularly homosexual ones—like dirt. While
putting Cohn in his place, Belize also displays both knowledge of AIDS
and its treatment and a peculiar empathy for the suffering of his despica-
ble patient. He advises Cohn to refuse radiation treatment "because radiation will kill the T-cells and you don't have any you can afford to lose,"
and to resist enrolling in clinical trials of anti-retrovirals because Cohn
may be randomized to placebos. "You're just a fucking nurse. Why should
I listen to you over my very qualified, very expensive WASP doctor?"
Cohn responds. Belize persists. Get the real thing, because if you don't,
"you'll die." He tells Cohn, almost hissing, "So if you have any strings
left, pull them, because everyone's put through the double blind and with
this, time's against you, you can't fuck around with placebos."[38] Throughout the rest of the play, he is remarkable for his knowledge, competence,
grit, and courage.

One also finds positive accounts of competent, intelligent nurses in fiction. In 1999 Peter Baida won first prize in the prestigious American short
story competition, the O. Henry Awards, for his remarkable entry entitled "A Nurse's Story." Baida, who had suffered from hemophilia
throughout his life and worked for two decades at the Memorial Sloan-
Kettering Cancer Center in New York, was too sick to attend the award
presentation. In his story a respected veteran nurse, Mary McDonald, is
dying in a nursing home. Sick and frail, she is nonetheless alert enough to
encourage the nurses taking care of her to join a union. As she tells them
that they deserve a lot more than they're getting, she recalls her own reluctant decision, years before, to vote for a union in her hospital.[39]

A positive figure in detective fiction is the heroine of novels written by
Echo Heron, a nurse who made her literary debut with two best-selling
nonfiction works about her experience as a nurse, *Intensive Care: The Story
of a Nurse* and *Condition Critical: The Story of a Nurse Continues.* Between
1998 and 2000 Heron wrote a series of four detective novels including
Pulse, in which RN Adele Monsarrat solves a series of crimes in the San
Francisco Bay Area.[40] The books are unique in the way they combine an
intimate look at nurses' working lives, the hospital workplace under managed care, and internal nursing politics in the standard whodunit formula.
Unfortunately, this series was discontinued by its publisher.

To find the most powerful nursing character in contemporary fiction,
we have to turn to Anne Perry's series of Victorian mystery novels. Best
known for her first mystery series featuring Inspector Thomas Pitt and

170   his indomitable wife Charlotte, Perry introduced another memorable character, Hester Latterly, in the first of her series of William Monk novels, *The Face of a Stranger*.[41]

Monk is a high-ranking police detective who lost his memory in a carriage accident. In the course of the next eleven novels, Monk loses his job in the police and ends up working as a private agent of inquiry. His partner in detection is Hester Latterly, a well-to-do woman who joined Florence Nightingale's band of nurses in the Crimea. When Latterly returns from the war, she finds that her parents have died bankrupt. Refusing to be dependent on her only brother's charity, Hester decides to put her nursing skills to use to earn a living.

With Latterly, Perry has produced one of the only accurate fictional accounts of what nurses did in the Victorian era and of the obstacles they encountered trying to do it. "What Perry's novels do is create a character who represents the link between useful work that women could do for pay and women's struggles to move from the domestic dependence to independence," says nursing historian Joan Lynaugh. "Nursing was good, hard work, which made it all right for women to do it for pay. Women could be virtuous and free at the same time."

Perry told me that she chose a nurse as one of her main characters because that was the only historically sound choice. "I wanted a woman who was independent, had courage and opinions, and would dare to speak them," Perry explained. "In that period it would have been socially anachronistic for that kind of woman to have stayed at home waiting to be married off. A nurse who was in the Crimea would have had these shattering life-and-death experiences. . . . She would also have been placed in the position where she was the only one with the ability and the responsibility to make major decisions."

Perry also wanted her heroine to be something of a crusader. "Being a nurse also gave her a cause and a crusade to fight for, because nurses were aware of what was going wrong and nobody would listen to them. Florence Nightingale spent her whole life after she returned from the Crimea, a lot of it in bed, we know, writing endless letters and reports to try and persuade people just to use common sense in nursing." Perry's own personal experiences with nurses also influenced her choice, she admitted. "When my mother had a serious heart illness and was sent home afterward, her greatest distress came from some of the side effects of medication, and nurses helped to relieve that."

In all the William Monk novels, Perry puts this combination of a crusading spirit, medical knowledge, and compassion on display. When Hester sets out to work in London hospitals, she is burning to reform hospitals through better sanitation and ventilation and to create an educated cadre of professional nurses. But at every step of the way, she encounters the same hostility from physicians and hospital boards that Nightingale and her real nurses met in the Crimea.

Although Florence Nightingale appears only once in the series, her spirit permeates all the novels. Nightingale never appears as an "angel of mercy" but always as the tough-minded, abrasive, but charming character she was. In *The Sins of the Wolf*, when Hester is accused of murdering a patient, Nightingale is a witness at her trial. Although it is a total invention, the scene is priceless. Perhaps believing the sentimental propaganda of the era, the prosecuting counsel makes the mistake of patronizing Nightingale, asking if Hester is "diligent, honest, and brave." When she answers in the affirmative, he asks, "Then, Madam, how is it that she is obliged to earn her living, not in some senior positions in a hospital, using these remarkable qualities, but traveling on an overnight train from Edinburgh to London, administering a simple dose of medicine to an elderly lady whose health is no worse than that of most persons her age?"

Nightingale moves in for the kill. "Because," she retorts, "she is an outspoken woman, with more courage than tact, thank God. She does not care for hospital life, having to obey the orders of those who are on occasion less knowledgeable than herself but are too arrogant to be told by someone they consider inferior." And when the prosecutor persists in maligning Hester's character, Nightingale tears him apart with an eloquent elaboration of just what nurses know and do. "And when you are ill, sir, vomiting and with a flux you cannot control, is there someone to hold a bowl for you, wash you clean, bring you a little fresh water, change your sheets? I hope you are suitably grateful, sir, because dear God, there are so many for whom there is not, because there are too few of us willing to do it, or with the heart and stomach for it!"[42]

The entertainment media conveys the message that the only central player in the care of the sick is the doctor. He—and now she—is the only hero. Health care isn't about teamwork. It's about a team of one. Recovery isn't a long and often painful process that depends on the skilled monitoring and judgment of nurses. Unencumbered by nurses, whose only function is to be mocked by, screwed by, or otherwise used by the doctor, patients leave the hospital and recover. Nurses don't have curiosity about science or play any role in the curative process. Even if one buys the erroneous notion that doctors cure and nurses care, few fictional nurses even administer a needed dose of TLC or fluff the odd pillow. This version of the nurse's job not only contradicts reality—where nurses in fact do much of the technical and medical work normally associated with physicians—it denies nurses even the narrow corner of expertise history has set aside for

172 them. On TV, in the movies, and in fiction, it is doctors, not nurses, who make the hospital "a place of joy," as the bishop of Rochester has said.

If people read and see doctors depicted as smart, important, and consequential, and nurses as handmaids, harridans, harlots, or harebrained, is it any wonder that today's bright young woman, asked to consider a career in nursing, feels that her parents are expecting too little of her? In fact, today it almost seems as though the culture, and the media that reflects and reproduces it, believe that to be a nurse is a demotion, a kind of gender backsliding that one would want to avoid at all costs. And why would a bright, ambitious woman want to be a nurse, when TV and Hollywood tell her that she really should be a doctor? Why would a man go into nursing when so few male nurses appear on the media radar and those that do, like the Ben Stiller character in *Meet the Parents*, are targets of a series of one-liners? Couple this with the journalistic media's depiction of nursing, and it's a miracle anyone wants to be a nurse at all.

7

Missing from the News

A couple of months ago, I was walking by Mount Sinai Hospital in Toronto. Located on University Avenue, one of the city's main north-south thoroughfares, it's in the heart of Toronto's business and political center. Although I'd passed Mount Sinai many times, this time when I looked up at the hospital entrance, I noticed three vertical banners flying in the wind. Read from left to right, they proudly hailed, "The Best Research, The Best Medicine, The Best Patient Care."

Like a Haiku, these three lines invite countless different interpretations. Some nurses, for example, might wonder why no banner with "The Best Nursing" was included. The average person walking by Mount Sinai might assume that nursing is present and accounted for in the banner "The Best Patient Care." Doctors, after all, care for and about patients. Aides deliver patient care. So do occupational and physical therapists and a whole host of other people. Given the historical framing of health care, you could easily read the banners from left to right and come to the conclusion that the best research coupled with the best medicine equals the best patient care. In this formulation, nursing would be lumped in with everyone else involved with the patient.

The hospital PR people and administrators responsible for these banners thus give us a very complicated story with multiple subtexts. The story gets far less complicated and has fewer subtexts when hospitals market themselves in publications strewn in waiting rooms and patient lounges, in newsletters and magazines, in newspaper ads, and in news releases and pitches sent out to the press and "decision makers" by battalions of PR personnel. When hospital PR staff define research, it's almost

173

174 always doctors who do it, as if nurses didn't participate in a great deal of that research. When they define medicine, doctors are the ones who deliver the latest cures without the help of nurses (and when it comes to medical matters, nurses, we've seen, tend to vacate the premises). Finally, when it comes to patient care, PR people usually portray doctors as the dispensers of the really serious care, while nurses do the fluffy stuff.

While PR staff in hospitals, medical schools and centers, and other institutions diligently promote physicians and biomedical researchers, they do little to promote nursing. Hospitals tend to leave nursing out of the picture in hospital advertising, hospital publications, and hospital public relations efforts.

Hospital Advertising

As managed care crested in the American health care system in the 1990s, hospitals increased the number of ads in daily newspapers. The template was the full-page photo of a band of white-coated physicians—sometimes as many as forty or fifty, sometimes as few as two or three—looking authoritatively into the camera. Below the picture, the reader learned the qualifications and activities of these physicians. Aside from vague references to the health care team, most ads don't specifically add nurses to the mix and certainly don't focus on the activities of nurses. HMOs and insurers also use this template. In a quarter-page ad on the *New York Times* op-ed page and in the *Wall Street Journal,* the Blue Cross Blue Shield Association advertised its services with a picture of a female physician looking into the ear of a child. "Diagnosed by one doctor," the copy going across the top of the page read. "Supported by thousands," it explained at the bottom.[1]

The same kind of iconography and message is depicted on hospital websites. In December 2003 I took a journey to a variety of United States and Canadian hospitals via cyberspace to check out whether nurses were absent or present and accounted for. The Massachusetts General Hospital's website informed me that its mission is "to provide the highest quality care to individuals and to the community, to advance care through excellence in biomedical research, and to educate future academic and practice leaders of the health care professions." The focus is clearly on medicine, and has little to say about nursing.[2]

A quick scan of the dozens of press releases the hospital sent out in 2003 reveals that few had anything to do with nursing. When one clicks on grand rounds and symposia, there is no indication that nurses are also involved in interesting presentations in the hospital.

The Harbor-UCLA Medical Center website had a bold headline, "Excellence in Biomedical Research," with a picture of a doctor leaning over a small baby preparing to listen to the baby's heart with a stethoscope. On the UCLA Medical Center home page, a small box told you to click here to get the latest news on the separated conjoined Guatemalan twins. If you did, a story updated you on their progress. Nowhere would we learn that these fragile babies have survived not only because of medical but also because of nursing care.[3]

Hospitals that are deemed to be magnets for nurses seem not to magnetize Internet readers with nurses' accomplishments. When I entered North Shore University Hospital and Long Island Jewish Medical Center I found that nurses don't seem to have much to do with making it into the top hospital ratings in the United States. Cardiology, cardiovascular surgery and renal care and breast health services were extolled. But there were no nurses in these advertisements or any other nonphysician members of the health care team.[4]

One of the most interesting websites is that of the prestigious Mayo Clinic in Rochester, Minnesota. On the clinic's website, a section entitled "The Tradition" attributes its history to the activities of two physician brothers. "Around the turn of the century, Drs. Charlie and Will Mayo organized medical professionals in a new way to better care for patients. . . . The system was built on the idea that two heads are better than one and five are even better."

If you click on history, the website tells you that Dr. William Worrell Mayo joined the Sisters of Francis in building the Saint Mary's Hospital, from which the Mayo Clinic grew. What this description leaves out, Sioban Nelson tells us, is the story behind the official history. As the website informs us, the Saint Mary's Hospital was built after a great tornado practically flattened the city in 1883. The nuns took the injured to the Academy of the Lady of Lourdes, their motherhouse. Recognizing the need for a hospital, they went for help to the physician William Worrell Mayo, Charlie and Will's father. What the website leaves out is that he insisted that the town could not support a hospital. The nuns persisted, raised the money, built the building, and got St. Mary's hospital going. When Dr. Mayo had nothing to do but walk through the doors, he agreed to work with the sisters of St. Francis who ran the hospital. As Nelson explains, "It took the sisters four years to raise the money for the hospital, which the Mayos made their own! Doctors sought the advice of the outstanding surgical nurse, Sister Fabian. For years the Mayos would not operate without her, but this is unknown outside of the community." The Mayo brothers later founded the Mayo Clinic.[5]

The Mayo Clinic has become an almost Lourdes-like shrine to doctors'

176 dominance and to faith in the power of heroic medicine, with nursing practically invisible to its reputation. Armed with reams of charts and sheaves of X rays, people travel to the Mayo Clinic from all over the world. Even nonmedical pilgrims immediately learn of its magical allure. When I went to Rochester several years ago, the cab driver ferrying me in from the airport boasted, "We've got the Mayo Clinic here in Rochester. It's the best hospital with the best doctors and the best medicine."

"And what about the best nursing?" I asked.

Hospital Publications

Internal hospital publications—newsletters, magazines, and educational materials—similarly tend to feature physicians and exclude RNs. I discovered a particularly illustrative example of this phenomenon when I spent a day with operating room nurses at Boston's Children's Hospital. Because a number of the cases I discuss in this book concern nurses who work in pediatric cardiology programs, I wanted to see what these nurses really do. As I was waiting to meet the OR nurses, I glanced at a publication called *Children's News*, which is published every week by the hospital's department of public affairs. The May 23, 2003, issue began with a front-page story called "Doctor for a Day." The article read as follows:

"On May 4, 300 pint-sized surgeons-to-be had the chance to play 'Operation' with real medical instruments in Children's operating rooms. The annual OR Open House was sponsored by the perioperative nurses as part of Nurses Week. 'This is a great way to help children to feel comfortable with the idea of the operating room,' says Michele Serino, RN, one of the event's organizers. 'And who knows—it might even inspire some future pediatric surgeons.'"[6] The photo accompanying the short article shows a nurse demonstrating equipment to a group of children and adults. The nurse is not identified, but the caption identifies an Asian doctor and her family, who are also watching the demonstration.

The occasion for this open house, Nurses Week (or Nurses Day), has been celebrated since 1974 all over the world to coincide with Florence Nightingale's birthday.[7] It's supposed to highlight nurses not doctors. So why, especially in the middle of a major nursing crisis, were nurses at Children's Hospital arranging for kids to come to be a "doctor for a day" and recruiting future pediatric surgeons?

As a group of Children's Hospital nurses and I were sitting in the lounge having coffee, I learned the real story behind this Nurses Week event.

As a memo written by nurses to the public affairs department explained, the nursing department and nurse Michele Serino had actually organized another event to highlight Nurses Week. Serino planned for an event with nurses "demonstrating techniques, equipment, doll hospital, pulse oximetry, and microscopes" to the children and their families. But somehow Nurses Day, in the hospital publication, became a de facto Doctors Day; the photographs the nurses took to illustrate nursing practice were not used; and Michele's hope that the event "might even inspire some future nurses or surgeons" became "inspire some future pediatric surgeons." It would be hard for anyone reading the article to imagine that the job of nurses is not only to assist doctors but to recruit new ones. They might even conclude that nurses didn't want to recruit nurses.

This reinterpretation, however, illustrates the paradox that is at the heart of Nurses Week, which manages to simultaneously celebrate and devalue nursing. Like Secretaries Day or Black History Month, it tends to be a low-budget reparation for the past year's neglect. Nurses are given free manicures, massages, or cosmetics and are regaled with showers of trinkets—heart-shaped key chains, hospital pens, or an inexpensive meal. To observe the event, some hospitals invite inspirational speakers to extol the virtues of nursing and encourage RNs to soldier on.

In 2000 I was asked to speak at the Dana Farber Cancer Institute's annual Nurses Week event in Boston. At the time of the invitation, the world-renowned research hospital, certified by the National Cancer Institute, had been buffeted by scandal. It was experiencing not only cost cutting and managed care but the continued reverberations from a major medical error that had occurred at the Farber in 1995, when a massive overdose of chemotherapy drugs ultimately killed two patients, one of them *Boston Globe* reporter Betsy Lehman.

When Susan Grant, chief nursing officer and vice president of Patient Care Services called to extend the invitation, she explained that nurses at the Farber definitely needed a boost. The hospital had, therefore, rented two galleries in the elegant Museum of Fine Arts. As the nurses sipped their predinner drinks in a Chinese sculpture gallery, Dr. David Nathan, the hospital's new president—accompanied by his physician team—breezed in to make a few brief remarks before leaving for a more important engagement.

Nathan stood at a microphone and related an incident that, he said, symbolized the meaning of nursing at the institution. It involved the mother of a young child who was being treated at the Farber. The child, no more than three or four years old, was critically ill. Realizing the child might die, the mother had introduced the subject of heaven and angels.

"What are angels?" the child asked.

"They are spirits who are always with you," she replied.

"Oh, you mean they're like Kristin?" the child said, naming a nurse.

178   "Yes," the mother agreed.

So did Dr. Nathan.

Nurses, he said, were the "angels of the Farber," and he thanked the nurses for always "being there" for patients. Then Nathan and his physician team left.

When I later asked him about his view of the profession, Nathan said he is a real fan of nursing. He talked enthusiastically about the nurses' critical role at the Farber. Along with pharmacists, he said, nurses run the hospital's experimental clinical trials. "Doctors may dream up the trials, but it is the nurses and the pharmacists," he explained, "who do all the work. They run the trials. They collect the data. They call the shots about when to withdraw someone from a protocol, because they know who's having the side effects."

Doctors are with patients about five minutes a day, Nathan continued. Nurses are with them eight to twelve hours each day, he said, carefully adding that it's the content of what nurses do with patients during those eight to twelve hours, not the minutes that make them up, that count.

In his Nurses Week speech, Nathan was clearly trying to thank his nurses. Yet, his pep talk did not allude to the nurses' role in the conduct of scientific inquiry or patient care or use any of the terms that physician administrators routinely summon when they are complimenting their own physician colleagues.

Other hospitals and health care organizations employ similar metaphors to applaud the work of nurses. The Cleveland Clinic launched a 2000 Nurses Week promotional and recruitment poster campaign designed to celebrate its nurses. The hospital held focus groups with nurses to find out how they viewed their job. The nurses told them that working at the Cleveland Clinic, a major research institution, meant that they had to learn and know a lot. But rather than showing nurses doing their work, the ad campaign featured mountain climbers, firefighters, and individual shots of runners, kayakers, and rock climbers. Inspirational messages scrolled underneath: "There are some people who don't worry about the odds. Nurses for example." Then followed words of institutional gratitude. The Cleveland Clinic "salutes" its nurses for their "courage, strength, dedication, commitment, talent, unselfishness, and more commitment." With a heavy emphasis on nineteenth-century virtues, there is not a single word about knowledge, brains, intelligence, skill, expertise, judgment, technical, or medical know-how, or even compassion and caring.

In 2003, Northwest Medical Center designed a recruitment ad to attract nurses to its Tucson facility, featuring a smiling nurse holding the hand of an elderly woman. Against a pale blue background, bold black letters ask, "Ever wonder how angels make a living?" To emphasize the theme, a pair of filigreed angel's wings shimmer behind the words "make **179** a living." When it comes to advertising the hospital itself, there is no mention of the angelic in the catalogue of services on its website.

The angelic depiction of nursing has become so commonplace in the hospital industry that it infects anyone who works with hospitals and nurses. For example, at a 2002 convention for Canadian nursing students held in Victoria, British Columbia, one of Canada's health care job fair companies invited hospital recruiters from both Canada and the United States to speak to the students about potential employment opportunities. The company decided to give the students a gift, complimenting them on their choice of career. The gift was a white tee shirt decorated with bold black letters across the front that read, "I didn't know angels flew this low!"

Hospital PR Staff and the Mainstream Media

When hospital public relations staff try to interest outside media—newspaper, radio, and TV journalists—they clearly aren't going to suggest that reporters meet with a bunch of angels. They usually suggest that they meet with doctors, and they produce reams of press releases and other materials with which they inundate journalists with doctors' accomplishments. Richard Knox, former medical writer for the *Boston Globe* and health and science correspondent for National Public Radio, notes that "it's rare to get anything from hospitals or medical centers that talks about what nurses do, innovations in nursing, nursing practice, research. We just don't hear much about it." Knox says that he and his colleagues may sometimes hear about nursing research if it's published in a mainstream journal like the *New England Journal of Medicine* or *JAMA* or if a nursing school like the University of Pennsylvania School of Nursing—an institution that has its own PR staff—does media outreach. As for hospitals, there is little outreach about the nursing research or practice that goes on inside.

That's why Claire Fagin, dean emerita of the University of Pennsylvania School of Nursing, originally hired a PR person to promote the work of researchers and practitioners in the school. When Claire Fagin went to the University Pennsylvania in 1977, the hospital made a commitment to help her promote the school in the city and country. "But the major goal of the public relations department at the hospital at the University of Pennsylvania was to publicize medicine and the achievement of physicians, so while the department was helpful in providing us assistance, it was clear that it wasn't enough to promote the significant nursing research and practice going on within the school. If we wanted the word to

180 get out about nursing, we realized the only way was for us to do it ourselves," Fagin told me.

Knox and other journalists say that when hospital PR staff promote new stories and developments, nurses tend not to be included among the spokespeople put forward by the institution. In spite of all the contemporary talk of the importance of the "health care team," hospital PR still reflects, as Knox puts it, "the power relationships within the hospital." Furthermore, when a new cancer treatment or surgical procedure is hyped, nurses are not described as participants in either cure or care. Unless the story is specifically about nursing, nurses will not be put forward as spokespeople—unless, that is, a reporter specifically asks to speak to a nurse. "If you ask to speak to a nurse, hospitals will usually be glad to provide one," Knox comments. "But nurses are not otherwise put forward as participants in studies or innovations."

The structure of the hospital hierarchy often limits a journalist's sources, explains Irene Wielawski, a former *Los Angeles Times* medical reporter who now freelances for that paper and the *New York Times*. "If I call a hospital PR person because I am pursuing a story at X hospital and want to know more about it, the hospital often steers me to a doctor or administrator and does not offer a nurse for an interview. I, the media person, am on the outside. I don't really know who the players are and I am dependent on that hospital to steer me to the appropriate people, and they may not include a nurse in that."

When she arrives at the hospital to interview the people the hospital has identified as key players, the presentation is "hierarchical." The journalist is corralled, as she puts it, in a room where typically "there's the hospital president, the chief of surgery, perhaps the inventor of a new medical device, and the nurse who actually knows the patient. She's the last one to speak and will usually say, 'I agree with what doctor so-and-so said.' From the nurse, there's a lot of demurring."

Both Knox and Wielawski add that today it is harder than ever to reach frontline workers. "Hospital PR has moved from the academic to the corporate model," Knox explains. "Hospitals want to more tightly control who they allow reporters to talk to. Ten or fifteen years ago, it was easier to develop sources and call them directly and have them respond. Now you almost always have to go through PR people who want to know who you are, what you are doing, why you are doing it, and what questions you want to ask. Sometimes they even ask to sit in on the interviews you are conducting. People who are doing frontline care are buried even deeper in their institutions than ever before."

Even when a journalist actually reaches out to hospital PR for a nurse, they may not get one. André Picard, who is the public health reporter for the *Toronto Globe and Mail*, has been covering health care in Canada for **181** over a decade. Picard, who wryly comments that there is "no lack" of press releases hyping physicians' work, says he gets "virtually nothing" from hospitals about nursing. "When I speak to nursing audiences I always tell them that hospital PR departments are their worst enemies."

Picard describes a typical dialog with a hospital's PR department. You call up and ask for an expert on diabetes. The PR person tells you, "I'll see if I can get Doctor So-and-so, but he's probably busy." "Well," you ask, "don't you have a diabetes clinic?" To which the PR representative responds, "Well, yes." "And isn't that clinic run by a nurse?" "Well, yes." "So, what about her?" you ask. "Oh," the PR person replies, "I'm sure you'd much rather speak to a real expert, the doctor."

Picard concludes, "The only time I've ever been pitched a story about a nurse is when it's a human interest story about a nurse who's been, say working for forty-nine years, and isn't this a lovely story."

These experiences reflect the strict hospital pecking order that usually defines the PR staff's job. Hospital PR staff are hired specifically to promote medicine and biomedical research, practice, and innovation. Nursing and other clinical disciplines tend not to be considered to be a part of that mandate.

Tony Swartz-Lloyd, former vice president of communications for the Beth Israel Hospital, explains that most hospital PR staff never receive the kind of mandate and education he enjoyed when he worked for Beth Israel in its heyday as the Mecca for nursing. When hospital CEO Mitchell Rabkin hired him, he was given a very different and unusual brief. "Mitch Rabkin met with me and specifically told me that the hospital was a nursing institution as much or more than it was a medical one. That's not to put down doctors," Swartz-Lloyd says. "As someone who'd been hospitalized before I took the job and has been hospitalized many times after, I know it's simply the reality of patient care."

Many hospital PR staffers, he says, view nurses as a quantitative not a qualitative variable in patients' hospital stays. "They understand that hospitals need enough nurses to keep the hospital running. They say having enough nurses is important so they can be there and be kind and caring and motherly. They say there aren't enough qualified nurses, and that nurses are overworked and underpaid. But their understanding usually doesn't go beyond that. They can't tell you why having an individual, highly qualified nurse is important."

This, Swartz-Lloyd says, is very different from a PR staffer's understanding of physicians. "A PR person can easily explain why it's important to have a doctor who's skilled and qualified. They'll explain that if you don't have a good orthopedic surgeon, he could attach your left leg to your right."

182   But, he says, they don't understand that to patients, nursing is equally important. "They don't understand the consequences of nurses not being able to do their work effectively or not being supported by their institutions. They don't get that you don't just want nurses there to 'answer the bell' but you also want them to do research and teaching and publishing and furthering their own education. This is a good thing, not just a ducking-out-of-work kind of thing."

Some physicians reinforce the notion that PR staff should not be promoting nursing. "Some doctors I've known have gotten upset if you give too much attention to nurses. They feel it diminishes them. Some doctors feel that giving attention to nursing trivializes their own work. They will complain about it to PR staff and hospital administrators," Swartz-Lloyd says. "Doctors, who have so much influence in some institutions, are key in minimizing the importance of nursing's role."

PR staff may become part of the feedback loop that reinforces traditional stereotypes of nurses and passes them on to patients. "Even though they've benefited from excellent nursing care, patients will reflect these attitudes. They'll complain because they haven't been able to see someone who'll take care of them, and then you ask them whether they saw the nurse and they'll say, 'Well, sure, the nurse just came by, but I really wanted to see the doctor.' They don't understand that the person who's critical to their recovery isn't always the doctor," says Swartz-Lloyd.

Maureen McInaney, senior public information representative at the University of California San Francisco Medical Center, explained that "most hospital PR staff are not taught that promoting nursing is part of their brief, and too few institutions make it part of their brief. They conceive of hospitals as buildings with patients and doctors in them."

Unlike many other public information officers, her job is to promote the work of nursing on the clinical side of the hospital while another PR staffer works with the school of nursing. This is because the dean of its nursing school and the vice president of nursing have pushed the public information staff to promote nursing in its PR efforts. Without that kind of internal pressure, and sometimes even with it, the tendency of public relations staff in hospitals and medical centers is to promote doctors and forget about nurses. McInaney paints a typical scenario. "A reporter will call in and make an inquiry for an expert on the new guidelines for evaluating blood pressure. That's a question that a nurse specializing in cardiology could easily answer. Or it might be answered by a nurse and a physician, or a nurse who does research in that area. But it's often shipped immediately to a cardiologist, internist, or physician," unless, she adds, someone in the PR office is educated to understand the role of nurses.

McInaney also has to educate journalists who might be reluctant to talk to a nurse. "You have to explain the breadth and depth of what research nurses do. I often have conversations with reporters who are quite resistant to talking to nurses," she says. "I say, look, you don't understand we've got nurses doing research in that area."

What it takes to promote nursing is thus an institutional commitment: PR staff devoted to finding out what is going on within nursing inside their own hospital, medical center, or nursing school, and time devoted to educating other PR staff and journalists. If this doesn't happen, nursing, McInaney says, will simply not be on the institutional radar. And if it isn't on the institutional radar, it's never going to make it onto the journalistic radar.

Nursing in the Mainstream Media

Hospital PR creates, reflects, and reinforces journalistic coverage of nursing. And journalistic coverage of nursing similarly affects a hospital's PR efforts. It's a tight feedback loop that produces a very skewed image of the health care universe. In the mid-1980s, when I first began writing about nursing during an earlier serious nursing shortage, the question of nursing's public image was a predictable subject of debate, analysis, and proposed remedial action. During that shortage, a group of nursing organizations called the Tricouncil of Nursing—with a large grant from the PEW Charitable Trusts—launched a project called Nurses of America (NOA) to attract high-quality candidates to the profession. The NOA also funded a major study of the journalistic media to ascertain whether journalists regularly sought out nurses to be sources of information for, or subjects of, their stories. Bernice Buresh and I worked with Nica Bell, a statistician, to analyze articles that appeared in the *New York Times*, the *Washington Post*, and the *Los Angeles Times* for the first quarter of 1990.

We wanted to know whether women were represented in news and analyses of health care and what were the occupations of those women who were covered. The goal was to determine whether the full range of women's roles and expertise was made visible in news coverage.[8] What we found was extremely sobering on all counts. Of the 423 articles analyzed and 908 sources directly quoted, 32 percent of the sources quoted were from doctors and only 1 percent (10 quotes) were from nurses. Sources from every other occupation or group connected to health care—researchers, business people, representatives of advocacy groups, attorneys, hospital administrators, patients, family members—were quoted far more than nurses. Even when the subject was about nursing, as in stories about nursing homes, nurses were not sources of information. Both female and

184   male journalists did, in fact, seek out more female sources of information, but like the TV producers who go for the gold, journalists interviewed female doctors, female hospital administrators, and female government officials, but neither female nor male nurses. Although female journalists wrote a significant number of stories for these publications, they "did not make any appreciable difference in the representation of nursing in the sample—a profession that is 97 percent female."[9]

The relative invisibility of nursing in the media continues to have a significant impact on public perceptions of nursing and nurses' work. Many studies have documented the power of the media in shaping public opinion in general and health care in particular. In 1997, two surveys, one sponsored by the National Council on Aging and the other cosponsored by the National Health Council and PBS, found that many Americans depend on the media for health care and medical information.[10] The National Council on Aging study reported that when it surveyed one thousand women between the ages of forty-five and fifty-four, over 80 percent said they relied on television, newspapers, and magazines for information on health care.[11]

The PBS/National Council of Health study reported that 60 percent of those surveyed considered the media to be their main source of health information. The elderly and people with chronic conditions tended to rely more on doctors for health information, but even these people said the media was their second major source of information. Large percentages of those surveyed believed what they heard in media reports.

More recent studies confirm these trends. Again focusing on the ever-present *ER*, the Kaiser Family Foundation published a study in 2002 documenting that many of those who watch the TV show *ER* on a regular basis learn about health topics and go to their doctors as a result. An earlier study found that children's strongest impressions of various medical professions were primarily derived from *ER* and other television dramas.[12]

Since the media significantly influence people's views of health care, it is understandable that few choose to seek information from nurses rather than or as well as doctors. Nursing groups frequently commission pollsters to survey the public about their impressions of nursing compared to other professions. Polls in Canada, the United States, and other countries show that many members of the public believe that nurses are some of the most ethical and honest of workers. But some polls show that the public won't consult nurses about major health issues such as sexually transmitted diseases, sex education, abortion, drug and alcohol use, birth control, or menopause and osteoporosis.[13]

The Breach Not the Observance

A closer look at how the journalistic media cover nursing reveals that nurses most frequently appear as angels or heroes, as killers, or as victims of serious workplace problems. With the exception of the rare angelic or heroic nurse, they are covered in the breach, when they are a problem or warn us of a problem. In part, this reflects the media's bias to report sensational events in scattershot bursts rather than probing a complex dynamic or process. But it also reflects the media's tendency to cover sources and subjects that it considers worthy and legitimate.

Newspapers will run the occasional story about the heroic or angelic nurse. In September 2002, for example, the Associated Press ran a wire service story on fifteen nurses who were honored by the American Red Cross and *Nursing Spectrum* for "risking their lives to save others." Many of these remarkable RNs rescued accident victims, and four were involved in rescuing victims of the World Trade Center and Pentagon attacks. The rest helped victims of traffic or other catastrophic accidents.[14] After the Bali bombing in October of 2002, a number of nurses, as well as doctors, who volunteered in a Bali hospital were featured for their courageous efforts.

In 2002 the *Toronto Star* ran a front-page story in its health care section on a nurse who had identified gaps in adolescent health care in Toronto and started a teenage health clinic. The headline of the story, "Angel in Our Midst," was followed by the lead-in "Meet nurse Ruth Ewert. She's kind, gentle and a hero to those whose lives she's touched."[15]

Other stories occasionally report on nurses involved in a particular field of health care, like hospice care, school nursing, or burn nursing. But these stories tend not to have what journalists call "legs." They are episodic, one-of-a-kind stories that offer little opportunity for follow-up. Stories may also appear when nurses challenge doctors—"Nurses Treading on Doctors' Turf" or "Nurses to Take Doctor Duties."[16] This theme centers on the competition between nurses and physicians for patients, and specifically on physicians' objections to nurse practitioners who make incursions on their turf.

Nurses receive far more coverage when they present a serious problem in the health care world. When, for example, there is a periodic nursing shortage, a spate of articles appears about its impact on home care, nursing homes, emergency rooms, and so forth. A short article in the *Boston Globe* describes on-line auctions that allow nurses to bid on different shifts in the hospital.[17] A related *Business Week* story, "How Much Do I Hear for This Nurse," carries a photo of a nurse wearing a 1950s nurse cap and

186 staring at a thermometer.[18] Similarly when there is a nurses' strike, the media may report on the workplace issues involved.

A nurse who kills a patient, mistakenly or deliberately, receives a great deal of coverage. A recent series of stories focused on nurse Charles Cullen, who allegedly killed over forty patients in his sixteen-year career.[19] Much of the newspaper coverage focused on the lack of any standardized system of monitoring either nurses' credentials or their employment histories. Cullen was able to move with impunity from hospital to hospital in two different states because, when an employer suspected him of harming patients, he simply resigned and took another job elsewhere with no further questions asked. Follow-up stories and editorials highlighted the fact that state boards of nursing are insufficient to provide serious oversight and demanded a better system of accountability for nurses.[20] Few, however, discussed the larger implications of the story. The fact that there is no standard system to make sure nurses are safe is a symptom of the lack of seriousness with which our society tends to view nurses and their work. As we will see, it also allows hospitals to use nurses as a cheap, disposable, and infinitely substitutable labor force; they hire temporary, traveling, or foreign nurses when the need arises, with little concern for their skill levels or employment histories.

Once again, these stories are noteworthy because they depict nursing as a problem, not as a dynamic and evolving field of practice and research. As Maureen McInaney observes, most journalists are unaware that there even is such a field as nursing research and few report on it systematically. When I first approached an editor at the *Boston Globe* about a decade ago to pitch a story on nursing research, her response was "nursing what?" Few journalists in America today know that the National Institute for Nursing Research exists and that it's part of the National Institutes of Health.

Nurses often appear in the news as anonymous or faceless. In photographs they may not be identified by name. Even when they are identified, they are not quoted. Images accompanying many stories still show us pictures or drawings of nurses in nursing caps, although the cap disappeared at least thirty years ago and nurses think of it as an archaic symbol.[21] When *Better Homes and Gardens* magazine did a story on the nursing shortage, the illustration was of a cartoonish nurse with angel's wings, wearing a white cap, and carrying a red cross.[22] Sometimes art directors seem so bereft of modern nursing images that they reach all the way back into the past and resurrect Florence Nightingale and her lamp. It would be hard to imagine the medical equivalent: contemporary stories of doctors showing them carrying foot-long thermometers or still wearing that strange headgear, a the band encircling the forehead with a light attached—as in the famous Norman Rockwell painting. Why can't art directors come up with a contemporary image of nurses?

In a *New York Times* story that ran during the anthrax scare of 2001, we meet an anthrax patient, Bud Richmond, in the process of diagnosis and treatment. The article describes a particularly harrowing moment when the patient is trying to get to the bathroom but "got so entangled and frustrated that by the time a nurse named Karen walked in, he was in tears." As the patient tells it, "Karen came in and said—she called me Bud—she said, 'Oh Bud, it's going to be all right.' "[23]

The physicians and even Richmond's daughter are fully identified in the article. Referring to the nurse simply as "Karen" is an interesting departure from the standard journalistic practice of either giving the full names of people they quote or not naming them at all. When I called the *New York Times* reporter to inquire about this story, I did not receive a reply.

In February 2004 the *Clarion-Ledger* of Jackson, Mississippi, ran a story on the front page of their Sunday Southern Style section about the positive experiences patients had with nurse-midwives. "Midwives making deliveries memorable," was the subhead of the story. It focused on the experiences of a new mother, Anita Wansley, who was attended by an anonymous nurse midwife. While it explained how midwives are trained and credentialed, it never named or quoted the midwife who delivered Wansley's baby. The story went on to quote a Jackson obstetrician-gynecologist, Dr. Freda Bush, who was a former nurse midwife. "I loved midwifery," said Bush, who left the profession because she had so much trouble with the physicians she worked with. The story quoted another obstetrician who talked about the problems physicians have with midwives. One short quote was allotted to a nurse midwife who is the director of professional services for the American College of Nurse-Midwives in Washington, DC. The story featured a photo of Wansley and Bush, but no working Mississippi midwife was either pictured or quoted.[24]

Newspapers print dozens of stories about medical education and training and the journey students make to become doctors. In spite of the nursing shortage, few if any newspapers and health reporters take us into the schools that produce nurses and explain the kind of issues and education student nurses receive.[25]

As we saw in Chapter 1, nurses are almost always left out of journalistic definitions of humanitarian groups like Médecins sans Frontières. A *New York Times* article on the problems of fighting malaria in Ethiopia repeatedly defines MSF as "an international doctors' group" or a "doctors' group," and the only sources quoted in the article are doctors.[26] When the *Guardian Weekly* reported on the role of pharmaceutical companies in

188   neglecting "forgotten diseases" like sleeping sickness in Africa, the reporter focused on the efforts of MSF, a "charitable organization that sends volunteer doctors to emergencies throughout the world. . . . Their doctors did not enjoy administering the fifty-year-old drug melarsoprol to sleeping sickness patients." In a box titled "Medecins Sans Frontieres: A Brief History" the group is defined as a doctors' group that has been successful in "capturing the imagination of doctors and volunteers across the world."[27]

Nurses are usually missing in stories about major catastrophes in which there were serious injuries. In October 2001 the *New York Times* ran a story about the terrible ordeal of Lauren Manning, a woman who had been severely burned in the September 11 attack on the World Trade Center. Although burn victims are kept alive by almost one-on-one nursing care, the story repeatedly leaves nurses out of the dramatic account. Seven of these patients, "including Mrs. Manning, remain in a deep, drug-induced sleep while doctors tend to their wounds," reporter Leslie Eaton tells us. "Her doctors would not talk, even in the broadest terms, about the treatment." The story, by implication, suggests that other clinicians will be involved in her care. We learn that "infection is a constant threat" (but not about who monitors infection—given the doctor-oriented frame, the reader would assume it is the doctor), and that "patients who survive face multiple skin grafts and months, even years, of physical therapy" (no word about who works to prevent the complications following such grafts or about the physical therapist who will be involved).[28]

Stories of high-profile patients who undergo medical treatment also routinely leave out the care of nurses. When Christopher Reeve had his dramatic accident, he was cared for on the intensive care unit at the University of Virginia Hospital for a month. While the surgeons certainly repaired Reeve's injuries, Reeve's recovery depended on of expert ICU nurses. You wouldn't have known this from media coverage. The only time a nurse was cited in the stories I examined was in a syndicated article in the *New York Post* that appeared in the *London Times*. An unidentified nurse exclaims that "the doctors are praying for a miracle." In an Associated Press study, another anonymous nurse briefs the press on details of Reeve's case (it's hard to imagine a press reporter with a physician spokesperson who is not identified). A 1996 story in the *Houston Chronicle* begins, "With his nurse at his side, actor Christopher Reeve told Texas home care providers via satellite link Tuesday they are the key to helping a patient recapture his or her life." But Reeve's home care nurses remain anonymous throughout the story. In an *Observer* story on Reeve's at-

tempts at recovery in 2003, we find that "while we talk, Christopher **189**
Reeve's nurse, Dolly Arro, applies his make-up for the photograph."[29]

Similarly, stories about the patients who received artificial hearts at the
Jewish Hospital in Louisville, Kentucky, in 2001 and about operations to
separate the Egyptian Siamese twins at North Texas Hospital for children
in 2002 include little or nothing about follow-up nursing care.[30] Since
these dramatic operations and procedures are surgically or technologi-
cally driven, it's appropriate for the lion's share of attention to go to surgeons and inventors. Nonetheless, these operations present a perfect opportunity for journalists to illuminate the role that nurses and other
clinicians play in innovation and cure, survival and recovery. With some
notable exceptions—including an excellent article in the *New York Times*
that brought attention to the role of burn nurses after the Providence
nightclub fire in 2003—those opportunities are rarely utilized.[31]

Nurses in Clinical Research and Discovery

Much of health care coverage centers on studies or reports on innovation,
progress, and refinement in treatments. Maureen McInaney explains how
these medical studies usually get reported by in-house PR staff. Who is
put forward, she says, is often a very "political decision" with lead authors,
who are physicians, as the primary spokespeople. Again, this is certainly
appropriate. In most reporting, however, journalists commonly ask other
experts in a field to comment on a particular study or issue. In a number
of cases, these experts could easily be nurses. Similarly, since nurses often
participate in the development and evolution of these studies, help administer the medications or procedures used in them, monitor and evaluate patients following them, and thus most closely observe how patients
tolerate experimental protocols, it wouldn't be odd to include brief comments from nurse researchers or bedside RNs. Few if any stories that are
not specifically about nursing research or nursing issues include nurses as
expert commentators. Similarly, stories that concern medical puzzles and
problems generally leave out or downplay nurses.

The *USA Today* website is an excellent example. Under its health topics
index, it lists dozens of stories that have appeared in editions of the national newspaper. The main topics are Women, Men, Children, and
Aging. Under "Other" one finds twenty-one different conditions or problems, including AIDS and HIV, brain, genetics, diabetes, exercise and fit-
ness, diet, and stroke, among others. When in the spring of 2004 I
checked how many of the stories that were not specifically about the nurs-

190 ing work force contained identifiable references to a nurse or credited a nurse as a source of information, I came up with a grand total of zero. Most of those quoted were doctors. But other sources of information included nutritionists, dieticians, drug company representatives, spokespeople for the government, the food industry, the meat industry, and a host of others.[32]

A 2002 article in the Health Science section of the *New York Times* offers an interesting example of the way nurses are often used in medical coverage. Jane E. Brody wrote a story about the vexing problem of prematurity. The story, which spans more than half a page, quotes one nurse, Cheryl Rolston, who also appears in the photographs illustrating the story. She tells us that "we're getting babies now at much younger ages, and now a lot more are surviving." The story then goes on to quote, at some length, five physicians, all of whom address the challenges of prematurity.

The story headline reads, "Premature Births Rise Sharply, Confounding Obstetricians." The pullout quote, in bold at the top of the rightmost column, informs us that "doctors can save most premature babies, but they haven't found a way to stop premature births." A large photo of Rolston with a patient in a neonatal ICU (NICU) has a caption that reads, "Cheryl Rolston, a nurse, tends to a small baby after a feeding."

The headline suggests that the problem of prematurity confounds only doctors, but not the nurses who help make sure these premature babies survive in NICUs. The pullout quote excludes nurses from the process of rescue. It reads "doctors can save . . ." not "doctors and nurses can save," thus conveying the inaccurate idea that in NICUs only doctors do the saving. Nurses are the tenders and doctors are the savers.[33]

So think about it for a moment. When it comes time to allocating health care resources, who are you going to give the money to? The tenders or the savers? If it's a question of entering a career in health care, who do you want to be, a tender or a saver?

This sidelining of nurses is so common that it is hardly ever noticed. The National Heart, Lung, and Blood Institute and the American Heart Association launched a recent national campaign to educate the public about the need to get to the emergency room if someone is experiencing symptoms of a heart attack. The press release announcing the campaign didn't offer any intimation that nurses—whether bedside nurses, ER nurses, nurse practitioners, or researchers—have anything to do with the care or education of potential or actual heart attack victims. This is in spite of the fact that nurse researchers have not only done major investigations of why patients don't go to the ER when they experience chest pain but have also devised strategies to remedy the problem.

The release reads, "A joint call to action urging physicians to educate **191** their patients about heart attack warning signs—and the importance of calling 911 immediately—was announced today at a news conference by the National Heart, Lung, and Blood Institute and the American Heart Association." *Act in Time* "targets patients and the general public as well as physicians and seeks to raise awareness about the need for fast response."[34]

So it's hardly surprising that the *Boston Globe*'s story on the campaign had as its headline "Doctors See Fatal Delays in Heart Attack Cases" and quoted only physicians.[35]

This absence of nursing in relation to cardiac patients is evident in many other journalistic accounts, including those that focus on health policy. In his 1996 book *Health against Wealth: HMOs and the Breakdown of Medical Trust*, George Anders catalogues the way that HMO policies have led to drastic cuts in the length of hospital stays for patients undergoing coronary artery bypass graft operations. Anders quotes Anne Billingsley, chief of cardiothoracic surgery at St. Francis Hospital in Lynwood, California. Most patients are "scared to go home after four days. . . . You have to get them out with a shoehorn. I come around and say, 'All right. It's time.' It's really bad. These poor old guys look at you. They're terrified. But they end up doing fine when they go home. There's nothing else we really do for them at that stage of the recovery. It's just babysitting and helping them walk up and down the hall a few times. Their wives can do that for them at home."[36]

What Billingsley didn't see, says one of the "baby-sitters," is the complexity of nursing care. Kathleen Dracup, a cardiac critical care nurse, is dean of the University of California at San Francisco School of Nursing and editor of the *American Journal of Critical Care*. "If a patient stays in the hospital after bypass, it's not because he's getting baby-sitting, it's because he's continuing to be observed for things like recurrence of respiratory difficulty, heart rhythm disturbances, or infection. And when it's safe to send him home, he may also need vigilant nursing care. With a new incision in his chest, a patient goes home and starts slowly to do exercise and recuperate. He could be on multiple medications. It's a slap in the face to his wife—not to mention the nurses who would have taken care of him in the hospital had he stayed an extra few days—to suggest that what she is doing is just baby-sitting."

One of the most interesting examples of this skewed picture of health care progress was a series of three front-page articles on experimental cancer treatments at the Dana Farber Cancer Institute in 2000. The writer, *Boston Globe* reporter Raja Mishra, spent eight months at the Farber following a patient, Adriana Jenkins, who was receiving experimental

192 cancer treatment for premenopausal breast cancer. The articles took up a section of each front page and two full pages inside the newspaper. In the first article we meet the patient and her chief physician, Eric Winer. The problem and experimental protocol are described. Nurses generally appear anonymously as recorders, not interpreters of data. "A nurse jots down insurance information, then takes her temperature."[37]

The next day's story zeroes in on scientific research. Here again, doctors are depicted as the only ones involved. "Hundreds of local doctors and scientists strive to advance medicine—and their careers—by running National Institutes of Health funded clinical trials." Mishra goes on to describe the hospitals and medical schools—Harvard, Tufts, Boston Medical Center—that produce such research (again, no mention of the nursing schools also involved in this enterprise).

In the section titled "The Doctor" we get a fuller introduction to Dr. Winer, who is described as a kind of lone ranger. Under the heading "The Results" (of the trial) there is no mention of any nurse—or social worker—helping Jenkins cope with her anxiety. When the side effects of the chemotherapy are described, Mishra tell us that "Dana-Farber nurse Kathryn Clarke brings in three syringes filled with a thick cherry-red syrup, Adriamycin. She hands Jenkins eight anti-nausea pills to take all day tomorrow."[38] Apparently, she doesn't stick around to see what happens or teach the patient how to take her meds.

For doctors, things get markedly more Olympian in the third and last of the series. Jenkins is having side effects. Should she continue on with the trials? Should she be withdrawn? Who grapples with these dilemmas? Who decides? "Doctors running clinical trials routinely engage in an ethical balancing act," Mishra writes. "When are side effects too much? When should a trial be stopped? There are no textbooks for this. Each doctor must decide alone. These are among the most difficult decisions made by the thousands of white-coated men and women in Boston's hospitals and clinics. And just such a decision would soon determine Adriana Jenkins's fate." Another anonymous nurse is mentioned when Jenkins has a heart flutter, but again the story goes on to tell us that "clinical trials mean risk. Doctors know it." And finally, we read that Winer is "engaged in his own moral calculus, through his own personal prism."[39] The result is that Adriana is removed from the protocol.

Coincidentally, I read the first two articles right before I called Dr. David Nathan, the Farber's new president, to ask him some questions about his speech at the Nurses Week celebration mentioned above. Nathan asked me how I liked the articles, which he thought accurately reflected nurses' roles. After I read the article, I sent him a letter detailing my concerns about it.

Although doctors like Winer are undoubtedly engaged in extraordi- nary work with great benefits, none of these articles give the reader any idea that medical research involves a team and that nurses and other clini- cians play a critical role in data collection and analysis, in evaluating side effects, and in deciding when patients should be withdrawn from the ex- perimental protocol. Nurses don't seem to be involved, curious, or even concerned about either the research or its impact on their patients. Be- cause they leave nonphysician clinicians out, the articles seem to miscon- strue completely the process of scientific research and inquiry. I won- dered whether the PR staff at the Farber had guided the writer to nurses and other clinicians.

Nathan e-mailed me back thanking me for my concerns. He told me he'd passed them on to the head of PR at the Farber, who had done his best with the reporter and who would surely call me to talk. He never did.

Television is no kinder to nurses. The stories about nursing strikes, nursing shortages, and nurses' complaints are not balanced by images of nurses advancing patient care on the job. Of the hundreds of medical sto- ries that run every year, few focus on nurses. One notable exception was a Discovery Health Channel series that aired in January 2001. The shows targeted different areas of nursing—critical care, obstetrics and neonatal ICU, oncology, and psychiatric care—at the Johns Hopkins Hospital in Baltimore, Maryland. This series was unique in its detailed attention to nurses' contributions. More typical of the image of the nurse in TV news was a four-part documentary that ran on ABC in August 2002, *ICU: Arkansas Children's Hospital.* The ICU, the narrator of the series informs us, "treats children whose hearts have failed them." The show is about the "doctors and nurses who save them." In fact, the series should have been called *OR,* and a more accurate description would be that it's about the doctor who saves them. Following the conventional medical superstar narrative, all the segments focus on surgery, not intensive care, and on one pediatric cardiac surgeon, Jonathan Drummond-Webb, plus a sup- porting cast of pediatric cardiologists. We see the miracles he performs on a number of infants, toddlers, and adolescents who have serious heart problems requiring heart transplants and other major heart repairs.[40] Some of these children die during the show's filming.

Tom Bonner, senior vice president of public affairs for the hospital, told me that the show began when he approached ABC's *Prime Time Thursday.* What was supposed to be a fifteen-minute segment eventually mushroomed into a four-hour miniseries. ABC crews stayed at the hospi- tal for sixteen months, Bonner told me.

Although the series does put nurses on air, and gives a prominent role to the cardiovascular OR nurse manager, Jean Ann Phillips, the portrayal

194   of these highly qualified and specialized nurses does not challenge the stereotypical view of the RN. The nurses occasionally explain something about a child's condition, and they are very concerned and caring. But the doctors invariably explain most of the medical problems and educate families about them. Since the new TV documentary spotlights the human foibles and problems of hospital staff, we discover that Phillips is on her third divorce and that nurses, like doctors, have trouble balancing work and family life.

The main function of the nursing staff, however, seems to be to serve as a cheerleading squad for the surgeon. Drummond-Webb obviously deserves credit for his many accomplishments. But the show almost deifies him and nurses play a major role in the process. In the lead-in to one show, a nurse appears in a small box saying of Drummond-Webb, "You can do anything. You're our hero." Jean Ann Phillips repeatedly extols Drummond-Webb's talents and virtues. "He's a good person," she tells us, and we see her massaging his shoulders. In another episode, Phillips says, "He's just brilliant. He knows what's going on in the room all the time. I mean what he's doing, what the circulators are doing, what perfusion is doing, what anesthesia is doing, he has the ability to know what everybody is doing and still concentrate on what he's got to do."

When a difficult operation is finished, Phillips exclaims, "What an amazing job he did. It was like I'd been witness to a miracle almost." She was so high after witnessing the surgeons at work that she couldn't sleep and had to call another nurse to ask her, Can you believe he did that? Working with such a brilliant surgeon, the narrator tells us, makes a nurse's personal sacrifices worth it, even the long hours away from her family.

Of course, doctors like this surgeon do extraordinary things and seem to be gods who hold life and death in their hands. That TV gives them air time is not the problem. The problem is that no one ever talks about the knowledge, skill, or even brilliance of the nurses. Indeed, the only significant decision that we see chief nurse Jean Ann Phillips make concerns a humorous gift the staff presents to Drummond-Webb for his forty-second birthday. As they prepare to offer him a cake decorated with "You da Man" in sugar icing, she and the staff wonder whether to dress a naked, life-size rubber doll—"Dirty Diane"—in OR scrubs.

Public affairs officer Tom Bonner told me that the show will help the public understand that nurses in the ICU and OR have special qualifications and are specially trained. "Some people don't understand that," said Bonner, who wanted to see nursing presented in a positive light. But from what we see on the air we learn nothing about the training of these nurses.

ICU does a disservice to more than nurses. It does a disservice to the public. The show fails to present what real high-tech medical treatment involves. Nurses serve as the early-warning and intervention systems in hospitals. On *ICU* babies, toddlers, and adolescents exit the OR with tubes snaking out of every orifice, with lines attaching them to a baffling array of monitors, and with a patchwork of stitches covering their torso. And then, a few minutes later, they leave the hospital looking good as new. The arduous period of recovery is left on the cutting room floor. When that happens, it's hard to understand why researchers like Aiken say that nurses are the early-warning and intervention system in health care. And it's hard to understand the risks that we, as patients, face when we sign on for surgery or other high-tech procedures.

As if to underscore the way the media often trivializes nursing, in the September issue of *Better Homes and Gardens*, an article explained to patients how they could have a "worry-free hospital stay." The secret? "Take individually wrapped chocolates, put them in a bowl with a sign that reads "Please help yourself," and leave them in the room. Word will spread and you can be virtually certain your loved one will be checked on regularly." That's because, according to the article, "nurses love chocolates."[41]

How Patients Write about Nursing

Any analysis of nursing in the media would be incomplete without looking at how patients write about their experiences with nursing. Although there are many books in which patients or family members write about the experience of illness, most focus on the role of the doctor. Two recent examples illustrate this phenomenon, Christopher Reeve's pair of books detailing his experiences after his accident and a book in which the famous "Central Park jogger" revealed her identity and wrote about her ordeal.

In his 1998 memoir *Still Me*, Reeve describes the riding accident in Culpepper, Virginia, that severed his spinal cord and required high-tech surgery at the University of Virginia Medical Center, which saved his life, and his arduous course of rehabilitation at the Kessler Institute for Rehabilitation in New Jersey. Reeve's every waking moment is a triumph of the art and science of care giving. His moving account of his new life adds much to any reader's understanding of the realities of illness. Unfortunately, his book also tends to reinforce some of the old gender-based stereotypes about who does what in our health care system and why. Although he identifies his main doctors by their first and last names, only

196   one of the core of nurses who played major roles in his hospital care is named, by her first name only.

Admittedly, a patient like Reeve may not remember much about his initial hospitalization. But, in this case, the author has clearly made an effort to learn a great deal about how his case was handled so he could recreate the details of it for the reader. Of the ICU nurses who kept him alive for a month he writes, "The nurses were so gentle. I still remember their sweet southern voices, trying to strike the correct balance between being sympathetic and being straightforward. One morning a favorite nurse, Joni, arranged for me to be taken up on the roof of the hospital to watch the sunrise."[42]

Empathy and comfort are, of course, key components of nursing care. But the nurses who tended to Reeve were not just nice people, they were experts in providing lifesaving critical care. They continuously adjusted medication and treatment to maintain his blood pressure, heart and respiratory rate, and his oxygen saturation and also acted to prevent complications like pneumonia and serious pressure sores. In an era when hospitals are laying off expert nurses, readers would have benefited greatly from learning about nurses' knowledge and expertise. Unwittingly, Reeve also reinforces the notion that caregivers work for love, not money. When he discusses the care giving delivered by his aide at Kessler he says, "That's his mission. That's why he's been there for fourteen years, earning eight dollars an hour. It's his service, his giving, his gift."[43] I actually think it's because he has never been given a raise.

Four years later, Reeve published another book, *Nothing Is Impossible*, in which he details his long journey toward what he hopes will be recovery. With arduous effort, he has, in fact, done what some considered to be impossible: move his little finger. In this book, he revisits his accident and his time in the hospital. The nurses who cared for Reeve would probably be quite amazed to learn that he attributed their many contributions to doctors. "The critical care," he writes, "was nothing short of miraculous. Dr. John Jane—arguably one of the best neurosurgeons in the world—achieved the nearly impossible feat of reattaching the base of my skull to my spinal column with wire, titanium, and bone grafted from my hip. Under his watchful eye, a team of internists and pulmonologists cured me of ulcers and pneumonia." And later, nurses might be even more surprised to see themselves further demoted from clinicians to adolescent family members when he comments, "I was like a child and the doctors seemed like parents, while the nurses became older brothers and sisters."[44]

Another high-profile case that received a great deal of media attention at the time, was the case of the "Central Park jogger," Trisha Meili. On the night of April 19, 1989, when Meili was jogging in New York's Central

Park, she was attacked, raped, savagely beaten, and left for dead. To pro- **197** tect her privacy, in the extensive media attention following the attack and in the subsequent trial of her alleged attackers, her name was kept confidential. In most of the media coverage in both the immediate aftermath of the crime and in follow-up stories, the focus was on the doctors who treated her many injuries.

For almost fourteen years Meili kept her identity secret. Then in 2003 she came out of her self-imposed anonymity and wrote an account of her long struggle to recover her life and bodily function. When she describes her first days in the hospital, she establishes the medical frame through which we will view her treatment and recovery. "And so it went, doctors working nonstop to save my life, neurologists watching for signs of understanding, my family by my side."[45]

Because Meili, like Reeve, was in a coma much of the time and cannot remember what happened to her, she had to reconstruct her treatment and recovery through conversations with those who cared for her. Her primary guide is Dr. Robert S. Kurtz, director of surgical intensive care, who cared for her during her seven-week stay at the hospital. When she was admitted to the intensive care unit, Kurtz tells her, her life was "hanging by a thread," and he had to make sure "nobody made any stupid mistakes." Is the implication here that, without his vigilance, the ICU nurses would have killed her? Kurtz also tells her he agreed to allow private duty nurses to care for Meili, because "they could do all those little extra things for you, massaging you, applying lotions, getting you into and out of bed, things like that."[46]

Meili seeks out one of her private nurses, Patricia Babb, to ask about the nurse's actions. Babb talks about the incredible skill and judgment she mobilized to care for Meili. "You were bruised and they had you tied to the bed," she says heatedly. "But I'm a hands-on nurse. You don't hurt patients, you do everything possible to ease their transition from illness into health. So I immediately untied you because you were fighting the restraints, and it seemed to me you were reliving the attack over and over. I told you, 'You're safe. It's over. You're not there anymore. You're safe now.'" To keep her safe, Babb made sure visitors didn't strain her and bathed her carefully so that she didn't develop bedsores or other complications. "The doctors couldn't understand how I could calm you, because I think they weren't listening to you. Patients know what's happening to them even when they're in pain or unconscious," Babb explains.[47]

While Meili is effusive in her praise of Babb, not surprisingly, given the cultural frame through which most people view nursing, she attributes these skilled judgments not to clinical knowledge but to her "nurturing."[48]

Fallout on the Public

Day after day, year after year, citizens of advanced industrialized societies are inundated with the media images about health care that I have described. Given the messages explicitly or implicitly delivered by the entertainment and journalistic media, would anyone who has not been hospitalized and benefited from nursing care imagine that such care is indeed a matter of life and death, rather than simply the gooey pink frosting on the medical cake?

While writing this book I got an intimate view of how patients and family members process these media and cultural messages about nursing. A friend of our family was diagnosed with multiple myeloma, a bone marrow cancer that attacked his kidneys. He received a potent chemotherapy regimen and thrice-weekly dialysis, but he remained very sick and became increasingly immobile and depressed. After about three months, he developed a blood clot in the leg and one of the most potentially catastrophic consequences of illness and immobility, a pulmonary embolus. A piece of the blood clot broke off from his leg, traveled to his lung and blocked the pulmonary artery, which could have killed him.

In these days of cost cutting, he had received fragmented nursing care both in the hospital and at home—with a dialysis nurse in the dialysis clinic, a chemotherapy nurse in his oncologist's office, and a "pump nurse," who would come and check the chemotherapy infusion pump that delivered his therapy while he was at home. When I learned that my friend had been admitted to the intensive care unit and was receiving treatment for this complication, I saw what was missing in this array of uncoordinated nursing care: a home care nurse who could have gotten him up and moving and overcome the resistance with which he'd greeted his wife's and daughters' entreaties, "Please, get up, Pop."

When I mentioned this to his daughter, she told me that one of the many doctors involved in his care had, in fact, suggested that he might benefit from home care nursing. But his wife refused. "That's just babysitting," his wife said dismissively. A former child care provider herself, she thought she could do a perfectly good job "baby-sitting" her husband. What she didn't know, and what her doctor didn't tell her (and what she has not learned from the mass media culture), was that nursing is not baby-sitting, that getting a sick man to walk may make the difference between life and death and requires knowledge, persistence, and sheer grit. This failure to understand the significance of nursing care almost cost her husband his life, complicated the process of his treatment, delayed what was to be, unfortunately, a very short remission, and added unnecessary

suffering to an already dreadful illness and a dramatically shortened life, **199**
not to mention adding thousands of dollars to the cost of his hospital bill.

What this suggests is that patients and the public do not "get it" by
simply watching nurses do their job. Many seem to believe that nurses are
nice—and yes, ever so ethical and honest—but nursing is not where the
challenge is. In part this is because of the media presentation of nursing.
But it's more complex than that. Nurses themselves are deeply ambivalent
about public communication. Recipients of strong social messages about
altruism and self-sacrifice, inheritors of a legacy of religious self-
effacement, put in their place by doctors or their own institutions, and socialized to deliver confused messages about who they are and what they
do, nurses themselves may unwittingly reinforce the public image they insist needs changing and, in this way, make the profession seem less important and attractive than it really is.

8

Unavailable for Comment

On the night of October 12, 2002, Barry Morley, his wife Kate Simpson, and their fourteen-year-old daughter Grace were in the Dewi Sri Hotel in Bali, where they'd gone to try to recover from the death of their twelve-year-old son Ben three months earlier. As the family of Australians was settling for the evening, at about eleven o'clock, they were startled by a huge noise and felt the building shake as something hit the side of the hotel and tore off part of its roof. A few minutes later there was another shattering blast and Morley and his family could see a red mushroom cloud rising above the area. Everything went silent and fell into total darkness. What they heard, of course, were the explosions at Paddy's Bar and the Sari Club in the terrorist attack known as the Bali Bombing.

After the blasts, the family quickly headed for the foyer of the hotel, where they found people panicking. Burn victims were already streaming down the narrow lane that led from the clubs to the hotel. Before they even realized the dimensions of the attack, they went into action. Both Barry and Kate were nurses. Burn victims, they knew, need to be bathed in water. But the water coming out of the hotels' faucets would be contaminated, so they put these burn victims in the chlorinated swimming pool.

Coincidentally, before he went to Bali, Morley had been the coordinator of Postgraduate Studies in Critical Care, a program that included disaster management. Although he had no hands-on experience, he knew the first thing he needed to do was to extricate people from the site.

When Morley arrived at the two clubs, what he found was, he said, inconceivable. "The Sari club was truly ablaze; you couldn't approach it. **201** The area between Paddy's and Sari's was a sea of blood, of burnt flesh and mutilation. A lot of people inside Sari's couldn't get out." Morley also worried that another bomb might be about to go off, and four cars were on fire and about to explode. Morley's first estimate was that maybe 50 people had died and there were 100 badly injured. He didn't know that 202 had died—88 of them Australians—and 400 had been injured.

The smoldering Paddy's Bar had been hit by a smaller bomb. The first floor had collapsed. There were no ambulances or police services, no fire brigade. People were in shock. They stood around and stared. About a dozen young men with shrapnel injuries were standing in front of the blazing club, hurt but able to walk. Morley immediately classified them as "the walking wounded," and they became his temporary assistants. "You and you," Morley commanded, "pick up that bloke there, and take him to the end of that lane. I'll meet you there shortly to treat him."

In the midst of the rescue process Simpson arrived. When she saw Morley she realized the extent and danger of the scene and said she would return to the Dewi Sri to receive patients. Of major concern in Simpson's mind was that they couldn't both risk losing their lives and leaving their daughter parentless. So Simpson stayed at the hotel to treat the victims and Morley returned to Paddy's. "The place was an absolute bloody war zone," Morley said. "The first floor was collapsing in on us. There were live electrical wires everywhere. I was tripping over people. Standing on people. Some of them were dead."

Within forty minutes, there were forty or fifty victims back at the hotel. But, as he exclaimed to his wife in frustration, they had no medical equipment or medications to treat them. "We didn't have an IV canula. We didn't have IV fluids. We had no intercostal catheters. We couldn't intubate and ventilate people." To which Simpson replied, "You've got to forget what we don't have and think about what we do have."

So Morley and Simpson organized teams of helpers—guests who didn't flee the hotel at the first explosions. The teams of assistants scoured the hotel for blankets, bottled water, sheets for bandages, and wood for splints. They searched for any medications they could find. Because skin is the major barrier to infection and keeps fluids inside the body, burn victims must be kept clean and hydrated. Because skin regulates temperature, burn victims must be kept warm to prevent hypothermia. Their newly recruited nursing assistants soaked the sheets in the swimming pool and bathed patients to maintain hydration. Blankets were used to prevent hypothermia. Many of the victims had open chest wounds, which meant they were at risk for a collapsed lung. So they searched for plastic bags and stuffed them around the wound cavity to prevent this potentially fatal

202   complication. Helpers applied tourniquets to severed limbs, compressed shrapnel wounds, collected bottled water to use for eye burns, or stayed with the terrified victims to reassure them. A cancer patient donated her oral narcotics.

At three in the morning the first ambulance arrived. But the drivers had to be taught how to handle the victims. Only two of their fifty-five patients died. One died, Morley fears, because the ambulance crew laid the patient down, against their advice. At five o'clock that morning an ambulance took the last victim to the hospital. Morley and Simpson closed their makeshift emergency unit.

As the authorities got word of the disaster, the media circus began. Although dozens of people lived because of their actions, Morley and Simpson more or less disappeared into the crowd. They talked to one large Australian paper and briefed police and government officials. That was all. A few other nurses who had worked on the helicopters evacuating patients from Bali to Australia, or who had been on vacation and volunteered at the hospital in Bali, had given press interviews. So did doctors. From a reporter's point of view, Morley and Simpson had, to put it mildly, a very dramatic experience. They were alone for hours helping scores of victims. Unlike their medical and nursing colleagues at the local hospital, they had no drugs or medical equipment, and they weren't working with teams of professionals. In a matter of minutes, they set up and staffed a virtual field hospital in a war zone. Yet, apart from the police briefing, the newspaper interview, and conversations with their closest friends, for a year and a half Morley and Simpson had not talked about the incident. When he talked to the press, he downplayed their contributions, attributing their actions to "common sense."

Common sense? I have plenty of that, but as I listened to his story, all I could think of was the incredible skill and knowledge it took to do what Morley and Simpson had done. Had I—or anyone who wasn't a medical professional—been confronted with a disaster of this magnitude, the immediate response would have been the paralysis of horror. Even if we were capable of action we wouldn't have known what to do without expert leadership. How many laypeople would analyze the sterility of the water supply and recognize that burn victims need to be put in a chlorinated swimming pool? I know I probably would have fainted at the sight of an open chest wound. Had I not, I certainly wouldn't have known that I needed to protect the wound with plastic bags to prevent a collapsed lung. I didn't even know lungs could collapse from an open chest wound until Morley told me.

Like most of the world, I learned about the two nurses' experiences only in 2003. That's when I gave a talk to three hundred nurses gathered

at a conference of the Royal College of Nursing Australia (RCNA), on **203**
Australia's Gold Coast. During the talk, I urged nurses to tell their stories.
Morley, it turned out, was one of the nurses in the audience. After my
talk, Barry Morley was scheduled to give a presentation himself. He decided to take that opportunity to tell the story of what he and his wife had
accomplished to his nursing colleagues and to the Australian public.

Why did these nurses shun the limelight? Perhaps it was because they,
understandably, did not want to relive a very traumatic experience. Morley said they were also concerned about the people they couldn't save.
They may have also wanted to avoid the media circus that resulted from
the incident. In an era of reality TV, sensationalistic talk shows, and
tabloids, the media sometimes appear downright threatening. Nurses may
legitimately fear the side effects of media attention—being quoted out of
context, being misquoted, or having one's story spun to fit a reporter's
agenda rather than the facts. Sometimes people don't want to talk to the
media because they had spent precious time talking to reporters without
ever seeing any of their views appear in the news. Morley undoubtedly experienced some of this. But he also told the RCNA audience that he did
not want to appear to be blowing his own horn. He had, however, decided
to tell his story—not for himself, he said, but for nursing.

These concerns aren't unique to nurses. Many other groups share these
fears, but doctors and lawyers, social workers, teachers, and many others
have overcome them. They understand that, in a mass media culture,
learning how to talk to the press is critical to professional survival. For too
many nurses these understandable concerns become insurmountable obstacles. Public communication seems to be synonymous with public exposure, and public exposure, many nurses seem to feel, will result in serious,
negative professional and personal consequences.[1]

This cultural and individual resistance to public communication adds
an important dimension to the problem of how nurses are depicted in the
media and why they are so invisible in the public discussion about health
care. Journalists and hospital PR people must take responsibility for not
seeking out nurses as subjects and sources of stories and insights. But
nurses' own fears of public exposure also make it difficult for members of
the media to construct a more accurate portrait of the profession.

Nurses and the Public

As I've thought about nursing silence over the years, I've often considered
what it would take to convince more nurses to speak about their work.
Why do people tell their stories? What encourages them to inform others
about their work and voice their opinions and concerns? As a journalist, it

204 seems to me there are certain nonnegotiable conditions that make voice possible. First, you have to believe you have done something, seen something, or thought something worth talking about. You have to believe that you have played a role in an event, that you're an agent in the action, and that you "own" your ideas, experiences, or insights. You also have to believe that you deserve credit for what you've done. It's important to believe that what you say, or write, will be received—someone will hear you, read you, or see you—and thus acknowledge your existence and actions. Although it's important to understand that some people may disagree with you, it's equally important to believe that someone will support you. (When I give a speech, for example, I always seek out the face in the crowd that's smiling and nodding and studiously avoid the one scowling or falling asleep.) It certainly helps to feel that you won't be punished for speaking out and to believe that even if voice involves risk, it will be a risk worth taking. It's also important to have role models and leaders who teach you that talking about your work is acceptable, even expected, behavior.

Yet, because of the history of nursing and its social downgrading, thousands, perhaps even millions, of nurses seem to lack this sense of agency, ownership, authority, and support. They fear retribution or punishment for speaking up and lack role models who would make it easier for them to talk about their contributions and concerns.

What I have come to think of as a publicly articulated "practice narrative" is, therefore, poorly developed in nursing. A practice narrative consists of compelling, credible stories—told in comprehensible, everyday language—that describe the routine activities and contributions of everyday clinicians as they make a difference to the people they care for. As I define it, a practice narrative would help the public understand why we need nurses at the bedside—wherever that bedside may be—by illuminating the complexity of what seem to be the simplest nursing tasks. It would explain why nurses are educated not born, why they need social resources to do their work, why they need good working conditions and decent collegial relationships, and why they need authority within their institutions. A fully developed practice narrative—the kind, for example, physicians routinely mobilize—would allow us to see why the bedside matters.

Instead, what one finds in nursing is a growing research narrative, an advanced educational narrative, or a protest narrative. The research narrative focuses on abstract scientific discussions of nursing work, as well as the statistical mapping of the nursing work force and its problems and contributions. It also investigates the efficacy of nursing activities and nursing treatments (here, I simply refuse to use the term that nurses have adopted, "nursing interventions") and recommends changes and refinements in the delivery of nursing care. This narrative is of course important and does not receive enough attention from the media.

The advanced educational narrative tells us what nurses can accomplish when liberated from the traditional constraints imposed on their authority and activity, and often focuses on how nurses are moving away from the bedside and toward medical roles. Again, this narrative is important in showing us the kinds of work nurses do. But it tends to be presented, as Sioban Nelson and I have written, in a way that creates discontinuity between nurses' past accomplishments and their present ones, and between nurses at the bedside and colleagues in "advanced" roles. For that reason, Nelson and I worry that it represents what we call "a rhetoric of rupture" which subtly denigrates the contributions of contemporary nurses' foremothers as well as those who remain at the bedside today.[2]

What I call nursing's "protest narrative" emphasizes the problems nurses have in doing their work, the difficulties they have on the job, and the resources they lack. This protest narrative has become very robust today as nurses face cost cutting and deskilling, and as nurses grapple with their poor public image and try to enhance it.

All of these narratives are critical and necessary. But they are no substitute for a practice narrative that creates a clear view of the continuity of concerns and progress within the profession, that brings statistics and scientific language to life, and that tells us why we should care if there are not enough nurses or if they are having difficulty getting a decent wage and better working conditions.

Because this practice narrative is so poorly developed, when you ask a nurse to describe his or her work to a reporter, or even to talk to a friend, family member, or neighbor, within seconds, too many nurses will tell you not what they do but why they can't talk about it. This is a worldwide phenomenon.

"How can I describe the essence of nursing?" an RN in Copenhagen asks, desperately struggling to describe everything every nurse does everywhere. (But when I ask her to describe what she actually does as an infection control nurse, she swiftly moves from painful inarticulateness to fluency—in English no less.)

"Nursing is so depressing. No one wants to hear about it," says a nurse in Toronto.

"Nursing is so intimate, we can't talk about our work. It's a sacred trust," says a nursing student at the University of Melbourne.

"Why do we need to talk about nursing at all? We do wonderful things. Patients will understand," a fourth-year male nursing student at Boston College argues.

206   "If we talk too much about what we do, doctors will get angry," a nurse in Reykjavik worries.

"I don't need public recognition for my work. All I need is gratitude in the eyes of my patients," says a nurse during a call-in talk show after I suggested that the press should give nurses more ink.

"We've taken a vow of silence when we go into nursing," a nurse informs me during a talk in Stockholm. "We can't talk about our patients because that would violate patient confidentiality."

"Who owns the story?" an army nurse in Washington, DC, asks when I suggest she and other military nurses talk about their accomplishments in the Iraq War. "Do we own it? Does the patient? The military? The taxpayer?"

Nurses everywhere: "If we talk about what's wrong with the system, we'll get fired." Or, "Who am I to speak for nursing? I'm not an expert. I'm just a nurse."

So long as nurses say they cannot tell you about their work because it is too mysterious (or sacred, ineffable, diffuse, tedious, extraordinary), or because someone else (the doctor, hospital, or taxpayer) owns it, they will find it difficult to give reporters and the public a clearer picture of their work.

The Nurse-Journalist Encounter

"Among nurses, there's a tremendous desire for a better image, but they all think that somebody else should make the change," says Anne Schott, describing her difficulties getting nurses to talk to the press during her sixteen-year stint as communications director at the New York State Nurses Association. "If I asked RNs to speak to a journalist and they said, 'Oh no, I can't do it tomorrow, maybe we could set up an appointment next Thursday,' I'd say, 'What?' It was difficult to convince nurses that the way to get on television is to be available now, when you're wanted. Getting more publicity for nurses takes effort, some outreach and collaboration, and someone being available, and they don't want to do it."

Schott says that even when she asked nurses to tell stories about how they made a difference to patients, what she often got were stories about how patients made a difference to their nurse. "They'd tell us how moving it was to care for various patients, how brave their patients were through all their sufferings. But that wasn't what we were looking for, quite the opposite."

"Even when topics were not controversial, like infection control, many nurses who were expert in clinical areas and who had published in research journals refused to be interviewed by reporters because they did not want to put themselves forward as experts or claim to be speaking for the hospital or the profession," Schott says. Generally, she adds, they didn't want to be connected to anything that appeared to be controversial or overtly political.

This fear of controversy, which has its origins in nursing's tricky relationship with church officials, is very pervasive. When Jack Kevorkian was busily assisting dying patients in dozens of suicides, I wondered why more palliative care and hospice nurses didn't take advantage of the media opening he presented. A number of palliative care physicians jumped into the fray to talk about their alternative model for the care of the dying. Why didn't RNs? When I posed this question to some prominent palliative care nurses, they said they had considered entering the debate but decided against it. Why? Because they didn't want their model of nursing care to be tainted by Kevorkian's physician-assisted suicide.

Whatever the reason, "a lot of times nurses don't want to talk to the press," says UCSF Medical Center's Maureen McInaney. "I call them up and say someone wants to talk to you and they say, 'Oh I'm sorry, I couldn't do that. Reporters always twist things.' They worry about being misquoted. They worry about taking up too much space or credit. A lot of time they feel they're taking attention from the physicians, who, unfortunately, they inaccurately see as their superiors. Doctors are more worried about what other colleagues will think. Nurses are more worried about what other providers will think, like doctors." Thus, she says, a call from a PR staffer inviting the nurse to speak about a particular subject might be met with "Oh, that should really be so-and-so's domain. He's really the expert on that."

Of course, she adds, some physicians don't like attention, or worry that their colleagues will think they are media hungry and thus not true research scientists. With nurses, she says, it's different. "They themselves don't value their profession enough. They undermine their own work. 'Oh, I couldn't possibly' is the mantra."

The result is that nurses may fail to create or take advantage of media openings. Consider Raja Mishra's story about the patient undergoing experimental treatment for breast cancer. Although I believe Mishra skewed his story in a way that ignored the role nurses and other clinicians play in scientific research, he may not have gotten much encouragement from nurses to include their contributions in his articles. When I interviewed him about his experience, he admitted that he'd focused on one doctor for dramatic effect. He added, however, that during the eight months he spent at the Farber, nurses—with the exception of a research nurse who talked freely—seemed wary of his presence and did not seek him out to explain their work. Mishra is only one of many journalists to note this phenomenon.

In preparation for a talk she gave to a nursing group, Madge Kaplan, then Boston bureau chief and health desk editor of Public Radio International's *Marketplace* at WGBH Radio, surveyed a group of journalistic colleagues who cover health care. She asked them what it was like to work with nurses. These journalists, she said, expressed several frustrations. Many commented that "nurses are fearful about talking with the press—especially if they're coming from nonunionized workplaces. There is sympathy and understanding for why this is the case—understanding that for many registered nurses, talking to the press could jeopardize their jobs. Still, relationships with the media are built on being able to speak out."

Reporters also found a lack of media savvy among groups that claim leadership in nursing. These groups, the journalists said, "don't pitch stories to reporters." Kaplan said she "heard that again and again."

The journalists she surveyed "pointed out that nursing groups or their public relations representatives don't reach out to reporters to find out how best to relate and work together. Reporters don't seem to know which nursing groups to pay attention to, or who the important nursing leaders are. And when stories break, reporters say, spokespeople are difficult to track down. This is in stark contrast to physicians, who by reporters' standards seem very organized and media savvy."

Kaplan acknowledged how difficult it is to "sell" editors on stories about nursing. The media "must take some responsibility for not covering issues relating to nursing." But so should nursing. "Nurses," she said bluntly, "play a role in making things somewhat worse . . . and undermine the interest that does exist in the media world."[3]

The veteran medical reporter Irene Wielawski's experiences reflect those of many of her colleagues. Wielawski has covered medical innovations, high-profile medical cases and events, as well as the problem of the uninsured in the United States. Throughout her career, many of the nurses she has interviewed have, she says, reinforced traditional stereotypes of what nursing work is about and who is important in the medical hierarchy. "Nurses," she says, "seem more concerned than any other health care professionals we routinely interview with not taking credit but instead modestly assigning credit to others. There's a lot of demurring and reinforcing of the traditional medical hierarchy. Nurses," she puts it colorfully, "are constantly lowercasing themselves."

Modesty is "a laudable professional trait," Wielawski acknowledges. However, "from a very practical standpoint, it complicates the interview." "Remember, a reporter is always working under some kind of deadline pressure. So if you ask a question and you cannot get a crisp answer—because the person spends the first three or four minutes saying, 'Before I answer that, I'd just like to say I'm very grateful for the opportunity to

work with such a wonderful staff and I couldn't have done this alone'—
this puts the reporter in a very awkward position. A journalist simply
doesn't have the time and opportunity, or even the good manners, to say,
'Excuse me, could you please speak up or talk to me specifically about the
unique nursing function?' You can't ask the question twice, or coax and
cajole people."

Wielawski gives a telling example of the concrete difficulties a reporter
can encounter when dealing with reluctant nurses. In February 2003 a
band playing in The Station, a nightclub in Providence, Rhode Island, illegally set off fireworks on-stage, igniting a huge blaze that killed or injured hundreds of young people. The *New York Times* asked Wielawski to
drive up to Rhode Island to write about how a small state—one whose
hospitals that had no dedicated burn units—dealt with such an over-
whelming influx of burn victims. Some patients were cared for at Rhode
Island Hospital, where the chief of surgery, who was, fortuitously, a burn
specialist, turned two ICUs into burn units.

Before she traveled to Rhode Island, Wielawski called the hospital PR
department to outline the purpose of her story. She said she wanted to describe the continuum of care for burn patients and asked PR to arrange
interviews with key players involved in the care of these patients. She also
talked with EMTs and firefighters about their experiences. They were all
very cooperative.

When she arrived at Rhode Island Hospital, the PR staff had arranged
for her to talk to the president of the hospital, who was a physician, and
the chief of surgery. Although she had requested all the key players, no
nurses were included. In the course of her interview, she asked the doctors
about the mechanics of maintaining fluid levels in bodies that were losing
a huge volume of fluid because of the loss of so much skin surface. People
were comparing this fire to the spectacular Coconut Grove fire in Boston,
when many patients died of kidney failure. Part of Wielawski's mission
was to learn whether new burn science was able to maintain kidney function and how. But when she asked for concrete details, Wielawski recounts, "The surgeon replied, 'That's really a nursing function. You need
to talk to a nurse about that.' Three times in the interview he deferred
without any ceremony to nurses."

So Wielawski did the logical thing. She turned to the PR staffer and
said, "Can you find me a nurse who is very expert in burn care?" Without
any hesitation, the PR staffer went into his office to fulfill her request.
Wielawski noted that there was a lot of talking back and forth on the
phone before the PR person came out and asked her if she could possibly
wait in the hospital for two hours, when the nurses were off their shift.
Why? Wielawski asked.

210   He told her that six nurses wanted to come down and talk to her, but they couldn't do so until the shift ended.

Wielawski took a deep breath and said, "No, I cannot do an interview with six nurses. I need one nurse who can speak to the problem and I need to do it now, because I need to leave for New York to write my story."

Recognizing the legitimacy of this request—she hadn't after all, talked with every doctor involved in the care of these patients—the PR person disappeared into his office and there were more phone calls. Finally, one nurse agreed to come down and talk to her.

When they met, Wielawski explained that she was on deadline and what she wanted to learn from the nurse. She told the nurses she needed to understand the problem of the loss of fluid through the skin in, say, a 50 percent burn victim. She wanted to know the exact quantities of saline solution you have to be pumping into this patient in order to get a certain amount of fluid output through the kidneys so you don't have kidney failure.

Instead of telling her what she needed to know, Wielawski says, the nurse was very uncomfortable. "She started by telling me that she really wants to give credit to the team. She wanted to talk about how wonderful it is to work under this doctor who's so knowledgeable. She said they were so proud of the care patients were getting and explained that it had been a tough but incredible experience. She led with all these emotional statements."

Wielawski pauses. "Although I recognize how intimidating it can be to talk to journalists, I have to tell you, I was starting to hyperventilate. I was so aware of my deadline. I knew I was going to be driving all night and had to start writing my story. So I said to the nurse I was interviewing, 'You know, I'm on a very tight deadline, and I urgently need for you to tell me about the science of fluid management.' "

Finally, the nurse told her what she needed to know. "When I put urgency into the question, she immediately started giving me all the science." The nurse explained why fluid management is a critical nursing function, gave her needed technical details about how its done and described the almost minute-by-minute monitoring patients receive from their nurses.

"She was brilliant," Wielawski concludes. "The knowledge was all there. The surgeon was correct in deferring to her. It ended up being a paragraph or a couple of phrases in a very complicated story that had interviews with people, many of whom were never quoted. But it was very important information that helped me present the issues to the general public and to explain the continuum of burn care."

We can understand why a nurse might worry when a reporter from the

New York Times comes to call. But nurses also balk when the person solic- **211**
iting their story is a nurse who wants to write a positive portrait of nursing work. In the late nineties, when nurse Echo Heron was working on a
book called *Tending Lives: Nurses on the Medical Front,* she experienced
similar frustrations.[4] Heron wanted to collect stories from nurses in a variety of fields and then present them to the lay public. Heron thought she
would have no trouble finding nurses who would agree to share their stories with her.

She was wrong. She talked to hundreds of nurses and told them the
same thing. "I told them I was writing a book about what it was like to
walk in their shoes. I invited them to tell me why they became nurses. I
asked them to tell me a story that's made a difference in their life. I was
looking for all kinds of stories, spiritual stories, that one story, that one
patient, that you will never forget, the one that made you grow as a person, the one you still pray for, the one that still makes you laugh."

No matter how much she emphasized the positive nature of her project, nurses were reluctant to cooperate. "Most of them were scared about
losing their jobs. 'If the hospital ever finds out that I talked to you and
that that's my story, they'll sue me, fire me.' I told them this is completely
confidential. I promised to change their name, the place where they work
and live. I told them I never reveal a patient's name." None of Heron's as-
surances seemed to matter.

With great difficulty Heron found thirty-eight nurses who would share
their stories with her. When they heard about her project, five nurses who
had cared for people during the Oklahoma City federal building bombing
e-mailed Heron and asked if they could be included in the book. With the
exception of these nurses and a few others, the majority of the nurses were
adamant that Heron not attach their names to even the most positive, up-
beat stories. So Heron made up pseudonyms—"Medlina W.," "Mildred
M."—to identify the nurses.

The kind of frustrations that Wielawski, Kaplan, and Heron describe
may explain why even more nurse-friendly PR staff hesitate to put nurses
forward as spokespeople in critical, breaking stories. The job of the PR
department is, after all, to help, not frustrate journalists. Because of
nurses' ambivalent relationship to the press, Maureen McInaney says, she
tends to save nurses for less frenzied moments. She will ask a nurse to
speak when the issue is nursing research, the nursing shortage, or the role
nurses plays in the science of care.

But if nurses' comments are limited to the nursing shortage, as McI-
naney herself points out, the public will view nurses "only as subject of
crisis, not as experts who can reflect on any issue." Similarly, limiting
frontline nurses' participation in the news cycle would also leave them out

212 of coverage of nursing research or other stories about advances in nursing treatment and science. While we certainly need to hear from more nursing researchers or advanced practice nurses, we also need to hear how that research translates into the practice of the person delivering nursing care. Frontline caregivers will not necessarily feel that nurse researchers or advanced practice nurses are their role models any more than they feel that physicians and biomedical researchers are.

If nurses—frontline nurses as well as more elite RNs—are to get more ink, they need to be included in breaking stories about medical innovation. These are the staples of daily medical reporting and, as we've seen, they almost always exclude the nurses who have participated in these breakthroughs and have actively contributed to the advance of medical knowledge.

Why Are Nurses So Afraid to Speak about Their Work?

That nurses feel so afraid to tell their stories, even positive ones that would enhance their professional image, has a great deal to do with their relationships with physicians, workplace experiences, and contemporary professional socialization.

Many bedside nurses have told me they hesitate to broadcast publicly the realities of their work because they fear physician anger or retaliation. As we've seen in Part One, this fear of doctors is based on real experience and on learned powerlessness. When, for example, I wrote my first story, "The Crisis in Caring," for the *Boston Globe*, I didn't include much about doctors at all. Yet nurses at the Beth Israel Hospital told me that some MDs complained because physicians were not in the story. Hildur Helgadottir, a nurse manager in Iceland, related an even more disturbing incident. Nurses in her hospital were taking care of a young woman who had breast reduction surgery. The surgery went well, but the next day, when a nurse was doing her morning checkup, she began to notice signs that the young woman was in trouble. "While she was in the room, the woman gradually got shorter of breath, paler, more anxious, and restless. The nurse called another nurse in for a consult and after having taken her vital signs and giving her oxygen, they called the physician and suggested the young woman was suffering a pulmonary embolism. She (the physician) agreed and thirty minutes later the patient was en route to the University hospital," Helgadottir recounts.

At the larger hospital, the patient was indeed diagnosed with a massive PE and was given aggressive treatment to try to dissolve the clot that had lodged in her pulmonary artery. The next day, the nurses and physician were talking. The physician seemed pleased with the call she had made.

When the nurses also expressed pride in the fact that they were the ones **213**
who initially identified the problem, the doctor became angry. As if the
fact that the nurses also got satisfaction from a job well done was somehow stealing her thunder, she announced huffily, "Well, I guess when
good things happen, everybody wants to take credit."

Nurses who encounter these kinds of responses will be hesitant to risk
physicians' displeasure by telling their stories. Some may worry that even
the most matter-of-fact descriptions of reality will be considered doctor
bashing. Others may seek safety in silence or confine their descriptions of
their work to the softer aspects of patient care that doctors seem unconcerned about claiming. Unfortunately, nurses may not get a lot of help
confronting these obstacles from hospital nurse management. Maureen
McInaney, for example, believes hospital PR can change, but only if institutional leaders change it. "If the vice president of nursing or the dean of
the school of nursing, or both, go to the public relations department and
tell them what's happening in the hospital or school, then nursing moves
onto the agenda, onto the radar screen."

A number of hospitals have such leadership and have injected nursing
stories into the news and public conversation about health care. But not
enough actively work with PR departments to push nursing forward,
while others inadvertently—even deliberately—silence their nurses.
When I recently spoke to a group of nursing executives in the southern
part of the United States, I gave them a short survey to try to ascertain the
level of their contact with their own PR departments.

The nurse executives in the audience were in hospitals large and small,
in cities and rural areas. I asked them if their nurses were represented in
the media and if they worked with hospital PR departments to educate
them about the role of nurses in the hospital. I asked if they'd supplied PR
departments with a list of nurses who could speak about nursing in the institution, if they had a media strategy and if they talked with the press
themselves.

Of the sixty people who filled out the questionnaire, almost all had a
nursing shortage in their hospital and most said their local and regional
media didn't cover nursing. But only fifteen said their hospital PR departments worked for nurses. Only ten out of sixty said they meet with PR
staff to educate them about nursing; eighteen reported supplying PR staff
with lists of nurses doing interesting work in their hospitals; and only ten
said their hospitals sent out press releases pitching nursing stories. In a remarkable statistic, only two out of the sixty said that they and their staff
met with reporters. Upper-level nursing leaders may also silence nurses
by eliminating some of the most assertive nurses as spokespeople, because
they may have internally criticized institutional policies.

214   Deciding who will make an institution look good is, of course, a highly subjective enterprise that can complicate the issue for nurses—particularly today. If hospital working conditions have eroded for so many nurses, hospitals may be concerned that putting a nurse forward to speak about new developments in health care would provide journalists with a story the PR department couldn't control. They may worry that a nurse who's asked to speak about the latest development in cancer treatment will also alert reporters to the latest problem delivering high-quality care to cancer patients. "PR departments were always afraid to feature nurses, except management nurses, because they were always afraid of what the bargaining unit nurses might say," Anne Schott explains. Nurses active in the union would, she said, be scratched from the list even if they were excellent clinicians.

Schott said that nurses' fears of speaking out also stem from management retaliation against nurses who overcome their sense of loyalty and try to protect their professional integrity by speaking with the media. "Everybody knows these days that in most hospitals most of the time nurses don't have the time to follow exactly the letter of the law," Schott explains. "Things are not done exactly the way they should be all the time or as the nurse would wish to do them. Nurses have too many patients, so they are always open to management criticisms that they are failing to do things that management knows they can't do. They are very vulnerable."

Middle-level nurse managers can also play an important role in either encouraging or discouraging nurses from speaking about their work.

In May 2003, I was invited to speak at a prominent U.S. teaching hospital for Nurses' Week, known for its innovations in medical technology and the care of seriously ill patients. At lunch, a group of nurse managers told me that a journalist from a prestigious publication was in the hospital following patients undergoing a variety of state-of-the-art treatments. The journalist, they said, was spending a lot of time on a patient care unit.

When I learned this news, my first response was, "That's terrific, now the nurses on that unit can get to know the journalist and help him understand the role of military nurses." Before I could express this sentiment and explain how nurses could make use of this opportunity, a nurse manager interrupted, practically boasting. "Of course, the managers have instructed the nurses to avoid the journalist and be very careful to protect patient confidentiality."

How ironic, I thought. I had been invited to talk to nurses about how to move from silence to voice and to tell their stories. These nurses had the perfect opportunity to turn their yearning for a better public image into conversations that might produce that public image. Unlike physicians who are schooled to talk about their work and how to talk about

their patients without violating patient confidentiality, it seemed that **215**
these managers had little education in dealing with and managing the
press. Lacking strategies that could help nurses protect patient confidentiality, their solution was "just say no."

What is true of silence seems also to be true of anonymity.

In my experience, nurse executives and managers and even academics
may inadvertently socialize nurses into the old religious notion that they
are part of a mass and should not, therefore, highlight their individual
contributions to either the patient or the health care team. In many hospitals, nurses have told me that managers often post signs proclaiming
"There is no 'I' in the word Team" on the walls of nurses' stations and
nurses' lounge rooms. In a recent article in *Advance for Nurses,* nurse leaders are exhorted to retain new recruits by encouraging teamwork, which,
according to the author and magazine, means "No 'I' in Team."[5] It's hard
to see how this advice represents an advance for nurses. In brandishing
these kinds of slogans to nurses, many of whom arrive in the workplace
having been long admonished to hide behind or inside the group, this peculiar definition of teamwork and collaboration risks muting their professional voice.

Self-Presentation and the Presentation of Nursing

In his classic book *The Presentation of Self in Everyday Life,* the sociologist
Erving Goffman analyzes the way in which people convey information
about their status, aspirations, and self-perceptions to others in what he
calls "definitional claims." Goffman tells us that a person conveys critical
information in "the expression he gives" and in "the expression he gives
off."[6] The first generally involves verbal communication while the latter
involves "a range of other actions," including how one dresses, body language, introductions, and how one generally acts on the stage of life.
Goffman spends a great deal of time dissecting initial introductions. It is
in these critical moments that the individual makes "definitional claims,"
that he "automatically exerts a moral demand upon the others, obliging
them to value and treat him in the manner that persons of his kind have a
right to expect." In order to be considered who they claim to be, Goffman
says, people try to refrain from what he calls "definitional disruptions," or
events that may occur "within the interaction which contradict, discredit,
or otherwise throw doubt upon" what a person says he wants another person to believe.[7]

Part of the process of making definitional claims involves professional
performances, and many of those that Goffman examines actually take
place in the hospital. These performances, he tells us, can either establish

216 or disrupt definitional claims. The management of initial impressions is central here, as it is in life. That's why, Goffman tells us, actors on the stage of life constantly try to exert what he calls "front region" control so that people accept the impression they say they want to give. No matter how private and intimate they believe their work, no matter where it is performed, Goffman would argue, nurses are always acting on a public stage. As Bernice Buresh and I explain, elaborating on Goffman, nurses' patients are part of their public.[8] So are patients' families and other health care professionals and workers. The patient for whom a nurse cares is both an actor, someone acted upon, and a spectator in the broader health care drama. Along with lessons on how to take their medication or change their diet, the patients are absorbing messages about status and legitimacy as they observe the intricate choreography of hierarchy that takes place around them. When subtle messages of deference conflict with the nurses' definitional claims, patients usually take notice, as do their families and friends.

When they are on the job in their professional capacity, journalists, TV writers and producers, playwrights and novelists, and even children's book writers are also part of the vast public audience that watches the health care performance unfold. Indeed, a journalist or political representative might also be a patient, or a patient's friend or relative. Nurses are thus constantly given the opportunity to confirm or contradict their own definitional claims as well as those of physicians and administrators.

Women struggling for their liberation realized the importance of this kind of performance and front region control of even the most subtle messages early on. Feminists recognized that it was crucial to change how people looked at women, talked about women, and referred to women—whether in public or private. We women knew that these changes would not just follow but would sometimes precede concrete changes in our social and work life. That's why we refused to allow men to call us "sweetie" or "cutie," give us the once-over on the street, or the "innocent" pat on the rear in the office. We insisted that newspapers identify us as "Ms." rather than "Miss" or "Mrs." because we insisted on an individual identity that was not linked to our marital status. We fought for the use of "his or her" and "humankind" instead of "his" and "mankind." We wanted to liberate ourselves from corsets and curlers and to do away with the claim that only one person could wear the pants in a family. How we dressed, how we walked, how we talked was, feminists recognized, political, and it upheld or contradicted our definitional claims.

In both private and public spaces, nurses' definitional claims to professionalism, however, seem to be constantly disrupted. Certainly without meaning to, nurses often present a confusing picture to the person who is **217** trying to take their claims seriously.

Journalists and the public receive other confusing messages about nursing. Consider, for example, the campaign around the movie *Nurse Betty*. When I first saw the movie, I recalled the protests that feminists launched against similar sexist films, or of the campaign that nurses waged against the TV series *Nightingales*. For devaluing nurses, *Nurse Betty* was certainly a close contender. Yet nursing organizations didn't protest the film. Instead, USA Films, the movie's producer, apparently convinced the National Student Nurses Association to work with it to bring more nurses to see the movie. For each of the first ten thousand nurses that went to see the movie by October 31, 2000, USA Films promised to donate one dollar to the NSNA's Nurse Betty Scholarship. The scholarship would provide financial support for undergraduate nursing education. The NSNA sent out an announcement encouraging nurses to go to the movie, instructing them to send their theater ticket stub to the Foundation for the National Student Nurses Association. "*Nurse Betty* epitomizes the universal values and ideals of nurses and nursing students," wrote Diane Mancino, executive director of the NSNA and FNSNA, in a message that was sent out to other nurses and nursing students. "With a serious nursing shortage developing throughout the United States (and internationally), the timing of this film has the potential for making a lasting contribution to the profession and society! . . . Don't miss a great film and a great opportunity to support nursing education!"[9]

Prevalent attitudes toward basic nursing work within the profession don't help nurses illuminate its importance. In an effort to combat the idea that nursing is made up of tedious work, many nurse academics and other professional leaders hastily dismiss the core activities that take place at the bedside as mere "tasks." Commonly expressed sentiments are: "Nursing is not the tasks, it's the critical thinking, decision making, management, and judgment." "You can teach a monkey to take a temperature, a blood pressure, or give a bed bath" and "teach anyone" to use complex medical equipment like ICU monitors or put in IVs. Nurses then teach each other to talk a jargon of theoretical functions and abstractions.

This understandable attempt to give status to nursing work ends up concealing it from those who have a need to know. As a journalist, for example, I've found it illuminating to discover that nurses take blood pressure readings, not to jot numbers down on a piece of paper that is put on a conveyor belt and delivered to the doctor, but because they need to know if the patient is at risk for hypertension or an internal bleed (which can lead to cardiac arrest and death) after surgery. It was, for example,

218 hair-raising for me to learn from an OR nurse that if she didn't position what is called a Bovie pad correctly under a patient having surgery, the patient could actually catch on fire or be electrocuted. (I knew you could get the wrong leg or arm cut off during surgery, but going up in flames is a risk that's rarely mentioned.) Dissing the "tasks" involved in nursing convinces nurses they shouldn't talk about them.

Presenting Definitional Disruptions

Nurses, as Goffman tells us, define themselves not only in the expressions they give but in what they give off—how they introduce themselves or dress. Again, many nurses subvert their claim to credibility in what would appear to be meaningless behavior. When, for example, nurse managers and academics allow or even advise nurses to identify themselves without using their last names and titles and to tolerate uniforms that make it impossible for patients, reporters, or, for that matter, anyone in the hospital, to distinguish a nurse from a janitor or other hospital worker, they are making it impossible for nurses to maintain front region control.

Interestingly, when I have raised this issue with nurse executives and lower-level managers, many agree. And then they throw up their hands in frustration, as if they can't possibly do anything to control the nurses in their employ. Since hospital employers, like all others, do indeed have a great deal of control over how workers dress and how they introduce themselves to clients or patients, one marvels at this claim of powerlessness.

In fact, since the advent of hospital restructuring, many hospital nurse executives have introduced—or tried to introduce—name badges that substitute the title RN, registered nurse, with some version of the term "patient care associate" or "patient care technician"—a title used to identify any person who delivers nursing services including licensed practical or vocational nurses and unlicensed nursing assistants. In some hospitals, nurse managers have replaced name badges that said "Sue Jones, RN" with badges that say "Sue—Nursing" (think of the medical equivalent: "Bob—Oncology"). Like those managers who allow OR nurses to boycott individual physicians, hospital nurse managers also seem to turn a blind eye when nurses reverse their hospital name badges or cover their last names with tape so that patients cannot identify them. (When I was recently at a local hospital, one pediatric nurse had a large teddy bear dangling strategically over her name tag so that no one could possibly read it—this in spite of the fact that a large sign in the waiting room advised patients that they had the right to know the full name, title, and function of the person taking care of them.) Similarly, managers commonly use **219** first names when they note who is taking care of a particular patient on unit assignment boards or on the panels over or near a patient's bed. So one sees the patient's name ("Mrs. Cameron"), the doctor's name ("Doctor Pereira"), and the nurse's name ("Joanie"). Which means that the nurse is the only person who is not fully identified as an individual.

In nursing schools, teaching students to use standard professional introductions—first name, last name, and title—is a haphazard affair at best. Some professors and instructors insist they teach students standard professional introductions. Some professors have told me they tell their students *not* to give last names to patients, because they are worried about safety or privacy. Some seem to consider the issue to be less important than how friendly or accessible the student or nurse appears to the patient. Nurse practitioners and other advanced practice nurses often confide that they don't know quite what to call themselves. We work with doctors, they explain, who introduce themselves as "Dr. Jones." So what do we do, call ourselves "Susan Smith, Nurse Practitioner"?

When I have suggested that to protect themselves and convey a professional image, nurses might want to introduce themselves with "Hello, I'm Nurse Smith" (perhaps adding, "You can call me Susan"), nurses find this idea very alien. Indeed, many nurses consider this form of introduction to be a veritable kiss of death. "If you use the title Nurse with a last name, that sounds just like Nurse Ratched," a professor in a Boston nurse practitioner program told the students I was talking with.[10]

Having heard this assertion so many times, I decided to conduct an informal survey of friends, neighbors, and assorted passersby to see if the dark angel of nursing has the same affect on them. Strolling around the street near my house on a pleasant summer day, I stopped several neighbors and asked them what they would think if they were in the hospital and a nurse introduced her- or himself as "Nurse Smith." My sample also included friends as well as a number of cab drivers I interviewed on the way to the airport. Most of the people I talked to were in their late forties or fifties. Some were in their twenties.

Of the thirty people I surveyed, particularly younger or working-class respondents, about half had never heard of Nurse Ratched. "Nurse who?" they asked. Regardless, every one of them told me that it would never have occurred to them to connect the specter of Louise Fletcher, in her winged hairdo and starched white cap, with a contemporary nurse concerned about their welfare.

"Wow!" said a sociologist friend, "I would never have thought of that."

"For pity's sake," said a lawyer.

"Oh come on, it wasn't the word 'nurse' that was the problem with

220 Nurse Ratched, it was her affect. If a competent nurse introduces herself as Nurse Smith, why on earth would I think of Nurse Ratched? Give me a break!" commented another friend, a molecular biologist.

Nobody thought it would be odd for nurses to introduce themselves by last name and title. One person thought it might sound a little formal but, like the others, seemed pleased that nurses might tell them their full names and functions.

"You go the hospital and you never know who's taking care of you. I don't think we ever knew who the nurses taking care of my aunt were, did we?" one of my neighbors asked, turning to her partner. "You didn't know their first names, you didn't know their last names, and you didn't even know if they were nurses. It was exasperating."

Definitional Disruptions and Caring

One way nurses claim social value and legitimacy is by highlighting their caring functions, the importance of the "nurse-patient relationship," and nursing's "holistic" approach to patient interactions. And indeed, all of these are critical skills a nurse learns in school and on the job. When nurses talk about caring, holism, and the nurse-patient relationship, they are pointing to the attention they give to the entire process of illness: treatments, cures, side effects, feelings and worries, family and friends.[11] This attention to how patients navigate through illness often—but not always—distinguishes the work of nurses from that of physicians, who are often taught to view disease states as if they were detached from the patients who have them.

Nurses are sometimes accurate and often shrewd when they define caring as the core of their work and use the term holism to contrast the nurses' approach with that of the physician. The emphasis on caring and holism gives nurses a platform, a moral high ground, and an important appeal in their efforts either to defend or promote their work and profession. For laypeople like myself who have often experienced the health care system as frightening and impersonal and some of the doctors who work in it as detached and sometimes even abrupt and impatient, the notion of caring and holism is particularly appealing. It offers the promise of someone on your side who will escort you through an alien, scary world and fight for you.

Caring and holism can be a powerful arguments for nursing, but they can also be double-edged swords. They may suggest that nurses mobilize female intuition, not skilled intuition, that their work is rooted in hormones, not in the mind, and that nurses aren't really holistic clinicians but "halfistic" ones who focus only on the psychosocial aspects of illness that the doctors leave out. Thus, holistic care can easily be interpreted as un-skilled kindness, the proverbial TLC that just comes with being—well, a woman, or a particularly sensitive guy.

When they pitch caring and holism to journalists, administrators, and the public, many nurses define these concepts in a narrow, almost antimedical, antitechnical way. When I was recently introduced at a conference of Canadian Emergency Room nurses, the nurse who introduced me said, "Suzanne Gordon appreciates us not for our technical wizardry but for what we give of ourselves to our patients." When I took the podium I had to demur. "With all due respect," I said, "I appreciate you for your technical wizardry and for what you give of yourself to your patients. And I have to admit," I added, "although I would prefer the total package, if I were admitted to an ER and a nurse told me I had a choice between what she gave of herself to me and her technical wizardry, I would say, please, technical wizardry any day."

In my work with nursing students (some of whom are working nurses going back for a BSN or master's or doctorate degree), I often ask them to write a short anecdote that would explain, to a lay audience, the difference that their routine daily activities make to patient care. Nurses' claim to holism is often based on a critique of the kind of Cartesianism that artificially splits mind and body. Yet, their stories are often permeated with a new kind of Cartesianism that counterposes nursing and medicine, the emotional and the physical. In a typical anecdote, an oncology nurse in a master's program wrote, "People may think the most important part of being an oncology nurse is inserting an IV, accessing a porta catheter, administering anti-nausea medication, or infusing chemotherapy. This is not true. The part of my job that makes the greatest impact is educating a patient to take care of himself safely and efficiently at home."

Since the cancer patient isn't going to make it home at all if his IV isn't inserted correctly, his porta catheter safely accessed, his nausea managed, his chemotherapy infused (indeed he could die if any of this goes awry), and the nurse knowledgeable about this as well as family dynamics, I wondered why the student didn't construct her explanation as follows: "As an oncology nurse I do a number of critical things. These include inserting an IV, accessing a porta catheter, administering anti-nausea medication, infusing chemotherapy, and educating a patient to take care of himself safely and efficiently at home."

Nursing scholars like Patricia Benner put caring on the nursing map. When, for example, Benner and her colleagues described "caring," they focused on the physical as well as on the medical and technical. But this emphasis seems to be shifting. When I was asked to work with students at one elite nursing school, the professor leading the fourth-year class

222   showed me a paper in which a student had described how nursing care makes a difference in patient's lives. The professor warned me that the paper was not at all good, not at all "what I was looking for." By this time, I recognized that professors and I sometimes have different views of a good nursing narrative, so I asked to see it anyway. The student wrote a concise, compelling story about walking into a patient's room, finding the patient lying flat on her back vomiting. Although the student was on a clinical rotation, she quickly realized that the patient was in danger of aspirating the vomit, which would go into her lungs and almost certainly lead to aspiration pneumonia if not to death. She acted quickly to save the woman from this potentially catastrophic—not to mention costly—complication.

What was wrong with this anecdote? I wondered.

"This isn't an example of holistic care," the professor snapped.

While these attitudes have long simmered within nursing, the increasing focus on caring seems to lead some nurses to believe that caring about whether someone goes to an ICU with pneumonia does not constitute real "care." Or that anything connected to a "doctor's order" is somehow not the core of nursing.

Similarly, nurses tell me that other nurses stigmatize them if they work in more technical areas of nursing where there is less opportunity for intense personal contact with patients over a longer term. Thus OR, ER, or endoscopy nurses report that their colleagues will insist they aren't real nurses, because they don't really care for their patients. Nursing students have told me that some of their professors urge them not to talk about the medical functions the nurse performs, because they should be seeking that elusive, exclusive niche that only a nurse can fill.[12] This means that students, when they graduate, may find it difficult to describe their full participation in the medical activities in which they are involved. They might also defer to the doctor, because they have been taught to respect rather than challenge the artificial barriers long ago erected between medicine and nursing activities.

Things become all the more confusing when one looks at the images that nursing groups often use to describe their work to the public. When nursing organizations prepare for the annual celebration of Nurses Week, they usually come up with a slogan that will define or describe the essence of nursing to outside audiences. Although the recent studies done by nurse researchers and often promoted by these organizations highlight the lifesaving nature of the care nurses deliver to patients, these Nurses Week slogans tend to focus on the touchy-feely. Thus, after September 11, the Nurses Week slogan of the American Nurses Association was "Nurses

Care for America," the words covering a heart made up of the stars and stripes. The next year, set against a white background, a gauzy, angelic pastel figure soared above a different slogan, "Nursing, Lifting Spirits, Touching Lives." A logo that the Canadian Nurses Association has used is "Nurses—Always There for You and Your Family." The association's 2003 slogan was "Nursing: At the Heart of Health Care," with a drawing of a jagged white heart superimposed over a collage of different nurses. In Quebec, nurses advertised nursing as "an Expertise of the Heart," and the Féderation des infirmières et infirmiers du Québec told the public that nursing is "The Noble Profession."[13] In 2000 the ICN picked a fluffy pure white heart to be the symbol of international nursing, and it now sells pins with these white hearts to nurses.[14]

Sioban Nelson and I have argued that these images try to capture an important part of nursing. Unfortunately, they do so in a way that reinforces the image of nursing as virtue work, and nurses as virtue workers, that was established in the nineteenth century. This virtue script in nursing may seem to bring nurses much-needed recognition, but it is recognition for a very limited, albeit extremely important, aspect of their work. It also perpetuates the idea in the public imagination that nursing work is not a matter of life or death but only a matter of TLC. It establishes a feedback loop in which nurses—recipients of a legacy of virtue—advertise themselves as virtue workers, which in turn leaves journalists, politicians, and even patients with the impression that being kind and nice and thoughtful is the primary function of the nurse. When patients like Christopher Reeve or Trish Meili—or journalists like Wielawski or Kaplan—turn to nurses to help them gain a picture of their work, the picture they give may not be as complex and detailed as their work really is.

When I interviewed Christie Berner, a nurse executive who has been the senior vice president of patient care services at Arkansas Children's Hospital for eight years, about the TV special *ICU*, she told me she was very pleased with how nurses were portrayed on the show. The show wasn't just about doctors, she said, it portrayed nurses as "real, important people in the care of patients."

When I asked Berner to explain how she describes the importance of nursing to patients, she told me that "the nursing impact on patients" is in "the things that aren't written by the physician as orders, the things that are inherent in the relationship between nurses and in our case patients and families." She explained "the anchors of the profession" are the "caring, the teaching, the being there because [nurses are] the ones that are around and not just there to carry out the physician's orders and deal with the technology. All of that's there and they have to do that," she said, but

224 she reiterated that the most important activities of the nurse, "the core values of nursing, are based on teaching support, their expertise, and just being there."

In these comments we see the complex legacy of the relationship of nursing and medicine at work. Berner did not emphasize that nurses are, in fact, masters of technology. She did not discuss how much nurses have to know in order to safely administer and monitor medical treatments. Nor did she seem to affirm that the technological competence of nurses is central because it keeps patients alive. Like many nurses, she downplayed—in fact, almost seemed to dismiss—some of the most important things nurses do. In the process, nursing and medicine become opposites not complements, and nurses lose the opportunity to explain that surgeons like Drummond-Webb can succeed only because nurses have the medical and technical skills to make sure patients' operations don't kill them.

Berner defined the core of nursing in almost sentimental terms as "the personal touch things." She told me that one of her favorite things in the *ICU* series was the shot of a toddler dragging around a red wagon filled with "ten syringe pumps . . . with all his blood pressure regulatory medications on it." He was terribly sick, yet the nurses were getting him up to go to the play room. "That's the important part of nursing that we have and do so well. And that really makes a difference."

While it may have been clear to Berner that nurses were the ones who got the boy his red wagon, the show, as broadcast, does not make this clear to the viewer. Nor does the viewer understand the skill involved in helping such a sick child maintain a semblance of normal life on an ICU. We see the little boy dragging around a red wagon filled with medications. That's it.

In an era when birth rates in industrialized countries remain low and greater numbers of people need care for longer periods of time, nursing will become attractive only if it is well paid and well respected. For nurses to be truly respected, the public needs to know what nurses really know and what they really do. The legacy of professional silencing and of nurses' individual self-silencing makes this difficult. In fact, it allows nurses to believe they are choosing silence rather than having it imposed on them. If virtue is supposed to be its own reward, and taking pride in one's accomplishments is a sin, then being rewarded with public recognition becomes unwelcome. If one is supposed to attribute one's agency to a higher power, then giving credit to those perceived to be higher up in medical hierarchy will be perfectly appropriate. If anonymity is prized and avoiding conflict and controversy are useful survival strategies, nurses will be reluctant to jump into the fray when a controversy erupts. Finally,

so long as angelic images promise safety and legitimacy, nurses will proj-   **225**
ect those images when they step out in public.

If this legacy, and the images it has produced, aren't overcome, nurses
will not be able to argue credibly for their work. Not to journalists, not to
political representatives and policy makers, and not to a public that needs
to understand how cost cutting in today's health care system jeopardizes
patients' lives.

PART THREE

HOSPITALS AND NURSING

As I was dozing off while reading one Saturday night in 1996, the ringing of the phone woke me. It was a critical care nurse at an important Boston teaching hospital.

Was I the Suzanne Gordon who wrote about nursing and managed care, she asked?

Yes, I answered.

"Oh, thank God, I need help," she practically sobbed. "I'm working tonight and it's impossible. We have too many patients. Since the hospital merged with another in town and bought up some suburban hospitals, they're feeding people from all over the state into our critical care unit. There aren't enough nurses to take care of these patients."

What prompted her call, she explained, was news that another patient from another feeder hospital was supposed to be admitted. "We don't have enough nurses to take care of these people," she pleaded. "You can't believe how sick they are. It's not safe." I asked if she'd told this to her nurse manager. Of course, she answered, but they just tell us to do it, to get with the program or leave. As we talked, I felt as powerless as the nurse. Sure, I'm a journalist, and she knew I'd been writing about the impact of managed care on nursing. But she didn't want an article that would appear in some newspaper or magazine in two or three weeks—or

228 months. Of course, I would try to write about her experiences. But she wanted help. Immediately.

That was not the first call I received since hospital cost cutting began in the early 1990s. In fact, the calls keep coming. A clinical nurse specialist in California recently phoned me with essentially the same story. Too many very sick patients, too few nurses. Hospital administrators who don't listen, or won't listen, or who—because they are so overworked—can't listen. I'd coauthored a book urging nurses to move from silence to voice. Well, here she was ready to use her voice. What should she do, now, to protect her patients? I asked her if she'd called her professional organization. Yes, she said, they were no help. I asked if she called the California Nurses Association—a nursing union that has fought for better staffing for nurses. "Well, no," she said sheepishly, "they're so political." In fact, she told me that a union had tried to organize her hospital but she'd voted against it. The managers told us having a union isn't professional, she said. We'd be just like truck drivers. We're professionals. They assured us that we're a family here. If you have a problem, just tell us.

Well, she did. She even wrote a letter to her CEO detailing the problems on the units. She got no reply. Now, she was calling me.

To me these phone calls were like mold growing in a petri dish—anecdotal evidence of a disaffection that would soon produce a national shortage of nurses and nursing care. Since, at that point, I had been writing about nursing for almost a decade, I recognized that these cries for help were very different from the conversations I'd been having with nurses at the end of the 1980s and in the early 1990s. Even though I began writing about nursing during a nursing shortage, the nurses I talked with then had a sense of growing optimism. Yes, they had their complaints—about doctors who wouldn't listen, about a poor public image, about managers and administrators who were too busy or too distant from clinical practice to appreciate their problems. But, underneath it all, nurses expressed a belief that things were moving in a positive direction. Many hospitals were developing primary nursing. They responded to the nursing shortage of the 1980s by raising wages (sometimes by as much as 22 percent), by providing day-care benefits and sometimes even on-site day care, and by giving nurses more flexible schedules.

In some academic institutions, nurses were given free tuition for their children. Many nurses felt secure in their jobs. They benefited from more in-house education and funding to attend outside conferences and seminars, as well as tuition reimbursement if they wanted to pursue higher education. More hospitals were also hiring unit-based clinical nurse specialists—nurses with special education and expertise in particular clinical problems, such as rehabilitation, diabetes, and oncology—who could serve as educational resources for busy staff nurses. Hospitals were also experimenting with clinical ladders—stepped systems of promotion through which nurses could gain raises and advance in their careers, while still remaining at the hospital bedside. This promised to remedy an age-old problem: the only way a nurse could earn more and advance in her career had been by moving away from bedside care and into management or academia. Finally, nursing management was gaining more power and authority inside hospitals, and some nurses at the highest levels were initiating experiments that empowered nurses lower down. In spite of tensions between labor and management, many of the unionized nurses I talked to also felt that there was great promise for the profession and that that their work at the bedside was challenging and dynamic.

And then came managed care and hospital restructuring. Advocates insisted that both would benefit everyone. Nurses would gain more freedom and autonomy, and patients would reap the benefits of a system that gave them more choice and better services. Would this promise be fulfilled?

In the mid-1990s, I had an opportunity to find out, when the American Association of Critical Care Nurses asked me to write a special supplement for their monthly magazine on what they termed patient-centered care. "Patient-centered care," I cheered mentally. "It's about time."

When I began calling critical care nurses to ask them how patient-centered care was being implemented on their ICUs, I was greeted with some very peculiar responses. The nurses I interviewed seemed less than enthusiastic—sometimes even hostile—about the concept. What was going on? Nurses always claim to be so pro-patient. Their professional jargon includes an almost devotional commitment to patient advocacy, patient partnerships, patients as unique individuals, and of course, patient-centeredness. Yet, I barely got the words "patient-centered" out of my mouth before these nurses practically jumped down my throat.

I didn't have to dig far before I discovered that patient-centered or patient-focused care was a central building stone in the restructuring and reengineering of health care. It was one of those Orwellian formulations used to describe its opposite. Under the guise of patient-centered, patient-focused care, nurses quickly told me, they were losing their ability to center on the patient and were increasingly asked to focus on profit.

In the late 1980s and early 1990s, when I spoke on radio call-in shows or talked to friends and acquaintances about the value of nursing, people would invariably respond by recounting a positive story about nursing. They recollected a forgotten nurse who saved their mother's life, or sat with them when they were in the hospital. In the mid to late 1990s, people began to change their tune. I began to hear many more complaints. The

230 nurses were rude, abrupt, and discourteous. Some of these people blamed the system. Since people generally don't understand the institutional underpinnings of nursing care, most blamed nurses. After all, whom would you blame if your wife couldn't get a bedpan during a hospital stay? If a nurse is telling your husband he's got to vacate his hospital bed? If your friend falls after outpatient surgery, and the nurse whom you call doesn't seem particularly concerned? As patients or family members, we don't usually meet the hospital CEO, the insurance executive, the government bureaucrat, or, in the United States, the employer who watches the bottom line and is really pulling the health care strings. It's the nurse who is the visible, audible representative of the system. She's the one who takes the heat for the entire system, which is why so many nurses complain that violence—verbal or physical—against them has increased.

In the next chapters about hospital and health care cost cutting, I describe problems in the system that make frightened, anxious patients feel that they are unwelcome interlopers in hospitals and other health care institutions, and that make nurses want to leave. Starting with a short historical description of the rise of managed care and hospital cost cutting, I explore the acute illness that has exacerbated chronic problems and produced the current shortage. I'll introduce some of the cheerleaders who led the way to hospital restructuring in North America and the West. Although health care consultants and social engineers also targeted medicine, doctors were not laid off in droves or replaced with completely unskilled personnel. While they attacked medicine with vigor, consultants and administrators also tried to buy off and mollify physicians, who are too powerful to alienate totally. Health care consultants and administrators—some of them former practicing nurses—seemed to have absorbed the steady diet of PR, as well as the medical myth that nurses are just handmaids and that any pair of hands, particularly female ones, will do when it comes to bedside care.

Health care downsizing at the expense of nurses and nursing care has not been limited to hospital nurses or to bedside nurses. As we will see, RNs in all areas of nursing have been affected. Indeed, one of the great ironies of the current crisis is that the nurse executives and managers who have been asked to implement restructuring and so-called patient-focused care have also been eliminated, as hospitals and health systems continue to cut costs. Health care cost cutting has also generated a stratum of temporary, traveling nurses whom hospitals use to plug holes left vacant by the nursing shortage. Because the nursing crisis exists in every industrialized country, I will also look at the explosion of nursing migration, particularly from developing countries to shortage-plagued countries in the West. All of these developments further fragment the nursing work force

and potentially undermine efforts to improve working conditions **231**
throughout the system. The nursing crisis has also produced an interesting internal migration inside nursing, which affects bedside care. Nurses
who are frustrated with their working conditions quickly move away from
the bedside and into advanced practice and nurse practitioner jobs, thus
further exacerbating shortages in institutional caregiving. Throughout
this discussion, I'll consider how tensions within the nursing profession
make it more difficult to create viable solutions that will make nursing a
sustainable career.

9

Mangling Care

Several years ago, at the height of the restructuring of American hospitals, I was speaking to about fifty RNs in the Midwest. The nurses were deeply concerned about their patients' well-being and their own ability to survive in their profession. One nurse who worked in a psychiatric hospital said she routinely cared for thirty-five patients on the night shift. Administrators insisted she could manage because they assumed that at night patients were all asleep. Amazing, she noted. Who was running the asylum?

OR nurses, orthopedic nurses, ER nurses, wherever the members of my audience worked, they described the same problems. Then a plump woman in her fifties stood up. She was no longer working in the hospital, she explained. She had tried to adjust to the new conditions of the nursing workplace until one recent night. As usual, she'd been assigned too many patients. One of them developed a serious complication, but her other patients also needed monitoring. The other nurses on the floor were as busy as she was. They couldn't help. Although none of her patients died that night, she felt they survived by sheer luck (like most nurses, she downplayed her considerable skill). When she returned home, she made up her mind. "I'm fifty years old. I just can't do this anymore. I quit." She paused, and then began to quietly cry. "I was a good nurse," she said. "I was a good nurse." But it had become clear to her that the system would allow her to be a good nurse no longer.

In gatherings like this around the world, nurses voice their thoughts about the fundamental realities that have produced the current nursing shortage. The nursing work force is aging. In 1983 the average age of

234   nurses was 37.4 years, and in 2000 it was 45.2.[1] But an aging work force is not the only reason why U.S. hospitals report 126,000 vacancies, or 12 percent of RN capacity, or why we will need thousands more in the coming decade.[2]

Nurses like the one who spoke in Illinois aren't that old. Under better circumstances, they could look forward to another ten or fifteen years of work. Moreover, nurses in their late forties and fifties aren't the only ones who want to bail out of a career in direct care. New nurses who go to work in hospitals say they've had it after only a year or two—sometimes only after a few months.

Whether young or old, nurses are disillusioned because they believe that health care systems guided by bottom-line concerns simply don't recognize the specificity of their work. Even at the best of times, nursing is a taxing job. First of all, bedside nursing, particularly for those who work at the hospital bedside, is physically exhausting. The average nurse in a hospital will walk miles in a single day. She will be turning patients—as the society gets larger, many of them may weigh over two hundred pounds—bracing them as they walk, lifting them, and picking them up off the floor if they fall. When in 2002 the Bureau of Labor Statistics ranked thirty-eight job categories according to the number of days lost at work because of nonfatal illnesses and injuries, registered nurses ranked twelfth; they had fewer days off work than laborers and construction workers but more than stock handlers and baggers.[3] Similarly, RNs had more days off work due to work-related musculoskeletal disorders than stock handlers and baggers and slightly less than construction laborers.[4]

Taking care of sick people whose needs do not fit the normal nine-to-five, clock-in-clock-out schedule is more demanding than many other professions or occupations. To keep a hospital open requires many more nurses than doctors willing to work nights and weekends and to give up holidays. More significant is the emotional toll nursing can take. Nurses, like doctors and other clinicians, work with the sickest, most vulnerable people in our societies. Nurses are dealing with people who are ipso facto not at their best. They may be in pain, depressed, sullen, irritable, anxious, and sometimes angry, maybe even violent. Nursing is hard emotionally and physically. This is so even under the best of circumstances: when there are plenty of RNs, when collegial relationships prevail between doctors, nurses, and other clinicians, when nurses have administrative support from hospital executives and managers, when clinicians know what's wrong with a patient and what to do about it, and when pay is good.

That's why Daniel Chambliss, in his book *Beyond Caring*, reminds us of the pitfalls of likening a hospital to any other business organization that processes goods and services. "In one crucial respect," Chambliss writes, "the hospital remains dramatically different from other organizations: *in hospitals, as a normal part of the routine, people suffer and die.* This is unusual. . . . Only combat military forces share this feature. To be complete, theories of hospital life need to acknowledge this crucial difference, since adapting themselves to pain and death is for hospital workers the most distinctive feature of their work. It is that which most separates them from the rest of us. In building theories of organizational life, sociologists must try to see how hospitals resemble other organizations . . . but we should not make a premature leap to the commonalities before appreciating the unique features of hospitals that make a nurse's task so different from that of a teacher or a businessman or a bureaucrat."[5]

The combination of difficult patients, taxing schedules, and arduous physical work means that nurses need a set of complex rewards. They must feel that they make enough money and benefits; they have to feel that they can enjoy a sense collegiality on the job; they need to feel that they are respected and that they have good working conditions; and, perhaps most important, they need to feel that they make a difference to the patients for whom they give so much on a daily basis. Unfortunately, policy makers, administrators, insurance company bureaucrats, and a slew of health care consultants have made precisely the leap Chambliss warns against, and as a result, nursing has become a job that offers fewer and fewer rewards. This creates a three-tiered shortage. There is, first, a lack of bodies willing to work at the bedside under current conditions and for current wages, which in turn sows the seeds for a future scarcity of nurses as the population ages and deals with more chronic illness. Both shortages are evident in quantifiable data: x number of missing bodies that an employer or society can count.

Cost cutting produces a third, more elusive, and—particularly for the patient—more significant shortage. Even when hospitals or health care institutions deem the available nursing bodies sufficient to fill the needs they are willing to pay for, cost cutting can lead to a shortage of nursing care that patients receive. We saw this kind of shortage in the mid-1990s, when hospitals were laying off nurses, and we see it today in different countries and settings. In the United States, for example, shortages exist in nursing homes (where employers have decreed they have enough RNs) and in home care, because insufficient reimbursement prevents home care agencies from hiring more RNs. So, in the society, we may have a lot of people with RN after their name but they can't give patients the care they need. Which means we have a shortage of nursing care.

Many observers point out that nursing shortages are hardly a novel phenomenon. When I began writing about nursing in the mid-1980s, we

236 were in the middle of one of the shortages of nurses that the United States has periodically experienced. Well, now we have another one, and it promises to be much more difficult to solve.

How has health care cost cutting contributed to this three-tiered shortage of nurses and nursing care? What has happened that has made working with the sickest, most vulnerable patients so frustrating for bedside nurses?

Although one can never attach a neat date to complex social phenomena, the contemporary shortage of nurses willing to work in direct care, particularly in hospitals, is intimately linked with new economic imperatives that began to wash over health care in the early 1990s. In the United States, employers who pay for health care for their employees in the employment-based, private insurance system began to rebel against escalating insurance premiums. Government payers, like Medicare and Medicaid, were also trying to control rising health care costs. Their target was an out-of-control, fee-for-service system of medical treatment and the inefficiencies that were rampant in the hospital system—the use of too much expensive diagnostic technology, of too many expensive drugs, or of too much medical equipment, and of too many expensive treatments and procedures. At the beginning of the 1990s, says economist Alan Sager, codirector of the Access and Affordability Project at the Boston University School of Public Health, the United States was in the midst of a stunning escalation in health care costs. "In 1960, health care spending was half of defense spending. By 2004, it was four times the amount of defense spending."

A quarter of the way along this trajectory of rapidly rising health care costs, Bill Clinton was elected president and tried to deal with out-of-control health care spending. He called his solution "managed competition." In this new system, employers, acting as proxies for their employees, would make consumer choices for them. They would push employees into health maintenance organizations that would operate according to market principles.[6] Managed competition, or managed care, would produce price competition—between insurers, between hospitals, between doctors, even between nurses, and this, Clinton assured the country, would control health care costs, provide universal access to health insurance, and enhance the quality of patient care.

Advocates of market-based managed care were quite clear about how the new system would work. Long before Clinton unveiled his plan, one of the major architects of managed care, Paul Ellwood, wrote that the health maintenance organizations, central to its implementation, "could stimulate a course of change in the health industry that would have some of the classical aspects of the industrial revolution—conversion to larger units of production, technological innovation, division of labor, substitution of capital for labor, vigorous competition, and profitability as the **237** mandatory condition of survival."[7]

The advocates of cost cutting were keen to follow the lead of for-profit hospital chains like Columbia/HCA which, Robert Kuttner writes in *Everything for Sale*, claimed to "increase efficiencies by centralizing administration, cutting waste, buying supplies in bulk at discounted rates, negotiating discounted fees with medical professionals, shifting to less wasteful forms of care, and consolidating duplicative facilities."[8] As David Himmelstein and Steffie Woolhandler have demonstrated, not-for-profits quickly began to emulate for-profit hospitals and HMOs.[9] Advocates of cost cutting argued that when health care became a market commodity, with business principles and efficiencies determining health care priorities, money would be saved and quality and access assured. Although functioning in different health care financing systems, governments in Canada, Western Europe, Australia, New Zealand, and other industrialized countries were under similar pressures to cut costs and were attracted to the same principles of market-based managed care.

Although the Clinton health plan ultimately failed, Clinton's attempt to introduce managed competition, market control, and price competition into health care helped to advance the increased corporate influence over health care.[10]

One of the cornerstones of managed competition or managed care was the micromanagement of doctors' practice patterns by health maintenance organizations and insurance companies. Insurers wanted to limit expensive procedures and medications and to shorten patients' length of stay in hospitals. Under other circumstances, curtailing waste in health care would have been an extraordinary advance. Given the problems of the health care system, efficiency is an essential goal, if it can be achieved without compromising the quality of care. The problem is that most latter-day HMOs—most of which were for-profit—wield the concepts of efficiency and productivity without defining them. What does it mean to provide health care more efficiently? Not wasting money on unneeded treatment so it can be invested in expanding the pool of those cared for, or saving money and redistributing it to CEOs? What is productivity? Enabling doctors and nurses to spend more time with patients, or getting them to see more patients? Is efficiency managing care or managing money?

Most managed care organizations were under tremendous pressure to manage profits, not care. They did this by scrutinizing physician practice patterns and forcing doctors or nurses to call 1-800-Mother-May-I lines (often staffed by nurses) to obtain approval for suggested procedures, treatments, and hospital stays.

238   Without the kinds of government controls Clinton proposed, employers nonetheless began to herd employees into HMOs. This was to be the first violation of the very market ideology that market advocates promoted. After all, in a true market system, it is the user of the service or product who decides what to purchase. But under managed care, as Kuttner and so many others have pointed out, it was the payer of the benefit, that is, the employer, who determined what insurance plan an employee could choose.[11] Most employees were offered only a few plans to choose from. Some employers offered only one, and the majority of employees made their consumer choice on the basis of cost, not quality. Advocates of market medicine insisted that consumers would have more choice, not less. But who was their ideal consumer? The patient/user or the employer?

Increasing competition between hospitals and reducing hospital length of stay was another cornerstone of managed care. The United States now has one of the shortest lengths of stay of any industrialized country in the world. Indeed, an influential early study in the *New England Journal of Medicine* concluded that virtually all of the savings achieved in HMOs were due to their ability to lower the number of days their patients spend in hospitals.[12] This has been accomplished by denying coverage for some elective procedures that insurance would have paid for in the old days (e.g., cataract surgery and bone marrow transplants for advanced cancer), while shifting many other procedures, which are covered, to outpatient settings. The final technique to reduce hospital days has been discharging hospitalized patients sooner.[13]

Lengths of hospital stays have, of course, been steadily decreasing over the past century because of more effective treatments and technologies. As a cost-saving device, government and private insurance systems have reduced them further. In 1983, for example, Medicare adopted a prospective payment system in which hospital length of stay was determined by what were called DRGs, or diagnosis-related groups. Medicare began paying hospitals a predetermined amount that would be assigned for each episode of illness, rather than reimbursing the hospital on the charges accrued for the actual amount an individual patient's stay cost. Average lengths of hospital stay would be given for each DRG—say, seven days for a hip replacement operation—and a sum of money would be assigned for the procedure. If a hospital could get the patient out before the seven days, it would pocket the money it saved. If the patient stayed in longer, the hospital received no money, unless the patient's diagnosis had changed. This created a perverse incentive to discharge patients "quicker and sicker," as the phenomenon was dubbed. As more health care services were bundled into prospective payment schemes, "patient throughput" (getting patients out of a hospital or nursing home, or discharging them **239** from a home care agency) became a major preoccupation.

In what the health economist Uwe Reinhardt has described as the American obsession with gutting the hospital, hospital lengths of stay were cut, and managed care companies outsourced patients and their nursing care.[14] Worried about its reimbursement rates, and competing against one another for managed care contracts, hospitals began to send recovering patients to a nursing home or rehabilitation hospital that would also receive a preset amount of money for their care. To save on the cost of care, the nursing home or rehabilitation hospital would try to discharge the patient quickly, sending him home where he or she might receive nursing care or personal assistance from a home care agency. But that home care agency would soon see its reimbursements cut and would limit services available in the home. Thus, nursing care would ultimately be outsourced to family and friends who would be asked to provide professional-level services to a loved one in the home.

Part of the move to get people out of the hospital came from a genuine concern for patients. Hospitals, after all, are awash with bacteria and viruses and are unhealthy places to be. Hospital stays in the past were probably too long. But with the help of consultants like John Miliman and Jane Robertson in Seattle, who compiled statistical averages of length of patient stay and assigned them to individual patients—a one-size-fits-all model became the rule.[15] Patients who might be unstable or lacked adequate support and nursing care at home were discharged sooner. In everything from bypass surgery to hip replacements to mastectomies, length of stay has shortened dramatically. Between 1980 and 1995, Reinhardt tells us, "total inpatient admissions per thousand population and average length of stay declined by 20 percent each; consequently, inpatient days per thousand population declined by about 40 percent."[16] The American Hospital Association has calculated that the average length of patient stay declined from 7.6 days in 1980 to 5.8 days in the year 2000.[17] (Reinhardt also explains that health care spending actually increased. "As track records go, this one is truly remarkable," he notes caustically.)[18]

With intense pressure to cut costs, hospitals competed fiercely to attract managed care business. The competition, Sager points out, was not about quality or compassion but about who could deliver services more cheaply. This meant that hospitals and other employers of nurses were faced with contradictory imperatives: maintaining an adequate supply of nurses, creating a decent working environment for those nurses, and cutting costs. But how were hospitals to reconcile these competing imperatives and at the same time provide nursing care to patients? Health care consultants, who imported downsizing strategies from manufacturing and

240 other service industries, were happy to provide hospitals caught in a tightening financial vise with some useful models of cost cutting, along with a number of helpful rationalizations for their actions.

Enter the Management Consultants

In the wake of the rebellion against managed care cost cutting, hospital executives at the turn of the twenty-first century often depicted themselves as victims of health care consultants and the business theories they espoused. In a 2003 article in the *Boston Globe*, Dr. Andy Whittemore, chief medical officer at the Brigham and Women's Hospital, blamed consultants for hospital's failure to provide enough beds for an aging population. "Consultants came in the early 90's advising us to downsize, which we dutifully did."[19]

But consultants didn't magically appear unbidden on hospital doorsteps. Nor were hospital executives, CEOs, and VPs of nursing the employees of consulting firms who had unaccountably become their masters. Hospitals invited consultants into their institutions because they wanted to cut costs—$20 million here, $45 million there, one former vice president of nursing told me—and they wanted to do it quickly. As another former vice president of "patient care services"—what used to be known as nursing—explained, hospitals hired these consultants because they wanted to effect rapid change in their organizations. While consultants would promise to tailor their particular business model to the needs of a particular hospital, what they would really do, she said, is "run your numbers through their model and tell you what you could do. . . . The dynamic of having a consultant come in and work with your staff keeps the administrator from having any kind of accountability." In other words, when staff complain about institutional policies, the administrator can say the consultant "made me do it."

The consultants that most hospitals hired—groups like Ernst and Young, Arthur D. Anderson, the Hunter Group, and American Practice Management—had a track record of cutting jobs, if not of actually saving companies money. The theories and models of business gurus like Michael Hammer and James Champy, whose best-selling *Reengineering the Corporation: A Manifesto for Business Revolution* became a corporate bible in the 1990s, were honed after years of working to downsize manufacturing and services industries.[20] Consultancy had become a multibillion-dollar industry that was netting $25 billion in annual revenues in the United States, and double that across the globe. The highest-paid consultants at the largest firms averaged $700 an hour, with the average partner earning $270 an hour and project managers and individual consultants earning $212 and

$166 respectively.[21] Hospitals paid thousands if not millions—between **241** $500,000 and $10,000,000 per restructuring, according to one estimate— to bring in these management experts.[22] Even so, hospitals desperate to cut costs felt their services were worth it (if they cut enough staff jobs, they could pay the consultants and still end up meeting budget targets).

Frantic to control expenditures, hospitals knew they had to target costs they could control. They had little influence over the cost of medications and durable medical equipment. Doctors were not their employees (at least not yet), but nursing budgets were something hospital administrators could control. Nurses receive the largest share of the labor budget, so nursing was a logical place to start cutting costs.[23] In fact, nursing was not only a logical target, it was an easy one. Doctors are well organized and visible, and their role in health care is well known, whereas few members of the public or the political community really understand what nurses do and how important they are. Many nurses feel that hospital and health care administrators share this ignorance. Nurses, as we've seen, haven't enjoyed particularly strong connections to the media, so their concerns would not be immediately registered or given much credibility.

Nurses are also poorly organized. Only about 10 percent of nurses belong to the American Nurses Association, and about 17 percent are members of labor unions.[24] During the 1990s, one began to hear nursing increasingly described as a "cost center" and a drain on hospital revenues, while doctors were still viewed as "revenue centers" or "revenue generators" who needed to be mollified while they were controlled. Ignoring the warnings of people like Chambliss, consultants redefined sick human beings as standardizable, predictable units of production and imposed another one-size-fits-all solution on a fundamental human service.

Typically a team of these consultants—usually junior employees in their late twenties and thirties managed by a senior partner in his or her forties or fifties—arrives Monday morning and leaves Thursday afternoon. Some consulting firms employ nurses or are even run by nurses. Indeed, whether as business owners, partners, or employees, this nursing presence was critically important in giving the consultant enterprise legitimacy—the presence of nurses sent the message that "we understand your core business."

Trish Gibbons, former vice president of patient care services at the Beth Israel Deaconess Medical Center, believes that "these companies, coming in to reengineer, co-opted physicians and nurses to join them. They did it with money. They paid them a lot of money to join firms like American Practice Management and to take the economic model and legitimize it with some clinical talk." Gibbons likens the phenomenon to physician participation in the broader managed care/HMO industry.

242   "The moment the HMOs got physicians in positions of power they could come in and make significant change, but they needed clinicians at the top."

Most of the consultants' work force on the ground was not, however, made up of nurses, or even of seasoned business people. The on-site consultants were often young MBAs with limited business experience, little knowledge of the realities of the actual delivery of patient care, and scant experience of being sick themselves. One public health professor laughingly told me that some of his students would graduate from school and then go out and get a job telling hospitals and nursing administrators how to do theirs. A vice president of nursing who'd been in hospitals for over thirty years talked about the galling experience of being confronted with young people who were learning about her "core business" while telling her how to change it. "There was little appreciation by the consultants or the rest of the senior management teams in most hospitals of the complexity of patient care, which is the core business of the institution," she complained.

In fact, both the hospital management and the consultants considered the failure to understand clinical concerns a strength. "I found their language quite interesting," Gibbons notes. "When they were trying to meet targets they would tell me that they were there to develop a hypothesis and it was my responsibility to prove that it wasn't possible. They give you a benchmark goal—an aggregate single number—and when you wanted to get more detail behind that number, in order to know whether it was truly comparable and whether or not it was a benchmark goal you could meet, that wasn't their job. Their job was simply to state the hypothesis that you could function with 25 percent fewer staff."

Using supposedly revolutionary principles, the consultants' templates were supposed to rework nursing care completely. In fact, the formula was age-old. They applied industrial models to health care, following Ellwood's recommendation twenty years earlier. Or to use Simon Head's recent formulation, they integrated health and human services into the "new ruthless economy" of the 1990s. They simply updated the theories of a host of early-twentieth-century "scientific" managers such as John Hall, Frederick Winslow Taylor, William S. Knudsen, and William Henry Leffingwell.[25]

Today, what Head terms "the four pillars of industrialism"—standardization, measurement, monitoring, and control—are guiding health care. Rather than controlling the labor of unskilled workers on the assembly line, the new industrialists "invad[ed] the territory of the skilled worker, with the reengineer trying to impose factory discipline on the work of even those classified by economists as 'very skilled.'"[26] They thus targeted physician practice patterns and other clinical and nonclinical areas. Analyses of what managed care has wrought in these areas has been and is still being duly chronicled.[27]

The goal of the scientific manager was to "achieve machine-like standards of speed and reliability with the routines of the workforce, whether of laborers, machinists, inventory clerks, purchasing agents, supervisors, or managers" and to "study the routines of all these employees, work out the simplest and fastest way for each to be done, and, finally, set a standard time for its performance."[28] The vehicles that allow Taylorism to be applied to the nursing work force are patient acuity systems, clinical pathways, and benchmarking, all of which, critics argue, initiate a widespread deskilling of nurses' work.

In developing systems to determine nurse staffing and skill mix—how many RNs are needed, how many licensed practical nurses, how many nursing assistants—consultants have accompanied or questioned registered nurses to find out how they deliver care. How many activities, they wanted to know, go into taking care of the average cancer patient, heart patient, diabetic patient, and surgical patient? How much time does it take to give a bed bath, walk a patient, or give out medications? Once this is determined, they create a program that allots an average length of time to the registered nurse to perform these activities. This is done through the development of computerized "patient acuity systems" that are sold to hospitals and that help them determine how many registered nurses to employ on a particular shift given the system's determination of the "acuity"—or intensity of the care needs—of the patient. Through standardized formulas that factor in patient acuity and correlate it with the time that consultants have deemed the task should take, hospital administrators can figure out how many nurses they need, not just on a weekly or even a daily basis, but on an hourly basis.

The pitch to hospitals from those who have developed these systems is that administrators can save money on nursing care. Thus, the website of Healthworcs, one company that sells patient acuity systems, proclaims, "Acuity systems save a lot of money over traditional staffing by patient counts. Acuity systems determine the right amount of staff according to weighted patient workload. When used each shift, the savings can be well over $150,000 per year for each patient care unit." That's because "every additional staff hour per patient day for 10 patients is over $110,000 per year." So the Worcsampling service can "quantify how your care staff spend their time as a baseline to your project."[29]

Trend Care Systems, which services Australia and New Zealand, tells prospective clients it will "measure patient acuity relating to clinical hours required for care; predict labour hours required; produce efficiency re-

244 ports (clinical hours); identify acuity and efficiency trends; provide acuity profiles for re-engineering rosters; facilitate the development of acuity based budgets; measure labour costs for specific episodes of care/DRGs; and facilitate benchmarking." Van Slyck and Associates "provides unparalleled strategies for the creation and use of patient and staff information to effectively manage patient care and the cost of that care" and helps hospitals "identify, per patient day, the cost of nursing care based on the patient acuity level."[30]

Luisa Toffoli, an Australian nurse, is researching the impact of patient acuity systems. She explains that nursing departments are now judged on "key performance indicators." Just as managed care organizations calculated their success in reducing what was known as the "medical loss ratio"—that is, how much money was spent on care for patients—nursing departments' "key performance indicators" are deemed to be satisfactory when there is a reduction in nursing care hours per patient day.

To reduce the number of nursing hours per patient day, consultants also "benchmark" hospital nursing care. They gather data on how much time is allotted to nursing care in different hospitals. The hospital that delivers the least number of nursing hours per patient day becomes the benchmark against which other hospitals must compete. "So if Podunk hospital can manage this patient population with 4 hours of nursing care, and you've got 4.5, Podunk has the best practice and you don't," Gibbons says.

Similarly, many consultants manipulated the laudable aim of developing evidence-based practices or best practices by developing clinical pathways or maps. These maps would chart the trajectory of a patient with a particular disease or undergoing a particular procedure and assign times that it would take the patient to execute his or her increasingly short march through the system. These pathways came to resemble the blue books that have been used to standardize work on Nissan factory assembly lines.[31] In the hospital, as in the auto plant, they chart what needs to be done and when, and how long it takes to do it. Again, hospitals bought into all of these ideas because the innovations promised to wrest savings out of nursing budgets. In 1994 representatives of American Practice Management boasted that since 1987 the company "has helped more than 80 hospitals trim a total of at least $1 billion in expenses." Just think of what you can save, APM advised. "In California, hospitals can save as much as $25,000 a year for each nurse's job that it converts to an aide's job."[32]

And Then Came the Nurse Cheerleaders

One of APM's chief health care consultants was, in fact, a nurse. Connie Curran attracted a great deal of attention in nursing circles in the mid-1990s, and she was involved in the restructuring of the Winnipeg Health Sciences Center that helped to create the institutional context of the deaths of the twelve babies in Winnipeg in 1994. When nurses in the Manitoba Nurses Union protested what APM and the Manitoba government were doing to nursing care in the province, one nurse, Maureen Hancharyk, then vice president of the union, got up and called Curran a "bounty hunter." "Nurses like to be nice," Hancharyk, who is now the union president, recently told me, "but Connie Curran and her company were being paid millions of dollars to lay off between twelve hundred and fifteen hundred nurses."

Curran, however, was not alone in her support for restructuring. Many prominent nurses became advocates of managed care, consultants, or academic advocates of market medicine and nursing.

When the Clinton administration first announced its managed competition plan, nursing organizations such as the American Nurses Association and the American Association of Critical Care Nurses gave it unconditional support. Although a number of nursing academics like the Boston College professor Judith Shindul-Rothschild, who was a former president of the Massachusetts Nurses Association, opposed managed care and spoke out about its potential negative impact on nursing, others supported it. Some, like ANA president Virginia Trotter Betts (who was a close ally of Vice President Al Gore, a fellow Tennessean), insisted managed care would provide greater access for uninsured Americans and give more opportunities to nurses. (In 1998, the Clinton administration gave Trotter Betts the prestigious job of senior advisor on nursing policy and senior health policy advisor in the United States Department of Health and Human Services.)[33]

Other nurses started consulting firms of their own. Tim Porter-O'Grady is typical of many nurse consultants. According to the CV published on his website, he was a staff nurse for two years—between 1973 and 1975. He then left bedside nursing and became a supervisor and then manager and then directed nursing services and patient care services at hospitals between 1975 and 1989. He also began to teach in nursing schools and went back to graduate school to get a doctorate in education and to study management.[34] In 1985, he set up Tim Porter-O'Grady Associates. In a voice-over on the introductory page of his company's website, we hear Porter-O'Grady inform us that "it's a new age for health care.

246   Strong leadership means engaging the issues of transformation. It means making change real for clinicians and making it happen in your organization."[35]

The website explains that Tim Porter-O'Grady Associates is a focused services health care consulting firm. The company provides "consulting services for hospitals, community and health care services in the midst of major clinical service transformation and restructuring. Consultants of the firm provide expert services in the areas of governance improvement, strategic and administrative leadership development, shared decision-making models, and crisis and conflict mediation and resolution processes."[36]

Earlier in his career, Porter-O'Grady explained the rules that govern the "new age for health care" and "the issues of transformation." In a 1994 article the *American Journal of Nursing* he ostensibly responds to nurses' concern that their profession was going through "another change for change's sake." In fact, he tells nurses, this particular change is nonnegotiable because "the driving force behind work redesign is economics."[37]

Economic imperatives dictate that the skill mix of nurses will change, and that many RNs will be laid off and RN duties shifted to either licensed practical nurses or even less-trained nursing assistants. But this is just fine, Porter-O'Grady argues, because "many services provided by highly educated individuals can be delivered by less trained personnel without sacrificing quality care. For example, nursing assistants can do basic treatments such as passive range-of-motion exercises or simple dressing changes."[38]

While less-trained people will be moved up, nurses will be moved . . . well, all over the clinical spectrum. That's because part of hospital redesign involves what is known as "cross-training." To prevent any downtime on the part of those providing care and to encourage patient "throughput," workers in various clinical disciplines (except of course medicine) will be cross-trained to perform duties outside their discipline. Thus, explains Porter-O'Grady, hospitals will be "deploying single-service providers, such as respiratory therapists, lab personnel, and assistive workers, in direct patient care on units rather than in centralized departments. They're cross-trained to perform specific tasks, such as drawing blood and conducting ECGs."[39]

Nurses too are "cross-trained to perform services previously done only by other disciplines."[40] But not to worry, the fact that you went into nursing to be a nurse and now find yourself being a respiratory therapist shouldn't trouble you, because, Porter-O'Grady tells us, RNs will still be in charge of nursing work. They will "retain the core responsibilities of assessment and patient teaching, and coordinate the work of care partners,"[41] which, although dissociated from the activities of hands-on care, will nonetheless remain in nurses' hands—or at least, so the consultants insist.

All of these changes are being made, Porter-O'Grady emphasizes, in the name of better care and better nursing. He quotes Gwynn Perlich, the clinical manager of a surgical unit at the redesigned Saint Vincent's Medical Center in Indianapolis. Perlich explains that nurses need to "broaden their perspective of their role and see themselves as coordinators and integrators of the activities of patient care rather than *just doers*. This is really important because nurses see the whole patient and the entire patient experience rather than just certain functions and activities."[42]

Yes it's true, the author admits, "redesign can mean fewer positions for nurses at the bedside, but it can also mean greater job satisfaction as it frees nurses from clerical and housekeeping tasks to care for patients." Besides, even if RNs do not accept restructuring, many will lose their jobs "with or without redesign." Given the new realities, he argues, it is better for nurses to adapt in ways that "enable hospitals to confront changing conditions while preserving or even improving quality patient care."[43] Since nurses have long been instructed in the arts of professional self-sacrifice, they are apparently supposed to lay down their jobs for their patients.

The drumbeat of inevitability, combined with similar promises of better patient care and a higher level of nursing practice, was the message of many other advocates of market nursing. In their *Reengineering Nursing and Health Care*, Suzanne Smith Blancett and Dominick L. Flarey assembled a roster of nursing devotees of Hammer and Champy. In her foreword, Barbara A. Donaho, former president and CEO of St. Anthony's Hospital in Florida, tells nurse managers that "the major shift to wellness, prevention, and a cost-effective health care plan requires a focus on cost-effectiveness across the total continuum of care, with health care professionals making every effort to use the most appropriate human and technological resource in the most appropriate setting."[44] And in the concluding essay Porter-O'Grady outlines what nurses are up against: high-intensity spending must be reduced as much as possible, and "there are no more permanent structures or boundaries."[45]

But again, why worry? The new health care universe, with its emphasis on disease prevention, health maintenance, and case management, will have plenty of room for nurses. "Hospitals will become triage centers with the primary objective of making rapid diagnoses and stabilizing patients. Most future inpatient units will be what we now know as critical status units; our typical medical surgical units will be virtually empty" of patients and nurses. But nurses will find plenty of work, since restructur-

248   ing of health services will usher in "many and varied health prevention programs. . . . Nurses will play key roles in patient and public education and many will practice in primary prevention practices."[46] The locus of care will shift from the hospital to the home and community where, presumably, nurses will follow patients as managers of the continuum of care.

Accompanied by an array of charts with overlapping circles, pentagons, and hexagons, replete with consultant jargon about visioning and dialoguing and even redialoguing, the various authors outline the tenets of restructuring: cross-training and the replacement of nurses by less-trained and less-expensive aides. Nurses are told that all of this will be worthwhile because restructuring will produce quality outcomes for patients and new opportunities for nurses. There will be "patient-centered" or "patient-focused" care (depending on the chapter). Nurses will work with a plethora of teams—the reengineering team, the patient care team, the operations improvement team, the process analysis team, the facilities management team, and the employee relations and public relations team. Teams will be self-directed and truly collaborative, and the physician will no longer be captain of the ship but just another team member.[47]

Nurses will serve as case managers, assuring continuity of care. Clinical pathways and care maps will help nurses chart the patient's journey through the system and make sure that practice is "evidence based." There will be fewer errors and a focus not only on acute care and individuals but also on the care of populations. In this way, the notion of health will expand beyond individualized considerations of health or illness and lead to a more community-based understanding of healthful living. The authors suggest that reengineering will allow for an emphasis on the social determinants of social problems such as "violence, poverty, homelessness, shelter, parenting, education, and a host of other social forces" and that under this new system they will be more effectively addressed.[48]

Another prominent nurse who believed in the market's ability to remedy many problems in the U.S. health care system was Peter I. Buerhaus. In 1996 Buerhaus and Douglas O. Staiger addressed the growing concerns of RNs who were losing their jobs or experiencing eroding working conditions. Buerhaus was then the director of the Harvard Nursing Research Institute, a center that had been set up by the vice presidents of the nursing departments of the major Harvard teaching hospitals. As early as 1992, Buerhaus had argued that turning health care into a market would succeed in rooting out inefficiencies and shoddy patient care, and would rein in the monopolistic power being acquired by hospitals, insurers, and professional groups.[49] In 1996 Buerhaus and Staiger's study on "Managed Care and the Nurse Workforce" was published in the *Journal of the American Medical Association*. He and Staiger concluded that nurses would in fact lose many hospital-based jobs. Citing a forecast of the Pew Commission on Health Professions, they seemed to suggest that "up to half of all hospitals will close by the end of the decade." Although they also acknowledged that nurses' wages were stagnating, they nonetheless concluded that nurses' concerns about managed care and restructuring were exaggerated. "We see no evidence that nursing personnel who have left the hospital settings are experiencing unusual trouble or delays finding employment in other settings; rather just the opposite seems to be occurring. Thus, there does not appear to be a need for intervention aimed at creating employment opportunities for nursing personnel."[50]

Following the lead of academics who have long tried to get a standard bachelor of science in nursing (BSN) degree for nurses, Buerhaus and his colleagues contended that policy action was indeed needed. The actions the authors proposed had little to do with what staff nurses began begging for as early as 1994—action directed to remedying the eroding wages and conditions in the hospital. Instead, the authors argued for action based on a recognition of the inevitable shifting of even more nurses out of the hospital setting. "Because managed care seems to be associated with a slowdown in nurse employment growth in hospitals and a shift toward nonhospital settings," and of the ability of baccalaureate programs to "prepare RNs for community and primary care settings, as well as acute care, it would be prudent for public policy to focus on shifting the capacity of nurse education toward baccalaureate programs." Or as the authors added, "policymakers should concentrate on actions designed to facilitate changes in nursing education that will enable students to acquire the knowledge base and practice skills needed to provide competent nursing care in nonhospital settings."[51]

No matter how many warnings nurses tried to express about eroding working conditions and poor patient care, many nursing academics and managers countered that nothing could be done to change the system, that bedside nurses were just being alarmist, and that change was inevitable and RNs had better adapt. Even as late as 1998, when evidence was mounting that patient care was deteriorating and a serious shortage of nurses and nursing care was imminent, Edward O'Neil and Janet Coffman argued in *Strategies for the Future of Nursing* that there was no alternative to a "more market oriented system that responds to the needs of organized purchasers," that "management will place the highest priority on cost reduction," that the hospital will be a place of the past as care moves into the community "in physical locations where low cost and high quality and satisfaction can be achieved," and that practice would now be "evidence based."[52]

In a concluding essay on "Nursing in the Next Century," O'Neil—who is a consultant and the codirector and founder of the Center for the Health Professions at the University of California, San Francisco—basi-

250 cally tells nurses they can like it or lump it, because nothing they do will change the march of progress. Or as he puts it, "Intervention by federal and state government policies and professional associations will not stop the transformation of the health care system. For-profit institutions may not dominate the health care industry, but they do set and will continue to set the standards for efficiency and consumer responsiveness. To remain competitive, community-based and nonprofit institutions will find it necessary to meet the standard set by the for-profits." Nursing, he insists, should respond "by adapting to change rather than resisting it."[53]

These arguments characterized the carrot-an-stick approach initially mobilized by those who promoted or supported market-based health care. In the name of leadership, nurses were told they should become followers and adapt to cost cutting, no matter what the consequences to their professional status. Given the prevailing view that there was no alternative to cost cutting and managed care, some nurse executives thought they could temper the severity of change if they tried to manage the managers of care and their host of high-priced consultants.

Some academics and leaders of professional organizations tried to find the proverbial silver lining. Nurses had long been concerned about continuity of care, and about organized medicine's focus on acute care interventions and its failure to deal with either chronic conditions or the health of communities. HMOs promised to take the name "health maintenance organization" seriously and deliver in these formerly neglected areas. The original prototypes, like Kaiser, Group Health of Puget Sound, and Harvard Community Health Plan, had in fact originally provided preventive services and instruction in health maintenance. Some nurses thus believed that growth in HMOs, even for-profit ones, would result in a greater focus on these important and long-neglected areas.

Other nurses were attracted by the promise that they would soon be managing care, functioning as case managers who followed the patient's journey through the health care system, and moving with the patient into the community. Indeed, this promise to shift the locus of care from the hospital to the home and community served a multitude of agendas. Since the late nineteenth century, as we've seen, the hospital has been not only the locus of care but also the locus of nurses' oppression by medicine. Perhaps some nurses viewed news that half of American hospitals will soon disappear as something not to worry about but rather to rejoice over.

Playing on the insecurities instilled in nurses since the nineteenth century and building on the long-standing disdain of some nurses for "tasks," consultants also promised that hospital redesign would catapult RNs to a higher stage of nursing. Thus, to some, giving devalued tasks to less-

skilled people may not have seemed to be a problem, but rather another **251**
form of liberation. Similarly, reconstructing the nurse as a manager and
supervisor of care seemed to elevate the status of the nurse in a culture
that devalues the care of the body and anyone associated with it. As one
nurse academic told me, nursing hadn't been able to sell the American
public on what staff nurses do at the bedside. Perhaps recasting nurses as
managers, rather than deliverers, of care was the ticket to long-sought-
after status. Finally, putting the nurse on the side of health maintenance
and disease prevention also allowed nurses to avoid the stigma associated
with caring for sick, vulnerable people who might never fulfill their social
obligation to become well and productive. As Western societies have
begun to focus more and more on people's responsibility for their own
healthful behavior—another cornerstone of market health care—health
becomes a "virtuous state" and those who are sick risk being stigmatized
because they have failed to be healthy.[54] Their caregivers run the same
risk by association.

Academics and other professional leaders who had long sought more
education for nurses and greater utilization of NPs were also drawn to
managed care. Since 1965 American nursing academics had fought for a
bachelor's degree and university education as standard minimum requirements for entry into nursing practice. With the exception of North
Dakota, no state in the United States had mandated university education
for nurses. The movement of nurses outside of the hospital, where the
role of the physician was less prominent, provided nurses with a perfect
opening to push for greater education. Nurses like Peter Buerhaus didn't
make the argument that all nurses needed the benefit of a university degree. Perhaps because that seemed an unattainable goal. What may have
seemed more pragmatic was to argue for education for an elite group of
nurses who would be "independent" of doctors and thus would more
clearly need to depend on an educated mind of their own. Finally, because
the original health maintenance organizations had employed a great
many NPs, increasing HMO membership (even against the will of most
patients) also promised to increase demand for NP services.

Unfortunately, the cheerleaders of market nursing asked nurses to ignore some fundamental facts. They also encouraged nurses to disregard
any warning signs that market-based managed care and its partner, hospital restructuring, might not actually be good for patients and would certainly create many professional problems for nurses. Concerned with the
limitations of government regulation, distressed by the power of medical
monopoly, and motivated by a genuine understanding of the inefficiencies
of fee-for-service medicine, they neglected to foresee that managed care
insurers might reproduce the very problems they were supposed to solve.

252   As many critics of marketplace medicine have pointed out, market theories are deeply flawed when it comes to dealing with the complexities of the care of the sick. The market is designed for healthy people, the kind who can stroll through Sears or Bloomingdale's or Circuit City in search of the perfect vacuum cleaner, three-piece suit, or computer software. Sick people, who are often angry, frightened, and in denial, do not necessarily make perfect customers who can act as educated health care consumers.

Market advocates ignored the fact that organized medicine was not the only sector in health care that could produce a monopoly of its own. Corporate regulation could mimic all the pitfalls of failed government regulation, and, absent a national health program, the well-intentioned and much-needed attack on the excesses of fee-for-service medicine could easily produce its opposite—what the physician Sidney Wolfe has called fee-for-nonservice medicine.

While many nurses were attracted to the laudable goal of managing care, some ignored what seemed probable to many of its critics (and I was certainly one of the latter): cost cutters were much less concerned with actually managing care than managing costs. From the point of view of nurses, advocates of market medicine and market nursing failed to see that cost cutters trying to wrest savings out of hospital budgets were unlikely to channel those savings (which, in an increasingly for-profit system, would now be directed to shareholders or to CEO salaries and marketing) to well-paid nursing jobs in the home and community.

Finally, the biggest failure of the market crusaders' "visioning" was their belief that laying off thousands of bedside nurses and closing thousands of hospital beds would be good for Americans who are, like citizens of other advanced industrial countries, not getting younger and healthier but rather older and sicker. These people would need more hospital beds and more care, not less. They would need more nurses—everywhere— not just more nurses delivering primary care. They would, of course, need well-educated nurses, not only in the NPs office, but at the bedside.

The stage was thus set to target nurses for massive layoffs, to deprofessionalize nursing practice, to jeopardize quality patient care, and ultimately to create a massive shortage of nursing care and the nurses who could provide it.

10

The New Nursing Universe

espite the promises of the restructurers, it took only a few years for nurses working at the bedside to recognize that hospitals facing a variety of financial pressures would try to solve them by downsizing the nursing work force and extracting as much productivity as possible from those who remained at the bedside. Nurses would soon be laid off and hospitals would not fill vacant positions. Since most hospitals lose between 10 and 12 percent of their RNs annually, the failure to fill vacant positions could eventually result in a significant reduction in the number of RNs. As promised, hospitals also changed the "skill mix" of RNs—that is, how many nurses are actually involved in hands-on patient care. This made perfect economic sense. In 1992 RNs earned an average of $37,738 per year, while the average staff nurse earned $35,212. Unlicensed assistive personnel (UAPs) may earn 20–40 percent less than RNs, and licensed practical nurses (LPNs) also earn less than RNs. Both groups may receive no decent benefits. In their restructuring many hospitals therefore replaced RNs with less expensive staff.[1] "In a cost-competitive system, persons with the lowest level of training who can do the job are employed, under the assumption that higher training leads to greater compensation."[2]

In 1984, 68 percent of all RNs in the United States worked in hospitals. By the year 2000 that figure had fallen to 59 percent.[3] One study cited in a report released by the Institute of Medicine in 2004 showed that the nursing staff in hospitals had declined by 7.3 percent between 1981 and 1993. Another stated that the "use of multiskilled workers who are not RNs to perform such activities as making beds, giving patients baths, positioning patients too ill to position themselves, performing electrocar-

254   diograms, and drawing blood was identified as a core feature of redesign initiatives by 61 percent of 360 hospital nurse executives surveyed in 1995."[4]

Nurses immediately began to worry about RN substitutes who were assigned nursing duties. No states regulate the education of nurse assistants. "No national standards exist for minimum training or certification of ancillary nursing personnel employed by hospitals. . . . Thus, they vary widely in educational attainments and in their training for simple nursing or quasi-nursing tasks. Furthermore, no accepted mechanism exists either to measure competency or to certify in some fashion that ancillary nursing personnel have attained at least a basic or rudimentary mastery of needed skills."[5]

The result? Someone with no high school diploma and few hours of on-the-job training could be changing sterile dressings, inserting urinary catheters, or cleaning tracheotomy tubes. The RN still on the job would have to supervise this nursing aide, while doing all patient assessments and documentation himself. Meanwhile the nurse's assistants would actually be practicing under the RN's license. Under state licensure rules, the RN can be held responsible for any mistakes made by aides working under his direction—and can lose his license as a result of those mistakes. Early in the restructuring process, Janie Storr, a member of the Service Employees International Union who worked at Providence Hospital in Seattle, Washington, expressed nurses' concerns about working with poorly educated aides. She described taking care of seven acutely ill patients with complex medical needs—one patient with an amputated leg, high blood pressure, and paralysis due to a stroke; another with Alzheimer's, back pain, and incontinence; an elderly alcoholic with a fractured arm—while struggling to monitor a certified nursing assistant who, after only forty hours of training, was asked to take the blood sugar levels of patients on the unit. One evening, the assistant was assigned to a diabetic patient. When he reported to Storr a few hours after he'd seen the patient, he causally remarked, "Oh, I forgot to mention this to you, but I didn't think it was important. The blood sugar in room such and such is relatively low, but that's okay because the patient is sleeping." In fact, the patient was in a diabetic coma.

Or there was the patient with a head injury who was admitted to Storr's unit from the ER. When he arrived in the emergency room he told staff that he wanted to die. Shortly thereafter, a nursing assistant brought him up to the floor where Storr works. Two days later, Storr discovered that the potentially suicidal patient had a stash of Tylenol, sedatives, tranquilizers, and psychotropic medications in a plastic bag in the drawer of his bedside table. How did these get here? Storr asked the patient. Oh, he remarked blithely, the patient had brought them with him to the hospital **255** and the nursing assistant who wheeled him up to the unit had simply put them in his drawer.[6]

Nurses aren't opposed to working hard or working with aides, Storr insisted. Aides are supposed to be there to help nurses by monitoring patients and advising the nurse of any significant changes in a patient's status. But how is an untrained aide going to recognize a significant change when he or she sees it? That takes years for nurses to learn.

Another element of restructuring—the cross-training that we discussed in the previous chapter—has also disturbed nurses. Again to save money, other hospital workers were trained, sometimes minimally, to pitch in and do nursing duties in their downtime. Thus when not busy with their primary job, maids, janitors, transport workers, kitchen workers, physical therapists, or other hospital staff would change sterile dressings or insert tracheotomy tubes. Similarly, if a nurse has a moment to breathe, she might be asked to do transport work, or social work, or housekeeping. At the same time, hospitals also laid off workers who actually helped nurses get through the day. Linda Aiken and her colleagues found that nurses were spending a great deal of their time giving patients food trays and then picking them up because food service staff had been laid off. Nurses were pitching in doing housekeeping duties because housekeepers were laid off or had to fetch blood products or lab specimens, or shuttle patients around the hospital because transport workers or lab staff were reduced.[7] If a unit secretary job was eliminated, then nurses had to answer the phone.

In 2003 I talked to one hospital vice president of nursing who told me that his hospital was now dealing with what he described as the "umpteenth" consultant in a decade of restructuring. This time the message was simple: don't cross-train or adjust skill mix, just eliminate nurses' jobs. He managed to convince the hospital CEO and CFO not to cut any more RN positions. Instead, they cut the jobs of one hundred housekeepers. "The place is a mess," he said, "and nurses have to do housekeeping work."

Whether they have been downsized or "rightsized," nurses tell us that their workload has increased and that they may be taking care of two or three times the number of patients they took care of in the past—perhaps ten to sixteen patients on medical surgical floors, and three or four patients on ICUs. In California, nurses lobbied successfully for safe nurse-to-patient ratios because they were able to document this increase in workload. For example, the Institute for Health and Socio-Economic Policy analyzed 18.2 million California hospital discharge records and other data collected from state agencies and the hospital industry. Be-

256   tween 1994 and 1997 there was "an 8.8 percent increase in the average number of patients for which an RN must care; a 7.2 percent decrease in the number of RNs employed; and a 7.7 percent jump in the number of patients per staffed bed between 1995 and 1998." Indeed, during this period California, a pioneer in managed care, ranked second-lowest nationwide (after Washington State) in the ratio of registered nurses to patients.[8]

"The nursing problem surfaced most dramatically in California," Alan Sager, a health care economist at the Boston University School of Public Health explains, "because California was near bottom of nurses per thousand people and has been cutting back on health care spending for past 20 years. Hospital spending was one-sixth, or 16.6% per person below national average, in 2002. In a state where the cost of living is very high, they're spending one-sixth less per person. The cost of living in Los Angeles is 42 percent above the U.S. average."[9]

In 1999 the Minnesota Nurses Association released yet another study confirming these trends. The report revealed that 70 percent of nurses surveyed said they were "unable to perform fundamental valuable duties of nursing . . . on a timely basis."[10]

When nurses complain about too much work for too few nurses, hospitals insist that the number of RNs working in the industry has not declined. One study found that between 1990 and 1996 the number of hospital nurses had actually increased by 15 percent.[11] But these numbers tell a complicated story. When hospitals count the number of RNs they employ, they include everyone who has an RN after their name, no matter where they are working. Administrators, utilization reviewers or discharge planners, nurses working in outpatient settings, clinical specialists, and nurse practitioners supplementing the work of medical residents—all will be listed on the books as part of the nursing work force, even though some are not delivering patient care on a hospital unit and cannot, therefore, help ease the burden of their stressed-out nursing colleagues on those units. "Hospitals now have a cadre of RNs who are taking care of the charts, not the patients," said Jean Chaisson, describing what happened when she was still working at the Beth Israel Deaconess during its merger. "On a floor with fewer RNs spread thinner, when I'm busy rushing one patient to the operating room, these case managers or utilization reviewers are not there to help make sure another patient isn't falling on the floor."

At the end of the 1990s, Jane Smith* gave me a detailed description of what it was like for nurses and patients in the restructured hospital. Smith is an orthopedic nurse who worked nights in a Southern community hospital. She told me she routinely cared for eleven or twelve, and sometimes sixteen to twenty, frail, elderly patients who had just emerged from the operating room after having total hip or knee replacements. Her patients **257** were completely immobilized and could do nothing for themselves. Some were in excruciating pain. Smith took frequent vital signs to make sure they did not develop postsurgical infections, pneumonias, or internal bleeding that could lead to cardiac arrest and death.[12] She helped them walk so they didn't develop blood clots in their legs and shifted their positions so they didn't develop bedsores, which is a serious risk of immobility for 11 to 13 percent of hospital patients under seventy-nine years of age.[13] She also drew blood for tests and, every one to two hours, pushed intravenous medications (such as pain relievers, or heart or ulcer medications) into their veins and monitored their responses.

Over the past decade, doctors and nurses have drawn attention to the scandalous underutilization of pain medication for postsurgical patients. Due to extensive educational efforts, most health care workers today understand that insufficient pain medication jeopardizes a patient's ability to heal. They also know that pain medication should be administered well before patients are turned, given a bedpan, or do their physical therapy. But Smith said, "If you have a really heavy patient load you don't have time to do it. They ask for pain medication and I tell them I'll be there as soon as I can. I recently had five patients in a row who needed meds, and I had to put them on a list. You run in there and give them meds, and get a pain scale, and ask if there's anything you can do and they'll say, 'You're too busy. I don't want to ask you.' "

Dr. William Marshall* works with Jane Smith and shares her frustrations. In fact Marshall, an orthopedic surgeon, was the one who introduced me to Smith and to the problems of nurses in his hospital. He had heard a column I did for Public Radio International when I was a commentator for its show *Marketplace*. Concerned about the nursing crisis in his hospital, he shared his experiences with me. Because nurses are so overloaded, "You order a unit of blood at six thirty in the morning and you find out that at five thirty in the evening it still had not been given. You find patients calling for medicine for pain and it wasn't given to them until an hour and a half later."

Marshall said "cuts to the bone" were driving individual nurses to despair. "There are people with whom I've worked for ten or fifteen years," he explained with mounting distress, "and I find them in tears, saying they can't stand it anymore, they're going to leave."[14]

Patient Acuity and Cumulative Workload

One of the things that makes the contemporary nursing workload so difficult to deal with is the fact that with decreases in patient length of stay

258 and pressure to enhance patient "throughput," nurses' duties have actually increased. This increase in intensity of nursing workload is created by a phenomenon called heightened patient acuity.

When patients stayed in the hospital for longer periods of time, they were generally easier to care for because they were less intensely ill. Over a decade ago, for example, a patient having surgery would be admitted to the hospital the day before his operation for tests, observation, and perhaps some education. After surgery, the patient would be permitted to convalesce before he was discharged. This meant that the average nurse might be taking care of one patient who needed little monitoring or pain and symptom management—the patient admitted the day before surgery or the patient fully stabilized and about to be discharged—as well as several patients who were acutely ill following their procedure. The nurses' caseload would be balanced with high- and low-acuity patients. Today, surgical patients are admitted the same day as their surgery. When they are out of the OR, they are discharged as soon as they no longer have a temperature or a tube inserted in their bodies. Thus patients in the hospital for all sorts of treatments have very intense needs.

Consultants who teach hospitals how to downsize nursing staff often insist that if patients are staying on a unit for shorter periods, it's only logical that they need fewer nurses to care for them. "When consultants crunched the numbers, they would tell VPs of nursing that a decrease in patient length of stay—from, say, five days to three days—for some particular patient population would mean that nurses could be cut from ten nurses for five days to six nurses for three," Joanne Disch, a former vice president of nursing, explains.

"Looking at it from a numerical point of view, the consultants, unfamiliar with the realities of patient care, saw a decrease of 40 percent in length of stay, which to them translated into 40 percent fewer nurses. What they didn't understand was that decreasing the length of stay could actually mean patients needed more nurses per day for the shortened stay. Cutting the length of stay involved cutting precisely those days in the hospital when patients needed less nursing care.

"Someone would say, 'But that's not how it works,'" Disch continues, "and the consultants would respond, 'Well, you're going to cut 40 percent of the work.' Then you explain that you can't apply lockstep financial analysis, and they would tell nurse executives, 'Well, you're just protecting nursing, you're being unrealistic, and you're not willing to change.'"

On its website, the travel nurse agency UltimateNurse maintains a variety of chat rooms. On one of them nurses posted their concerns about patient acuity systems: "Don't you just LOVE those acuities!! I work in the ER, and if a patient states he/she has arm pain, its a low acuity, even if this arm pain turns out to be a massive MI [myocardial infarction, or heart attack]. They take their numbers/acuity from the stated complaint vs the final diagnosis!! Keeps the staffing ratio down."

A labor and delivery nurse explained that "we do 800–900 deliveries a year, and so are fairly busy. Our staffing is based on our acuity system. Approx. a year ago, our hospital incorporated the Van Slyke model of acuities. Since that time our nurse/patient ratio has taken a turn downhill! It is so frustrating! When we complain to the nurse managers that our acuities do not adequately reflect what is going on, we get a 'canned' answer of: 'Yes it does, the time studies you did prove that.' The time studies were done prior to initiating the Van Slyke model. . . . I am so afraid that something bad will happen with the bare bones staffing we have the majority of the time! . . . I have been in nursing 20 years, and this is the worst it has ever been!"[15]

These nurses believe that systems for measuring patient acuity don't reflect the realities of contemporary patient care. In the United States, at least, "data on all Medicare hospital admissions for 1985–97 showed an annual increase in the complexity of cases treated in acute care hospitals as measured by the Medicare case mix index, while a review of patient data for all payers and all acute care general hospitals in Pennsylvania during 1994–97 revealed that the severity of illness of patients admitted to those hospitals increased in the aggregate by 4.5 percent over the four-year period."[16]

When length of stay is truncated, the hospital and other health care facilities become like a Midas Muffler shop. Norrish reported patient turnover rates sometimes as high as 40–50 percent over an eight- to twelve-hour period.[17] For the nurse, there is thus no downtime in the day and no ability to get a few minutes to catch one's breath, take a lunch or coffee break, or even go to the bathroom.

Erica Wilson* works in the oncology clinic of a prestigious teaching hospital in the Northeast. She describes how increased patient acuity has affected her working life. In her clinic, the same numbers of RNs now see more patients. Half of Wilson's patients are on experimental treatments. She must spend a great deal of time reviewing treatment plans and double-checking calculations of drug dosages. Because the side effects of experimental drugs aren't well known, drugs must be infused more slowly. She must also monitor patients closely, so that she can respond to any hint of an adverse reaction, and then go over with the patient the complex schedules for administering chemotherapy.

A great deal of medication administration is now outsourced to the home, and patients are now instructed on self-administration of highly toxic drugs that nurses used to administer in the hospital or clinic. If pa-

260   tients have side effects, they call the clinic. Wilson must leave her patients to respond to these calls. At the same time, patients who have been discharged from the hospital while they are still ill are bringing more serious problems to the clinic. The increased volume of sicker patients also leads to more clinic emergencies like cardiac and respiratory arrests.

As a result of the volume and acuity of patients, "Things are being missed," she says. "Bloods that need to be drawn aren't. For example, you didn't realize that the patient needed a specific blood draw that day and they didn't get it even though the study required it. If we aren't making major mistakes, it's by the skin of our teeth."

Nurses thus complain that they cannot attend to basic patient needs. They have trouble getting medications to patients on time, and they can't get patients to the bathroom or walk them as they should. They do not have time to make sure that the patients are not lying in feces or urine, which puts them at risk for skin breakdown and bedsores, and they do not have time to manage patient's pain adequately. In 2004 a nurse in Pennsylvania told me that she and two RNs and two LPNs share twenty-nine patients on a multipurpose unit that mixes geriatric patients with pediatric patients. She recently was responsible for a woman with a raging blood infection who had permanent feeding and breathing tubes and was in four-point restraints because she kept trying to pull the tubes out. To turn her or bathe her required at least three nurses and at least a half an hour. But how could three nurses find the time to do this when they had to care for twenty-eight other patients, all equally sick and demanding?

Nurses often tell us that they don't even have time to take one of the most important measures used for infection control—hand washing. This is a particularly significant and alarming problem. It's estimated that about two million patients a year in the United States develop hospital-acquired infections and about eighty thousand die of those infections.[18] Hand washing is one of the most important ways that nurses and doctors and other health care workers prevent the spread of infection inside the hospital.

Proper infection control doesn't just involve sticking your hands under the faucet and slapping on a little soap. Nurses are supposed to wash their hands thoroughly before and after patient contact. Atul Gawande, a surgeon, describes the process. "First you must remove your watch, rings, and other jewelry" (which are notorious for trapping bacteria). "Next, you wet your hands in warm tap water. Dispense the soap and lather all surfaces, including the lower one-third of the arms, for the full duration recommended by the manufacturer (usually fifteen to thirty seconds). Rinse off for thirty full seconds. Dry completely with a clean, disposable towel. Then use the towel to turn the tap off."

If you become an ace and manage to do all this in a minute, imagine, **261** Gawande and hand-washing experts ask, how many times you touch a patient and how much time you'd have to spend washing your hands. Not to mention the damage that all this contact with strong soap does to the skin of the nurse or doctor. Although hospitals are now using alcohol rinses and gels, which may be somewhat quicker and less irritating, each additional patient the nurse cares for increases the hand-washing burden. Do nurses all wash their hands in the appropriate manner? When Gawande checked out his hospital in December 2003, he found that even with the new gels, 30 percent of the staff were not complying with hand-washing routines.[19]

More patients to care for. More meds to monitor. More time spent washing your hands. Sicker patients to comfort. These aren't the only extra burdens nurses bear today. Shortened length of stay also increases what researchers Barbara Norrish and Thomas Rundall call nurses' *cumulative* patient load. "A typical nurse may come onto her unit at seven in the morning and take care of seven patients with an aide," says Norrish. "But four of those patients are discharged at noon, and four new patients are admitted at 1:00 p.m. The nurse manager who sees the patient at 1:00 p.m. will argue that the nurse only has seven patients. But she doesn't. She has eleven."

What is true of the speeded-up process of care for each individual nurse also applies to the unit itself. With more admissions and discharges, activity on the unit also escalates. Units feel more chaotic because with more patients, there are more people taking care of them. Nurses will have to deal not just with one or two doctors per four or five patients, but with multiple doctors dealing with multiple patients, all having different and sometimes contradictory suggestions about what to do about the patient. (The cast of characters is even larger in teaching hospitals with their interns, residents, fellows, and postdocs.) Nurses will have to confer with more social workers and more occupational, physical, and respiratory therapists. There will be more discussions with nutrition staff, and with transporters, pharmacy techs, and unit secretaries, if the unit still has one. Nurses will spend more time talking to home care agencies, rehabilitation facilities, nursing homes, or family members negotiating the handoff of the patient. Hospitals argue that there are now "case managers" or social workers to manage the patient's discharge. But nurses have to provide them with the information needed to care adequately for patients leaving the hospital. And of course, more family members and friends will ask nurses pressing questions about their loved one's condition.

Many nurses have told me that when they raise these issues with nurse managers or higher-level hospital administration they get little support.

262 "The business people have taken over and they staff strictly by the numbers," said one nurse in the Midwest. "When you express concerns that patient acuity is higher, they say, 'You have six patients and two RNs, what's the problem?' If you point out that there are problems when there are more admissions or acuity rises, and ask what will happen if . . . , they say, 'We don't staff for what-ifs.' "

Enforcing Throughput

While nurses are juggling all these demands, they are under escalating pressure to get the patient out of the hospital—or discharged from a rehab hospital or even home care. Indeed, nurses today are asked to become enforcers of the very "throughput" that they feel jeopardizes the patients they care for and makes their job so frustrating. When length of stay is truncated, it is not the insurance company executive or utilization reviewer, hospital administrator, government bureaucrat, or MD who actually gets the patient out of his hospital bed. It is the nurse.

Marie Heartfield, a senior lecturer in nursing at the University of South Australia, has studied the work of nurses on short-stay units. Heartfield began her study because of intellectual curiosity and personal experience. She herself had had surgery and was sent home far earlier than she would have been in the past. She found that she had much more pain than she'd anticipated and that nurses were not much help in managing that pain.

What is happening to patients and nurses in this new environment? she wanted to know. So she turned her investigative lens to a short-stay surgical unit in Australia, as well as to the preadmission unit where patients were given education prior to their surgery. Heartfield found that in both preadmission and on the actual short-stay unit, nurses were being asked to ignore the totality of patients' needs and responses in the interest of throughput. When they talked to patients in their preadmission interviews, Heartfield says, nurses often treated patients who were anxious about surgery or anxious about their potential diagnoses (if they were having breast cancer surgery, for example) as though they were not really sick at all. "It was as though the nurses were processing goods in a supermarket rather than engaging with people who were having surgery and who were understandably nervous about it."

Heartfield says she found the same thing on the short-stay unit. Nurses were constantly manipulating filled and unfilled beds, not patients. Patients would come in and go to surgery and the bed they were in was freed for another patient. The nurse would then get another patient who might then go to surgery, and another would come in. If patients returned from surgery to the unit, they were expected to stay no longer than two days. They were defined as short-stay patients, not as people with a particular condition or problem. If the patient expressed concerns about the length of their hospital stay, Heartfield says, the nurses were not encouraged to consider those concerns.

"One man in my study was middle-aged. He had come in to have surgery on his shoulder and was only supposed to stay for one night. He made it quite clear that he didn't think a one-night stay would be very good for him because he would have limited mobility after the surgery. He told the nurses that he lived by himself and felt that a two-night stay would be more appropriate. After the surgery he was in a lot of pain, and had virtually no mobility in his shoulder."

Under the new model, this patient was not defined as someone with a complex set of physical needs, who would face difficulties once he was outside of the hospital. "Because it was just a shoulder he shouldn't be requiring any hospital services. His problems had been localized to his shoulder and did not include living his life after having surgery on that shoulder."

To keep their jobs, nurses have adapted to the model. Privately, however, many complain about these issues to their unit managers and top-level administrators. Most say they get nowhere. Work smarter, not harder, they are told. Learn to delegate and prioritize. "How do you prioritize between a patient in shock and someone in ventricular tachycardia, or a patient in ventricular tachycardia and one who's in cardiac arrest?" an ICU nurse asked.

RNs also worry about what happens to patients when they are sent home. They know that patient care is now being outsourced to ill-equipped relatives—family members who are now asked to provide professional-level nursing care in the home. As a number of studies have shown, family caregivers of the elderly and chronically ill often pay for providing help to their loved ones with loss of income, loss of job, and sometimes loss of their own health and well-being.[20]

The Disappearance of In-House Education and Support

The stresses that nurses experience today are further aggravated by cutbacks in the kind of clinical education and staff development that hospitals often provided both veteran and new RNs. Like physicians, nurses need a period of apprenticeship or orientation after they graduate from nursing school to help them master the complexities of actual practice. Our society doesn't build a standard period of apprenticeship training— an internship or residency stage in the workplace—into nursing educa-

264 tion, as it does for doctors. Two reports, in 1996 and 2001, indicated that a majority of RNs had not been sufficiently prepared to take care of patients' needs in a rapidly evolving health care system in which there were constant advances in technology, treatment, and medications.[21] Because of this, hospitals must provide some sort of orientation and ongoing education that allows novice nurses to develop a high degree of competence.

Rather than throw them directly into the fray, many hospitals used to provide new nurses with a period of orientation—perhaps six, eight, or twelve weeks in which they attend orientation sessions and work with a more experienced nurse (in nursing jargon that RN is called a "preceptor"). If enough experienced nurses were employed on units, and patient loads permitted, nurses could also expect help from more experienced nurses with whom they can discuss patient care issues.

In many hospitals busy staff nurses, whether novices or experts, also received help and support from clinical nurse specialists, nurses like Marion Phipps or Jean Chaisson. These nurses had master's degrees and specialized in a particular area of nursing. They would often run staff development programs and educational sessions for floor nurses. If they were unit based, they were available to give nurses advice and seek out the latest research on a variety of different clinical issues.

Like physicians, nurses also depend on continued education to stay abreast of new developments in both nursing and medicine. They have to learn about new treatments and medications and about new research produced by both disciplines. Indeed, in order to maintain their licenses, nurses are required to collect a certain number of continuing education units (CEUs) every year. Many nurses benefited from hospital "in-services"—education provided in the hospital, sometimes even on their unit—that helped them keep current.

In order for nurses to take advantage of educational opportunities, hospitals not only have to provide teachers and speakers, they have to give nurses time off to attend educational or professional meetings. This, in turn, depends on the indirect resource of adequate nurse staffing levels on a particular unit. Doctors are able to attend a grand rounds or a conference outside the hospital because on-call doctors cover for them and because nurses remain behind to take care of their patients. But who will replace nurses who leave the bedside to advance their knowledge? Certainly not doctors. Other nurses will. If there are not enough nurses on a unit to replace a nurse who wants to go to an educational session, she won't be able to leave. Similarly, if hospitals don't allocate resources for clinical specialists, there will be no unit-based help for the busy nurse.

Cost cutting has led hospitals to eliminate not only nursing staff but also staff education and development programs. Many hospitals have scaled back their orientation programs for newly hired nurses and ongoing in-service training and continuing education programs for nurses as a result of financial pressure.[22] When hospitals were under pressure to cut costs, nurse executives and managers felt they were in a terrible resource bind. "Nursing leaders faced with draconian budget targets felt they didn't want to cut direct caregivers or nursing assistants," explains Joanne Disch, a former nursing executive and a current professor of nursing. "Faced with these kinds of budget targets that were pretty dramatic, a lot of people felt that it would be better to cut educational resources than to cut staff."

What happens when nurses don't get properly educated or oriented? The first days Carol Lincoln* spent on the job are an example. After graduating from nursing school, she took a position as a staff nurse at a major hospital in Toronto. Lincoln was sent to a unit that was short-staffed. No one expected or welcomed her. Most important, no one had time to orient her. She felt that the nurse who was assigned to introduce her to the unit was furious that she had to take on this burden on top of all her other responsibilities. "And she let me know it in no uncertain terms," Lincoln says.

Just to get this novice out of her hair, she sent her off for her first on-the-job patient contact—preparing dead bodies for shipment to the hospital's morgue. "I had never seen a dead body," Lincoln shuddered. "We don't do cadavers in nursing school. I had no idea how to provide postmortem care. I didn't know how to wrap a body and no one told me and I couldn't find any protocols that could help me. So there I was, in this room with one dead patient on a bed, and one live patient behind a flimsy hospital curtain. I had to battle to try to lift and shift this literally dead weight without alarming the living patient who was only a few feet away."

Although the more experienced nurse finally took pity on Lincoln and suggested that she help her with lighter tasks, her day didn't get any better. What was "light" to her was heavy to a novice like Lincoln. She was asked to set up the intravenous pumps that deliver fluids and patients' medications. But she didn't know how they worked, and the experienced nurse was too harried to give her the comprehensive lesson she needed. She didn't understand the Cardex system used to record patients' medication needs and care plans. As her shift was coming to an end and she was ready to breathe a sigh of relief, the nurse asked her to fill up a tub for a man who was dying of AIDS. She went into the bathroom only to discover that she was dealing not with a normal tub but a special hydrosonic tub whose sides had to be covered with gel before the patient bathed in it.

When she mastered that maneuver and began to fill it with water, the nurse peeked in the door and asked her to help with another patient.

266 Leaving the room, Lincoln shut the door behind her. "The unit was a madhouse," she says. "I went with her to her patient. And then on to the next thing. Phones were constantly ringing, nurses were being paged every which way. As the chaos increased, we answered one phone and heard a frantic voice on the other end of the line. It was the cardiac care unit, the unit just below ours. 'What the hell's going on up there?' they screamed. 'The ceiling down here is falling in and water is flooding the unit.'"

"Oh my god," Lincoln thought, as she hung up the phone and raced over to the bathroom. "I opened the door and water streamed out into the hallway. I had left the tub on and shut the door and forgot about it because of the crush of other responsibilities. I was . . . well, how can I describe it? mortified, humiliated. And also very, very angry." "You don't come out of nursing school ready to start on an understaffed unit. I should have been oriented," Lincoln says. Training was what she determined to get.

The next morning, Lincoln went to the nurse manager and begged her to let her spend the next five shifts with no patient load, following a veteran nurse and just absorbing and learning. She agreed, with one caveat. "She told me they couldn't pay me, that I'd have to work for nothing." The two came to an agreement: Lincoln would work seven shifts and get paid for only two.

With that week of training complete, Lincoln felt more secure. Over the next eleven months her skills improved, but the situation in her hospital deteriorated as more nurses were laid off and patient loads increased. Since Canada was experiencing widespread hospital "restructuring," Lincoln was unable to find more satisfying work. Lincoln followed many other Canadian nurses who went to the United States during the 1990s because of the lure of better pay. What she didn't understand was that positions in U.S. hospitals were vacant because similar hospital restructuring was taking place in the United States. When she spoke to the vice president of nursing in the U.S. hospital trying to woo her down to Texas, Lincoln was surprised to learn that she was being interviewed for a head nurse position on the cardiology unit. She told the nurse executive that she'd had less than a year's experience as a nurse with none of it in cardiology. Lincoln's reservations were dismissed, and she was told that the hospital would provide her with a few weeks of training for the position. She nonetheless refused to take the job and was hired as a staff nurse on another unit.

For years, nursing students have complained about the education they receive from veteran nurses in the clinical setting. Restructuring only exacerbates the problem. And the rudimentary introductions new nurses receive in the restructured workplace don't bode well for future retention. Many hard-won new recruits to nursing—students in nursing schools—report that generally they are not warmly welcomed when they enter hospitals, long-term care facilities, clinics, and other health care settings for clinical experience and contact. During these "clinical rotations" or "clinical placements," students are supposed to watch and question experienced nurses and help them care for patients. Today, these experienced nurses have little time to teach students and respond to what seems to be a relentless barrage of questions.

Teaching, like orienting the new nurse, is something a nurse racing between multiple, increasingly sick patients can ill afford, and many nurses make it quite clear that they do not appreciate this extra load. They aren't paid extra for teaching students, and their caseloads aren't adjusted accordingly. Harried nurses who lack teaching experience may not bother to conceal their resentment about this extra duty that has been placed on their shoulders.

Katherine Harris, who is now a labor and delivery nurse in western Massachusetts, says that when she was a student she had some nurses who were nice to her and a lot who weren't. "You go in there and think that you're there to help them out. But in fact, I see—now that I'm a nurse myself and work with students—that students aren't a help. They're an extra burden. They have nothing but questions and take up nothing but time." A student at the University of Toronto School of Nursing echoed these sentiments. What she found was not help but a disgruntled nurse who made her feel completely unwelcome.

When I was recently asked to lecture to a fourth-year class of bachelor's students at a nursing school at a state university in New England, I asked the students to write about their experiences learning to be nurses. The question was entirely neutral and did not specifically solicit negative comments. While many of the students remained committed to their choice of career, the majority were disheartened by their workplace encounters.

"My experience on a med-surg (medical-surgical) floor last semester was very difficult," one student wrote. "All of the nurses, and I mean all of them, were not open and understanding with us. We students received negative attitudes and a lot of harshness every time we went to clinical. This really impacted the way I worked with my patients because I was constantly thinking about how, for example, one nurse yelled at me earlier or gave me a dirty look after I asked a simple question. I was always nervous on the floor and scared to death to ask questions or ask for help. I would get nauseated before each clinical day because I knew what the response would be from the nurses when we arrived in the morning."

268   What is perhaps even more disturbing are the lessons that students learn about the realities of patient care in the era of cost cutting. Nurses, by their example, cannot teach students how to give patients thorough evaluations, take needed time to deliver and monitor treatments and administer medications, and—this is particularly distressing to students—take the time to educate them and listen to their patients' concerns and assuage their anxieties. What nursing students seem to learn is how to rush in and out of rooms and deliver just the basics in the shortest amount of time possible.

In an interesting essay, one of the students described her own experiences as a patient when she'd recently had her appendix out. She felt she got good care because the nurses in the hospital had worked with her when she worked in the same hospital as a nursing assistant. What stunned this young woman was the way the nurses treated her roommate, a patient who required much more care than she did. "Most of the staff ignored her call bells but would come running as soon as I rang mine. Eventually I would ring in for her as well. I could easily sense the impatience in everyone's voices when they spoke to her."

One student summed up the frustration her classmates conveyed: "I have often had to rush into a room, do the care and rush out. Not stopping to talk or do the extra things. I have often gone home crying because I could not do all I wanted, all I thought these elderly patients deserve."

These new nurses and nursing students would have benefited greatly from the assistance of clinical nurse specialists. The clinical specialist was one of the great innovations of the 1970s and 1980s, when nursing academics and hospital management recognized the need for unit- or hospital-based education and support for working nurses. This particular nursing job, however, was one of the casualties of cost cutting and restructuring. During the 1990s, clinical specialist positions were either reduced or eliminated. Indeed, in the mid to late 1990s, it became almost a vogue for clinical specialists to go back to school to become nurse practitioners.

"In the mid-1990s, with the advent of HMOs and consultants like the Hunter Group, clinical specialists were laid off in huge numbers. No one had ever before experienced anything like this," says Kathleen Dracup, who was a cardiac clinical specialist and professor at UCLA School of Nursing during this period. "People looked around and saw that the promise was that nurse practitioners were going to have the job security of the future. So schools of nursing developed post-master's programs for people who had master's degrees, such as clinical specialists, so they could get an NP degree. In 1995, there were about twenty-five thousand NPs in the United States; now there are over a hundred thousand. Part of that was fueled by clinical specialists transforming themselves into NPs."

Medicare also helped fuel the exodus, Dracup adds. At about the same **269**
time clinical specialists were being laid off, Medicare began to reimburse
nurse practitioners for their work. All of this, she comments, sent a big
message that nurse practitioners could find employment and reimbursement while clinical specialists couldn't even get a job. The message took.
"There was galloping motion toward NPs," Dracup explains.

The problem, Dracup says, is that the role of the NP is very different
from the role of the clinical specialist. "Clinical specialists are defined as
supporting systems of care. They work with nurses to support nurses, do
research, and help hospitals gear up for Joint Commission accreditation.
(The hospital accreditations that Medicare requires are done by the Joint
Commission on Accreditation of Healthcare Organizations.) Nurse practitioners spend their days doing very different things. They work one-to-
one with patients, often as physician substitutes or sometimes in collaboration with physicians."

Jean Chaisson's professional voyage over the past decade illustrates
what has happened to the role of clinical nurse specialist. When I began
to write about Chaisson for my book *Life Support*, she was practicing at
the Beth Israel Hospital in Boston. Chaisson spent four days a week working as a clinical specialist, teaching nurses about the latest developments
in medical treatments and nursing care and advising nurses and doctors
about how to provide better care for patients. Because she wanted to be
close to nursing practice, she spent one day a week delivering direct care
to patients. When her hospital merged with the New England Deaconess
in 1996, the cost squeeze was on.

Unit managers had been instructed to cut costs. They felt, Chaisson
said, that having a nurse available to teach and support RNs was a luxury
they could no longer afford. So clinical specialist positions were cut and
nurse managers, whose workload had also increased (a typical nurse manager would, under restructuring, manage two or perhaps even three units
rather than one), would be asked to provide clinical support to nurses
while simultaneously doing twice as much managerial work.

Chaisson didn't immediately lose her job as a clinical specialist. Instead
the balance of her work week shifted. She worked one day a week as a
clinical specialist and four days as a staff nurse. During what soon became
known as the "mangled merger" between the two hospitals, the newly
combined institution was hemorrhaging money. More and more clinical
specialists were laid off. Chaisson stopped doing clinical specialist work
and worked as a staff nurse.

The hospital had always used clinical specialists to run educational sessions. With money drying up for staff education and clinical specialists
losing their positions, there was less and less emphasis on education,

270   Chaisson explains. And the hospital began to cut back on the kind of day-long programs it used to run. These dealt with important subjects like skin and wound care, arrhythmias (irregular heart rhythms), renal failure, and other clinical issues. The hospital also offered lunchtime seminars—for example, a seminar for a geriatric interest group where nurses could come once a month and get an hour's worth of CEUs. With the departure of the clinical specialists, those programs began to disappear. Floor nurses were so overloaded with patients that they might be unable to attend the more meager fare that was offered instead.

By 2003, when I visited the Beth Israel Deaconess, a new nurse administrator was trying to reverse some of the problems caused by the merger and was starting to rehire clinical specialists. From conversations I had with the clinical specialist on the ICU as well as with a new staff nurse, it seemed, however, that the mandate of the clinical specialist had changed. Rather than planning care and conducting ongoing education to refine and expand nurses' knowledge, the nurse educator's role seemed to be far more limited. Her mission, said the clinical specialist, was to orient new nurses quickly to the ICU and get them out on the floors as speedily as possible.

In its 2004 report, *Keeping Patients Safe*, the Institute of Medicine (IOM) states that nurse education in hospitals and other health care facilities has suffered during cost cutting and does not provide the ongoing support nurses need. And if hospitals have skimped on training for nurses, who at least had a basic education in nursing school, what was even more alarming was that they were also failing to educate the nursing assistants who were now being asked to do many nursing tasks. The IOM report also noted that in the reengineering schemes not enough initial training and retraining was given to the nursing assistants who were supposed to lighten the load of the registered nurses that hospitals employed.[23] How then could nursing assistants—who may not even have had a high school education and who were not covered by any state or federal regulations—be safely left with significant patient responsibilities if they didn't have the training to fulfill them?

In fact, because nursing education and staff development has been so truncated, some unions have stepped in to fill the gap. Dorothy McCabe, the director of the Department of Nursing and Career Services of the Massachusetts Nurses Association (MNA), which provides continuing education for RNs, says that before cost cutting the MNA offered sporadic continuing education programs. "Now we now offer about twenty courses on clinical subjects, like lab values and cardiac arrhythmias, and many of them are filled—and not only with nurses who are MNA members. Fifty percent of the attendees are not MNA members. They're com-

ing because so many hospitals have done away with staff education de- **271**
partments and clinical specialists. In fact, I worry about RNs and their patients when our courses are filled."

Working Longer

In the spring of 2004 I went to visit an exhibit at the American Textile
History Museum in Lowell, Massachusetts. The museum is a monument
to American fabrics and to the workers whose sometimes backbreaking
labor produced them. On display were photographs of female workers
who toiled in the textile mills of Lowell during the latter part of the nineteenth century. One glass case exhibits a letter written to a mill official in
1867 and signed by dozens of mill workers. It reads as follows: "To the
treasurer of the Appleton Corporation. We, the undersigned operatives in
your employ, believing that 11 hours a day is inimical to our best moral &
physical interests, would most earnestly request you to reduce the term of
labor from 11 to 10 hours per day & your petitioners as in duty bound will
ever pray."

This petition, written over a hundred years ago, captures the struggle
workers have waged—and thought they'd won—for the eight-hour day
and the forty-hour week. While workers in other countries are fighting
for even greater reductions in the workday and workweek, nurses are
being asked to go back more than a century in time and devote more and
more of their weekly—and daily—waking hours to their work. A paradoxical combination of employer demand, nurses' fear of retaliation and job
loss, failure to pay nurses an adequate wage, and nurses' own voluntary
accommodation to poor working conditions has resulted in an epidemic
of overwork in the North American nursing profession. This epidemic includes four interrelated phenomena—so-called voluntary overtime work,
longer shifts, mandatory overtime, and lack of flexible work schedules. All
of these problems are another way that the new ruthless economy, to use
Head's term, is infiltrating nursing.

In the new global economy, when cost cutting and downsizing take
place, those who remain on the job are asked to work longer and harder.
Indeed, some form of overtime work is a central cost-cutting strategy in
the world of downsizing. That's because, in the "rightsized" workplace,
only the labor force—not the amount of work itself—has been rightsized.
The amount of work actually remains the same or increases. When, for
example, the automobile work force was downsized in the 1990s, the
number of cars that workers were expected to produce didn't diminish to
accommodate the reduction in force; the worker was asked to produce
even more with much less. Similarly, in spite of predictions of huge num-

272 bers of hospital closings and diminishing numbers of patients, the hospital and health care work place is dealing with more patients, and, as we've seen, more acutely ill patients.

Using overtime as a routine way to staff a hospital floor enables employers to increase worker productivity while simultaneously cutting labor costs. They do this by encouraging employees to work more overtime or by mandating them to do so. After all, it's more cost-effective to ask one worker to spend more time on the job doing the work of two or three workers than to hire those extra workers and incur the costs of their salaries, benefits, and job training.

As cost cutting proceeded during the 1990s and into the twenty-first century, hospitals cut their nursing budgets and many other expenses. "Some of the efforts to squeeze hospitals have been justified by evidence of wasteful practices," Alan Sager says. "But most hospitals today are run in a pretty lean way and on a pretty lean mixture. Nonetheless they are still under pressure to continue cutting costs." Sager and other critics of market medicine, like physician researchers David Himmelstein and Steffie Woolhandler, argue that this is because cost-cutting efforts have not addressed the real sources of waste, which "are clinical and administrative—unnecessary surgery, incompetent care, defensive medicine, all of which raise cost without clinical benefit. Then there are all the mountains of unnecessary paperwork," says Sager, "which also raise costs without clinical benefit. Again, those two forms of waste are not under hospitals' control, so hospitals squeezed on the revenue side continue to try to squeeze the costs that they can control—e.g., nursing."

Like other workers in the United States, nurses usually agree to take on large amounts of overtime work because their real wages have stagnated and they simply can't make it on their salaries. Thus, Michael Smith has argued, "the decline of real wages partially renders moot the question of whether an employer actually requires overtime; many workers consider overtime mandatory because they need the extra pay to maintain their standard of living."[24]

In addition to financial concerns, nurses' socialization makes them particularly susceptible to overtime: it is difficult for them to resist appeals for self-sacrifice. When a manager insists that their patients need them, or they know their refusal to work will add an even heavier burden on their colleagues, it's hard for them to say no. When workers don't accept overtime work on a voluntary basis, many employers mandate them to work an extra few hours or an extra shift. If workers refuse, they may lose their jobs or face discipline. With mandatory overtime, Smith writes, "workers lose the ability to weigh the loss of leisure and family time against the added income. Instead, they are often forced to chose between working **273** overtime and losing their jobs."

Here's how it works in the hospital. After an exhausting eight- or twelve-hour shift, a nurse may suddenly learn that she has to work an additional eight or twelve hours. For a largely female work force with child care and family responsibilities, this is particularly onerous, not to mention unsafe, because a weary nurse will be far less alert. "The problem is worse for us at night," explained Kate Maker, a nurse at UMass Memorial Hospital in Worcester, Massachusetts. "You work from three in the afternoon to eleven at night. You have arranged for someone to take care of your kids till you come home. So at ten o'clock, you're told you have to work mandatory overtime. Well, just like the hospital can't pull nurses out of the sky to suddenly work eleven to seven, we can't pull baby-sitters out of the sky at eleven at night to take care of our kids. So we're put in the terrible position of having to choose between abandoning our patients or abandoning our children."

In some states, if RNs protest that mandatory overtime assignments are unsafe for their patients, they may be told that any refusal to accept the assignment will constitute "patient abandonment." This is a particularly cynical use of a serious and important category of work place violation. To protect patients, a nurse who accepts a patient assignment by reporting to work can be disciplined and potentially lose her license if she walks off the job and thus willfully abandons her patients. This charge can lead to a disciplinary action by the state Board of Registration in Nursing. But patient abandonment only exists when the nurse has accepted the patient assignment and then abandons her vulnerable charges. It is a retrospective, not a prospective act. If she says, "No, I am too tired to work tonight," thus refusing mandatory unscheduled overtime, she is not abandoning a caseload of patients she has accepted.

Even nursing students learn how dangerous it can be to refuse a mandated extra shift. One nursing student described an incident that occurred while she was doing her clinical placement. When all the nurses gathered for report, she expected to hear them discussing medical and nursing diagnoses. Instead they were talking about a colleague who'd been fired. What had happened to this woman? she wondered. The nurse had been ordered to work mandatory overtime because another nurse had called in sick. The nurse refused. "Even though she needed to pick up her kids from daycare, the supervisor fired her, saying that she wasn't a 'team player.' Apparently a year earlier that same nurse had been instrumental during a code. Not a team member, what does that mean?"

Given these pressures, it is not surprising that nurses report an epi-

274 demic of overtime, both mandatory and voluntary, over the past decade. When the American Nurses Association surveyed 4,826 nurses in 2001, almost 70 percent said they work mandatory or unplanned overtime each month, some as many as three or four times per month. When they were asked about planned overtime, "the total percentage of nurses working some form of overtime rose by more than 10 percent. . . . More than half of the nurses (51.7 percent) work anywhere from one to sixteen hours of overtime, and only 20.2 percent work no overtime at all." Many said they work between forty and sixty hours a week, with the average nurse in the survey working as much as ten hours beyond the usual forty-hour work-week. Almost 12 percent said they worked sixty-one to eighty hours a week.[25]

In another report "61 percent of nurses surveyed said they had noted an increase in overtime or double shifts during the past year. Forty-eight percent said that 'the amount of overtime required' had increased."[26]

The use of mandatory overtime has added to nurses' discontent and fueled the exodus of nurses from hospital work. This in turn created greater demand for fewer nurses to work harder and longer. In an ever-downward spiral, hospitals found it harder to attract new recruits. Mandatory overtime as a solution to nursing shortages only exacerbated the problem.

And Longer Still

Overtime work is such a serious problem in part because of longer shifts. Ten or twenty years ago, most nurses in hospitals worked eight-hour shifts. To give twenty-four-hour care to patients, the standard hospital working day was divided into three eight-hour shifts. A group of nurses would arrive at seven in the morning and work until three. Another group of nurses would arrive to relieve them and work the evening shift, from three until eleven. These would be relieved by the night shift, who would work from eleven to seven.

Because they have to juggle work and family—or because they found the work so unsatisfying and preferred to get it over with as quickly as possible so they could have more free time for themselves—some nurses have turned back the clock on a century of labor law reform (as well as a growing body of literature documenting the relationship between fatigue, error, and poor judgment, not to mention irritability and poor communication in the workplace) and work three back-to-back twelve-hour shifts. Before cost cutting, some hospitals would pay them a full-time salary for thirty-six hours of work.

Today, studies and surveys have shown, fewer and fewer nurses work the standard eight-hour day, and more and more are working three back-to-back twelve-hour shifts. Whether they choose these schedules volun- **275** tarily or not, many find they are staying at work even after their shift is over because they simply have too much work. The American Nurses Association survey found that the majority of nurses were now working between forty-one and sixty hours per week, with some working as much as eighty hours a week.[27]

Anne Rogers, a sleep researcher at the University of Pennsylvania School of Nursing, is the principal investigator of a study funded by the Agency for Healthcare Research and Quality to investigate the impact of nursing working hours on patient safety. In the heated debate about resident and physician working hours, Rogers explains, there have been many studies (about thirty) on physician work hours. Data on hours have been correlated with patient safety problems such as errors in medication orders, operations on the wrong limb, and poor judgments about patient care. There have been no studies, however, of nurses' work hours. "We don't know what hours nurses work, nor do we know the effect on patients," Rogers comments.

To rectify this problem, researchers asked four hundred nurses randomly selected from the American Nurses Association, and five hundred from the American Association of Critical Care Nurses to keep a diary for twenty-eight days. They were to note when they slept, when they worked, when they were scheduled to work, if they made errors, if they were drowsy at work, if they fell asleep, if they worked overtime, and why. Researchers have collected data on ten thousand shifts.

Rogers explained that data on the first 5,300 shifts worked by the ANA nurses revealed "the majority of nurses no longer work traditional day evening or night shifts. About 60 percent of nurses in the first sample worked twelve hours. In the sample of critical care nurses, 86 percent were on twelve-hour shifts. Since hospitals are no longer willing to pay nurses who work thirty-six hours a full-time salary, they are also asking nurses to come in to do an extra four-hour shift to make up the difference."

But twelve hours, the researchers discovered, is not the full duration of many nurses' working day. Some nurses—a small minority—were scheduled to work twenty consecutive hours. More troubling is the fact that most nurses simply can't get their work done during their scheduled shift. "Every nurse in our sample," Rogers said, "worked extra at least once during the twenty-eight-day period. Only one out of five days could they count on getting out on time. The nurses are averaging fifty-five minutes extra every single day they work."

Although these nurses were staying late to finish their work, they were probably not being paid for this overtime. The Fair Labor Standards Act

276   mandates that workers be paid overtime, but workers have to put in for that overtime in order to receive their pay. Rogers and others report that nurses are not going to their employers and requesting their overtime pay. According to Rogers, one study has shown that some don't want to ask managers for extra pay because they worry about some form of employer retaliation or feel they'd be accused of being "too slow." In the latter case, the inability to finish work would not be blamed on the characteristics of the workplace—increased workload and patient acuity—but on the characteristics of the worker. Some nurses may simply be unaware of labor laws mandating that they be paid for anything they do in the workplace: reporting on the condition of patients to another nurse taking over for the next shift, documenting their work in a chart, or finishing up with phone calls or other patient care activities after they finish their shift. "All of this is working time," says labor lawyer Robert Schwartz, author of *Your Rights on the Job*.[28] "Reporting time, charting time, that is working time." But it will only be paid as working time if the employer exercises his or her rights.

Hospital workloads also lead nurses to contribute their unpaid labor to the hospital bottom line, as they increasingly work through breaks and lunch. Again, under state and federal laws and union contracts, nurses must be offered breaks and cannot be required to work through them. The nurse can volunteer to work through her breaks, but then the employer has to pay the nurse for those breaks or she must be permitted to leave work thirty or forty-five minutes earlier, depending on the amount of break time allotted.

Today, however, most nurses are working through lunch and getting no compensation for it. "On 63 percent of shifts, nurses didn't get a lunch break or a break relieved of patient care. They may have had a lunch break but they spent it answering call lights. Ten percent of these nurses didn't get lunch breaks at all, no matter how long their shift," Rogers reports. Ten states have laws stipulating that workers have to have a thirty-minute lunch break, but nurses in those states were not getting their legally mandated breaks and lunch periods. In forty states there are no laws mandating lunch breaks, but laws do stipulate that if you work on your lunch break, you should be paid. These nurses were not paid for the time they took from their breaks. In June 2004, after an investigation by the U.S. Department of Labor, the UMass Memorial Medical Center was forced to pay 367 of its nurses $614,449 in back wages because the hospital didn't pay them wages for their breaks even though they worked through them.[29]

"So," Rogers comments, "middle-aged women (the average age of nurses in the sample, like nurses in general, was forty-five) are working

eight, ten, twelve hours without any break from patient care responsibili- **277**
ties and then staying when their shift ends because they can't get their
work done."

Not surprisingly, Rogers adds, many of these nurses were sleep-
deprived. Some nurses didn't get enough sleep because they were doing
other things. Some had heavy family responsibilities at home. Many of
these nurses, for example, were taking care of elderly relatives, young
children, or both. Many reported not getting enough sleep, being drowsy
at work, or even falling asleep at work. While this is often a problem for
nurses who work at night, many nurses were having trouble staying awake
during the day.

Not only are nurses working without being paid for it, but their salaries
overall have stagnated. Although nurses have not been encouraged to
focus on the monetary rewards of the profession, the stagnation in wages,
at a time when the job has become more hectic and demanding, has contributed to a flight from bedside nursing into administrative positions and
even into other professions. "Since 1992," Julie Sochalski writes, "nursing
wages on average have done no better than keep pace with inflation in the
general economy. After adjustment for inflation, RNs saw no increase in
purchasing power of their annual earnings during most of the 1990s."
Similarly, Robert Steinbrook reports that "in recent years, wages for registered nurses have been relatively flat as compared with the rate of inflation. In 2000, the average annual salary of a registered nurse employed
full-time was $46,782. Between 1980 and 1992, real annual salaries for
registered nurses increased by nearly $6,000. Between 1992 and 2000,
however, they increased by only about $200."[30]

During the early 1990s, when demand for nurses was low, it is perhaps
not surprising, Sochalski notes, that nursing wages didn't rise. But even
after hospitals started chasing nurses, "RNs who did not seek additional
education or promotion to higher positions received wages that rose at
decreasing rates with experience. Wages paid to hospital staff nurses who
graduated twenty years earlier were only 10 percent higher than wages
paid to those who came into nursing ten years earlier." This pattern,
Sochalski speculated, would encourage new candidates to the profession
to view bedside nursing as a career trap and to believe that "the only way
to realize salary gains is to pursue more education or leave the bedside for
other jobs, such as administrative positions."[31]

Economist Barbara Bergmann has done some research on the issue of
nurses' salaries. Like Sochalski, she wondered why, in a market economy,
nurses wages haven't risen enough when there is a recognized shortage.
One reason, she believes, is that hospitals in many metropolitan regions
implicitly agree not to compete with one another to raise wages. Hospi-

278   tals do this, Bergmann argues, by informally exchanging information about the salaries they pay nurses, which essentially limits wage increases. Indeed, in 1994, the Department of Justice brought an antitrust suit against the Utah Society for Healthcare Human Resources, an organization controlled by Utah hospitals, for doing just that. "In 1996, the Federal Trade Commission issued a joint statement of policy outlining what kind of information sharing hospitals may engage in, so as not to violate antitrust laws," Bergmann says. "It would be interesting to know whether these guidelines are being followed. I suspect they aren't."

Nurses' wage stagnation is part of a larger pattern of the stagnation of middle-class wages in the United States. Simon Head argues that there is a connection between broader reengineering in the economy and the income inequalities that the United States experiences. "Data for the economy as a whole provides strong circumstantial evidence of a causal link between technological change in the form of reengineering and ERP (enterprise resource planning), and the stagnation of most U.S. wages and benefits."[32]

Hot and Cold Running Nurses

Nurses' morale has also plummeted because of the increasing use of floating—another hospital staffing practice nurses have long deplored. "Floating" means moving nurses from the unit where they usually work to another nursing unit that is short-staffed. For example, if a nurse calls in sick, is out on vacation, or on maternity leave, managers will send an oncology nurse to a cardiac unit to replace her, or a cardiac nurse might be floated to a surgery unit. While floating a nurse on an occasional basis to deal with patients that she is relatively unfamiliar with may not be a terrible burden, floating as a routine practice is part of a larger deskilling of educated professionals that decreases morale, and, nurses say, is unsafe for patients. "Would you ask an ear-nose-and-throat doctor or dermatologist to cover cardiology for the day and expect high-quality care?" Jean Chaisson asks.

This is precisely what many hospitals ask nurses to do on a daily basis. Over a decade ago, nurses would usually work on units that specialized in a particular health problem. Hospitals might have a float pool of nurses that would supply a nurse to another unit in an emergency. Today, hospitals use floating as a routine staffing strategy both to avoid hiring additional permanent nurses and to deal with the shortage the lack of new recruits creates.

Susan Davis* told me how nurses in her teaching hospital are constantly floated between units. Davis, a nurse manager, said that the hospital tries to match the nurse's skills to the unit to which he has been assigned. But sometimes a nurse may be asked to work with an unfamiliar group of patients. "A nurse coming into the hospital to work won't know where she may be working," Davis said. "She knows where her home base is, but if that floor isn't too busy, he or she may be floated to another floor. The possibility of working with people you don't know, patients you don't know, and units you don't know is always there."

Today, hospitals want the flexibility not only to float nurses but also to float patients. If a unit has a full complement of patients and nurses, but a new patient needs to be admitted to that unit, the patient may be sent to a floor where a bed is free and a nurse is available to staff it. Davis explained that decisions about patient placement are based on available resources rather than patient need. Either the patient may be sent someplace where nurses have little expertise but a lot of free beds, or the nurse may be sent to a unit where there is a surplus of patients about whose conditions she has little expertise.

Again, this reflects the nineteenth-century notion that a nurse is a nurse is a nurse. It also suggests that managers may assume that nurses don't need any expertise of their own because they can always rely on the expertise of the physician, or can get a quick catch-up on how to care for an unfamiliar group of patients by checking the clinical pathways or care maps. Nursing work is destabilized by another practice that hospital restructurers have imported from manufacturing industries. Like just-in-time supplying of auto or stereo parts, we now have just-in-time staffing in the hospital. "Every manager who's responsible for living within a budget wants the budget to be as flexible as possible," Alan Sager explains. "In health care that means as the amount of care you have to give goes up you can hire more people and buy more IV solution, and as the amount of care goes down you can adjust your costs accordingly. Today no hospital wants to pay to staff beds that are empty, that don't have patients in them. Managers want to match staffing and cost to patient census and therefore revenue. If the patients are there, they are generating revenue. They don't want to staff empty beds which are not generating revenue."

Just as health care managers try to control the length of patient stay in the hospital, they also try to control the duration of the length of a nurse's stay in the hospital. They do this by denying many RNs the predictability of a fixed schedule. Using patient acuity systems, nurse managers are told that they have to "flex" their work force up and down as patients either fill or vacate hospital beds. At midnight before the following day of work, nurse managers check the midnight census of patients on a particular unit. Then they look at planned discharges and predictable admissions. With the help of computerized patient acuity systems, they decide how

280   many nurses they need for the next day. If the patient census looks like it might be low, a nurse who was scheduled to work might be called at home and told not to come in to work. She is told to take a vacation or personal day and absorb the loss of income. This is a reversal of the scheduling of vacation and personal time, which is usually chosen by the worker, subject to the employer's okay. If the patient census looks like it's going up, managers will frantically call nurses and beg them to come in and forego whatever plans they may have made for their day off. No matter how senior she is, the nurse is vulnerable to these appeals.

"They count your volume at midnight, which is your lowest volume, and you're staffed to your average daily volume," oncology nurse manager Maureen O'Keefe* explains. "So my midnight census might be eighteen. But you can be pretty sure that from nine in the morning till seven at night I might have twenty-one. Then you play with the numbers and say, this is the amount of discharges I'm going to have over the unit. How many am I going to assign to each unit and therefore how much staffing is going to be built on it? You have this much money in the budget. How are you going to divvy it up?"

According to Susan Davis, "On our unit, we go over with physicians on the day before how many patients we think are going to need dialysis and how many apheresis (a blood treatment process) and we try our best to identify those who might need it. Then we always have four or five patients who come in unexpectedly. If those four or five patients don't materialize, nurses have to go home early. Yet if we get ten unexpected patients, we stay until they're done, which means we may stay till midnight. We are expected to flex up and down, but we are never allowed to breathe a sigh of relief and say, 'Okay, now maybe we can get a chance to go over policies for the future, or do some education, or just some reading to improve our own knowledge.'" Under this new system, Davis says, the nurses she works with are conceptualized as machines connected to a bed with a person in it. If the bed no longer has a person in it, then, of course, the tool should be turned off so it doesn't consume any more electricity.

In this case, the tool is of course a human being who is paid by the hour. When the tool goes home, it's not paid. "Nurses are given an option of a day without pay, vacation time, or comp time," Davis explains. "But we experience bumps in census on a daily basis. In fact, we can experience low census for a month at a time so it's possible for a nurse to lose a day a week." She says that when she and the nurses she works with raise their concerns to upper management, "their response is, 'Don't complain, we could float you to another unit.' If we say we don't know how to work on another unit, they say, 'We'll teach you.'" "In how many minutes?" she asks.

This doesn't happen only on a daily basis. Sometimes it can happen on **281** an hourly basis. Luisa Toffoli, a nurse manager in Adelaide, Australia, is conducting a study of the use of flexible schedules and their impact on nurses and managers. In their attempt to shift nurses in and out of the hospital, Toffoli says, start times will be staggered, nurses will be asked to leave the hospital, or managers will implore a nurse to come in for only a few hours. "Please come in and help the patients," the manager begs. "Most times it's 'Please come in and help your colleagues, they're really up against it.' Sometimes, depending on how the manager relates to staff, it's 'Come and help me, I'm drowning.'"

And managers literally are drowning, she says, because the number of nursing hours per patient day is constantly being benchmarked downward with hospitals arbitrarily reducing nursing hours per patient day. The number, she says, never goes up.

In response to these pressures, nurses may adopt a shift-work mentality toward their employment. In the early stages of her study, Toffoli says, she found that nurses started to talk about their work differently. Before the new restructuring, only managers or administrators spoke about nursing hours. "All of a sudden nurses on the ward were talking about nursing hours and actively seeking to reduce the hours. They'd ring up and say, 'Oh look, the place is quiet, I'll go early. Get someone else to start later and I'll start earlier.' So all of a sudden the nurses at the ward level were organizing their lives in terms of nursing hours. I found that disturbing. Nurses were still talking about patients, but patients were in the background now. Nursing hours came to the foreground."

Rather than viewing the nurse as a shift worker, this reconfiguration of nursing, as a mathematical calculation of predictable hours per patient in a bed, turns the nurse into an hourly worker. She is not a professional who can determine how she controls her working day once she arrives in the workplace. She becomes a mechanical robot fulfilling a certain number of predetermined tasks, set not by the doctor but by the patient acuity system or clinical path. If the clinical path or patient acuity system determines that X patient gets only so many hours of nursing care, the nurse is not free to decide that the patient needs a little more of this—say, more teaching about how to take the twenty-four medications he may be going home with, or how to adjust his diet to newly diagnosed diabetes. Or maybe she needs a little bit more of that—a conversation about her anxieties because she just lost a breast to cancer and is concerned that her husband will no longer find her attractive.

Nurses don't have time to do this because they no longer have any

282   downtime. This, in spite of the fact that downtime, as any nurse will tell you, is often some of the most valuable time in the workplace. Just because nurses don't have direct patient duties, or occasionally empty hands, doesn't mean they have empty heads. They could be learning about new treatments and research. They could be sitting on committees planning or improving care. They could be doing one of the most important things of all—meeting with doctors and other clinicians or health care workers to develop interdisciplinary teamwork. But none of this can happen if the nurse is scurried out of the hospital the moment a patient is discharged. When nurses had more predictable work schedules, they could try to plan when to run errands or take care of family responsibilities. Now their work and professional lives are both unpredictable, which may leave them little energy for planning care or further study.

This trend is exacerbated by a so-called innovation that some U.S. hospitals are using to convince nurses that they have a more flexible approach to nurses' shifts. In some hospitals, managers are now running on-line auctions on which nurses can bid against each other for the shifts they would like to work. The Spartanburg Regional Healthcare System in South Carolina began an on-line auction that allows nurses to bid on extra shifts. Nurses bid against one another and the one who bids less gets the shift. The hospital says this gives nurses better pay and more control over their work and cuts down on the use of temporary nurses.

How, one wonders, can nurses sitting at a computer betting against one another claim the status of a professional? How can managers confronted by a constantly shifting cast of winners—and losers—plan the mix of expertise and experience necessary to staff floors? In this kind of scheduling, some nurses may receive more favorable shifts than others, but is this the best way to equitably distribute the shift work involved in patient care? Rose Ann De Moro, executive director of the California Nurses Association argues that these kinds of "innovations" treat patients like "widgets on an assembly line and nursing as casual labor," while Virginia Treacy, the executive director of District Council 1 of JNESO in New Jersey, said of the bidding program at Our Lady of Lourdes in Camden, New Jersey, it's "Keep them down. Keep them dumb. Keep them divided."[33]

When I asked Patricia Benner, a nursing researcher, about this trend, her first comment was a distressed "Oh my god!" Then she explained her response. "This is a logical extension of the market model. There's no vision of a community of practice where people are assigned because of how well they work together, where they can learn from one another, it's all

like these interchangeable parts and you create an institution that's inhos- **283**
pitable, or alien to the complexity of the work."

Given the nature of nursing work today, it is perhaps not surprising that so many newly graduated nurses and nursing students say they are profoundly discouraged by the lack of encouragement they receive from veteran nurses. New nurses as well as nursing students uniformly report that the experienced nurses they work with tell them they're crazy to go into nursing. Often discouraged because their friends and families have questioned their decision to go into nursing rather than medicine, they find it difficult to deal with the fact that bedside nurses seem to be rein-forcing broader societal attitudes toward the profession.

One of the reasons experienced nurses are having so much trouble in the workplace is that it's hard to find nurses who want to work in hospitals or giving direct care in other settings. If new recruits are discouraged from sticking around, that won't help already stressed-out veteran nurses. Yet, it's hard to tell overburdened experienced nurses to contain their dis-affection when they feel so overwhelmed and often betrayed, not just by hospitals but also by nursing management and somehow nursing itself. As one nurse put it, if you feel the hospital thinks you're just another shovel, then why not shovel yourself right out of the institution—the profes-sion—altogether? Which is precisely what a lot of nurses are doing. They believe the crisis is so deep and so pervasive that there is nowhere to run and nowhere to hide.

11

Nurses on the Ropes

I met Marion Phipps when I was working on my book *Life Support*. I watched her work with patients and with their clinical nurses and have listened to her talk about patient care and nursing for about a decade. Over her thirty-three-year career, Phipps is one whom nurses have repeatedly called on, whether they are struggling to deliver care to a frail old woman or a morbidly obese man. How do nurses shift the position of a woman whose bones are so brittle a gentle touch might break them? What is the best way to bathe a seven-hundred-pound gentleman or help him walk? How do they protect themselves while doing it?

The major portion of Phipps's career was at the former Beth Israel in Boston, and then continued at the newly amalgamated facility. In both, she worked throughout the hospital, caring for individual patients, advising and guiding nurses as they confronted tricky problems with patient care, and making the kind of system-wide improvements that allow nurses and doctors to give better care.

Ask Phipps to describe her days, and she'll tell you about the team she assembled to develop standards of care for preventing aspiration pneumonia in people who have swallowing problems after strokes or other illnesses. Or she'll describe one particular case—perhaps the quadriplegic patient she cared for a few years ago.

This patient, we'll call him Tom, had broken his spine between the fifth and sixth cervical vertebrae. Although he was wheelchair bound and couldn't move his arms or legs, he did have some use of the muscles in his arms and shoulders. With the help of adaptive devices, he could feed himself, shave, and write. After he finished his own course of rehabilitation, Tom got a job, **285** married, and adopted a child.

One afternoon a couple of years ago, Phipps recounts, she was working in the hospital when she got a call from Tom. He was in the hospital lobby, said he wasn't feeling well, and that he needed help. Phipps went downstairs to find him. "He looked like hell," she recalls. "I called his internist and we immediately admitted him to a medical floor."

Tom's wife had just gone in for an operation at another Boston hospital. Tom wanted to be with her as much as possible. When he realized something was wrong with his lungs, he ignored it, for far too long. So he arrived at the BI with a "walloping pneumonia."

"When someone is a quadriplegic," Phipps explains, "their interthoracic muscles have so little power that they will be much sicker than an ordinary person." The nurses knew that Tom, if he tried to breathe with the extra burden of pneumonia, might use up all his reserves of strength. He would then have no strength left to breathe on his own and could go into respiratory arrest. When that happened, he would have to be intubated—have a tube inserted into his lungs—and put on a mechanical ventilator, only available on ICUs. Without such equipment, he would die. Getting Tom to the ICU in full respiratory arrest would be much more taxing and traumatic than treating him on an ICU.

"On that particular day we had a very young cast of interns and residents," Phipps explains. "They had never taken care of a quad before. They looked at him and saw only a case of ordinary pneumonia." For doctors dealing with uncomplicated patients, pneumonia is pretty routine. You don't automatically send a patient with pneumonia to the ICU. Not surprisingly then, they insisted he wasn't sick enough to go to the ICU.

Because Phipps and nurses at the hospital were so well respected, they eventually prevailed. Tom was admitted to the ICU. Thirty minutes later, Tom could no longer breathe on his own and was intubated.

But that wasn't the end of the story. "The evening of his admission, his wife called from the other hospital," Phipps continues. "She was terrified that he was going to die and that she wouldn't be with him. She wanted to know if she should come by ambulance to the BI to see him. We talked with the internist, and we all felt that he would make it." She didn't race over to the hospital, and he survived the night.

Although his survival was no longer at risk, his ability to function was. With ICU clinical specialist Jeannie McHale, Phipps and Tom's ICU nurses worked to prevent bedsores and make sure he didn't lose what precious muscle function he had managed to salvage over the years.

"When someone is immobile, their muscles lose length and don't

286 stretch. They risk developing what are called contractures," Phipps explained. Those clawlike, twisted hands, the tortured, rigid limbs one sees on stroke patients in nursing homes—those are contractures. To make sure that didn't happen to Tom, the nurses had to move Tom constantly and exercise his legs and arms.

None of this, Phipps tells me, was easy. Imagine getting a large, tall man, who is essentially dead weight, out of bed without hurting him or the five or six nurses involved in moving him. "I don't think most members of the public understand how dangerous ICU nursing can be to the ICU nurse," says Phipps. Hundreds of ICU nurses develop serious back injuries. That's why, in dealing with the needs of patients in the hospital, Phipps's job is also to make sure nurses don't themselves become patients.

Tom made it out of the hospital, not only because of expert medical but also because of expert nursing care. Unfortunately, when I spoke with her in 2003, Marion Phipps had left Beth Israel Deaconess. Eventually, administrators decided the hospital didn't need hospital-wide specialists, and Phipps was laid off. Months later, she got a job at the Massachusetts General Hospital, where she worked on two units in a much more limited capacity.

Marion Phipps had loved her colleagues, loved Beth Israel, and loved her job there. "Nursing is so wonderful," she says, her voice practically vibrating with pride. "It can be a wonderful career. It involves you intellectually, spiritually, creatively. Sometimes it's sad, but it's also funny and uplifting. If you have the leadership and the tools, it's all of that. At the BI we had all that. And then they took it all away."

Phipps was fifty-six years old. With her thirty-three years of experience she is precisely the kind of nurse that administrators should bend over backward to keep in their hospitals and in the profession. Not only because she has such an extensive repository of knowledge and skill, but because she is an important teacher of younger, less experienced nurses. When, immediately after she left the BI, I asked Phipps how long could she envision staying in nursing, her reply was as disheartening as her demeanor.

"If I had the leadership and the tools, I could do it forever. Without those things," she says, her voice dropping, the enthusiasm draining away, "I'm going to try to make it to sixty-two. But I wish I could quit tomorrow."

Phipps echoed the sentiments of nurses all over the United States. It is not surprising that so many nurses report that they are dissatisfied with their work, feel burned out, and would like to leave their current position or nursing altogether. As we've seen, cost cutting has changed what many nurses have been taught to believe is the very core of their job. Their pri-

mary job, they feel, is no longer protecting patients from the risks and **287**
consequences of illness and its treatment but rather protecting insurers,
governments, and hospitals from the financial risks and consequences of
caring for patients.

For the past decade, dozens of studies and surveys have recorded the
disaffection of the nursing work force. A report by Linda Aiken and her
colleagues in a 2003 issue of the *Journal of the American Medical Association*
found that patient loads correlated with burnout and job dissatisfaction.
For this study, 10,184 staff nurses were surveyed. Of those who reported
that they felt burnt out and who complained of job dissatisfaction, 43 percent said they would leave their current job within twelve months. Aiken
and her colleagues compared this with nurses who say they are satisfied
with their job and found that of the latter group only 11 percent said they
planned to leave their position within twelve months.[1]

In 2002, Peter Hart and Associates surveyed RNs and found that, because of working conditions, 50 percent had thought about leaving patient care in the past two years. Of those surveyed, 21 percent said they
planned to leave within five years. The job was too stressful and physically
demanding, their schedules were unsatisfactory, and they didn't receive
enough money to make the job worthwhile.[2]

In a study in *Health Affairs*, Julie Sochalski analyzed the 1992–2000 National Sample Surveys of Registered Nurses. She reported that 81,000 of
those nurses *not* working in nursing were aged forty-three or younger.
Some of these were women with young children. But "the most common
reasons for working in other fields were better hours, more rewarding
work, and better pay." Interestingly, Sochalski found that "virtually across
the board, men are less satisfied in nursing than women are, regardless of
setting or position." Of new nurses, men were leaving nursing at twice the
rate of women. In 2000 "a surprising 25 percent of new nurses employed
in other fields, both men and women, said they had never worked in nursing. . . . In fact, 57 percent of new nurses working outside of nursing in
1996 had no experience in nursing."[3]

What was behind many of these findings was "sagging job satisfaction."
"Among all nurses, 69.5 percent reported being at least moderately satisfied with their jobs. In comparison, according to the General Social Survey conducted by the National Opinion Research Center between 1988
and 1998, 86 percent of workers in general and 88 percent of professional
workers reported being satisfied with their jobs. Nurses working in nursing homes and hospitals were among the least satisfied with their jobs,
with one of every three nurses in these settings reporting dissatisfaction."[4]

Nurses report that what Claire Fagin has called the "burden of care"
has increased significantly.[5] One of the major problems nurses articulate

288 is that their workplaces have become unmanageable, chaotic environments, so unstable that their workdays and work lives—and the delivery of patient care—have become impossible to predict or control.

Creating Chaos out of Order

One of the great innovations of nursing was to bring order to the chaos of the nineteenth-century hospital. By instilling order where the sick are cared for, nurses addressed a central and immutable fact: sick people are predictably unpredictable. Nurses and doctors know that a patient can destabilize in a matter of minutes. People who seem to be on the road to recovery can get an infection, or a heart that is beating can suddenly stop. To rescue patients from the innumerable threats that assail them, the environment in which a nurse works has to be stable. Which is why, in nursing scholar Donna Diers's well-known formulation, "nursing is two things: the care of the sick and the tending of the entire environment within which care happens."[6]

When the environment in which care is delivered also becomes permanently unstable, that's too much instability for anyone to bear. This sense of unrelenting turmoil in the workplace helps explain the comments nurses make when they talk about their jobs. What are episodic concerns for every professional become constant worries. If they haven't made mistakes, they say, it's only "by the skin of their teeth." They talk about "skating on thin ice," "dancing on the edge of chaos," "leaving work and worrying all night whether they'd forgotten or missed something." They cannot get their meds out in time; they don't know what the aide is doing, seeing, or interpreting; and they feel under constant pressure to compromise on care and, as one vice president of nursing told me, to do just the minimum.

Paul Duke, an emergency room nurse, described the process in a *Newsweek* column: "On an average day I have ten to 12 patients. Once I even had 22. On that night I was feeling swamped, so I went to the charge nurse for help. She was as busy as I was, so she told me to take the five sickest patients and keep them alive, and get to the rest when I could. Now, here's a question: do you want to be one of the five sickest who get attention right away, or one of the others who have to wait maybe seven, eight, or even ten hours before someone gets to you?

"That night I staggered home grateful that nobody had died. But I wondered, do I really want to do this job?"[7]

Veteran nurses feel that the chaotic environment in which they work turns them from experts into novices. In his column, Duke talked about how skilled he and his colleagues are. In this kind of environment, he added, skill cannot take you far enough. "Don't get me wrong," he wrote, **289** "my colleagues are some of the hardest-working professional nurses you will find. But when you're given 20 patients when you should have six, well, you're only so good."[8]

Jean Chaisson echoes this sentiment. "You can't do what there is no time to do. All the expertise and experience in the world doesn't allow you to help patients if you can't get into the room to evaluate them."

Sadly, hospital executives don't seem to recognize the value of expertise and the dangers of turning experts into novices. In an op-ed in the *Boston Globe* Charles E. Cavagnaro III, CEO and president of Wing Memorial Hospital and Medical Center in Palmer, Massachusetts, presented the management position against nurses' attempts to legislate safe staffing ratios in the state. Government regulations of nurse staffing would mean, he lamented, that managers would lose the flexibility to move a maternity nurse to a "busy ICU."[9] As Karen Higgins, president of the Massachusetts Nurses Association commented in a letter to the editor, it's not a very good idea to ask a maternity nurse to work on an ICU where expertise in complex technology is essential to keeping patients alive.[10]

While we take medical expertise for granted, we somehow consistently miss the point when it comes to our understanding of nursing expertise. That's why Patricia Benner wrote her groundbreaking book *From Novice to Expert*. Benner traces how a nurse acquires skill in stages after graduating from nursing school. The undergraduate is a "novice." In the first job, one is a "beginner." From there one moves to the stage of "competent," then to "proficient," and finally to "expert." Not every nurse, she explains, attains expertise. When it happens, the whole process usually takes about five years. And it involves not only attaining a sense of mastery in a particular area but also understanding limits, that you as an expert nurse aren't expert in everything.

Expertise, Benner explains, can't really be fast-tracked. Moreover, Benner says adamantly, it cannot overcome environment. "The most expert nurse will perform suboptimally in an environment in which he or she is denied resources, which is chaotic, and which is plagued by problems of shortage. . . . Even expert nurses cannot heroically overcome the odds. Practice needs to be supported by institutions. But today our institutions aren't just not supporting good practice, they are undermining good practice. In fact, the whole dialogue about health care has changed."

Lowering Standards of Care

Years ago I found that nurses often presented their work as an antidote to the impersonal medical world in which they functioned. Nurses often

290 insisted that, through their language, their behavior, and their priorities, they tempered medical discourse, medical attitudes, and medical demeanor. By presenting themselves as the antithesis of medicine, nurses found a place of their own. Today, cost cutting has made it more difficult for them to inhabit that alternative space. In fact, nurses are asked to integrate themselves into what Benner calls "the business dialogue" and obey the institutional imperatives. The result is that "nurses are required to lower their standards," Benner says. "The business dialogue," Benner says, "is to ask how many injuries, failures to rescue, rehospitalizations can we afford in a population in order to save money." Nurses, she says, are being asked not just to follow the rules of the marketplace but to promote this business dialogue and to embrace the system that has generated it. While this instruction is waning in some places, it was rampant during the height of consolidation and managed care.

This trend is reflected in a variety of studies and in the comments of working nurses. When Marie Heartfield studied nurses on short-stay units in Australia, she found that nurses were asked to adjust their vision of the patient to fit the time allotted rather than accommodating their schedules to fit patients' complex needs. Like those Heartfield described in her study, many nurses and managers almost seem to turn against patients who request much time and attention. Patients who have genuine needs are classified as too "needy" and "demanding." Because it is much harder to attack the real enforcers of a bad system—who sit in offices in the administrative wing of the hospital, or much farther away in Washington, Canberra, or Ottawa—nurses may subtly delegitimize the very real needs of their patients, who become the symbols not of illness and its tragedies but of relentless demands that have become impossible to acknowledge, much less fulfill.

Loss of Teamwork and Collegiality

Although the new watchword in health care today is teamwork, nurses and their managers describe a workplace that is made up of a shifting cast of characters constantly on the move. Models of care appear and disappear. Nurses can't get to know their patients because they're in and out too quickly; they are assembly-lined through the system as relentlessly as their patients. It is difficult for nurses to get to know one another, establish trust, work out practices and policies, refine care, pursue intellectual or clinical interests, or gain a sense of mastery over a particular subject, research issue, or basic patient caseload. If individual mastery is hard to attain, a sense of intraprofessional, collective cohesion seems ephemeral

at best, while significant interdisciplinary cohesion and collaboration is an **291**
even more unrealistic goal.

Maureen O'Keefe, an oncology nurse manager, told me she was rarely
able to get her nurses together for meeting when her hospital restructured. "There is no real group discussion. It is not a unit effort, because
the pace is that frenetic," she said. Nurse manager Susan Davis told a similar story. When she began her career over a decade ago, Davis and her
staff had the usual scattering of busy days when nurses barely had a
chance to catch their breath or make a pit stop in the coffee room. Those
heavy days, however, were balanced out by lighter days. "If you discharged a patient in the middle of a shift, you weren't forced to make a re-
calculation of how many nurses you were using and force someone to go
home. You could do some education, do some planning, do some things
that are necessary just for the day-to-day running of the unit." Things
have totally changed, she said in late 2003. "The whole idea of planning
care, that's gone out the window."

For nurses delivering direct care, loss of collegiality is also evident in
strained relationships between nurses and their nurse managers and high-
level nursing administrators. Of course, tension between labor and management is nothing new. Nurses have always sparred with managers and
matrons about wages and working conditions as well as professional authority. Since nursing's nineteenth-century makeover under the watchful
eyes of Florence Nightingale and her followers, nursing management has
often been hierarchical and authoritarian.[11]

During the brief honeymoon at the end of the last nursing shortage, as
I've said, these tensions seemed to abate somewhat. As restructuring advanced, many nurses said, they felt they had no support from their nurse
managers on the floor or from higher-level nurse executives. These
people were supposed to be their leaders, but they seemed to be missing
in action or as shell-shocked as the nurses they were supposed to lead.

Many staff nurses have told me that their managers are no longer available to them because they themselves are rushing from unit to unit.
When they are present on the ward, they are more preoccupied with
managing beds and bodies—frantically finding nurses to work when a
census goes up or pushing them off the unit when the census is down—
than supporting or developing staff. Oncology nurse Erica Wilson told
me that her nurse manager was hardly even around. This particular manager was responsible for the nurses on the inpatient unit, the outpatient
clinic, and the breast cancer clinic, and for research nurses doing clinical
trials.

"We no longer have regular staff meetings because she just isn't available," Wilson said. Just the other day, Wilson recounted, another nurse

said she has come to the conclusion that it just doesn't pay to raise concerns to this nurse manager because "she isn't listening to us." "I don't know who she is listening to. To the hierarchy? To the physician group? Maybe, but she is not listening to us."

Anita Stevens* is an RN at a hospital in the Northeast that was merged with another local hospital and then bought by a for-profit hospital chain. Stevens explained that the main thing she got from her nurse managers was pressure—pressure to get patients out. Stevens remembers the day a colleague was caring for a very sick patient who had been admitted to the unit. The patient became a Do Not Resuscitate and was clearly going to die in a few hours. Stevens's manager wanted to move the patient out of the unit to make room for other admissions. But the nurse put her foot down and said no. She would not move the patient because she wanted to support the family during the remaining hours of the patient's life. "This kind of pressure is typical if the census is high," she says. When she persisted with her complaints, she says the manager told her to find another job. Stevens did, but not in a hospital, for fear she would relive what she had experienced.

Nurses who persist with their patient advocacy run the risk of being fired as an unwanted "troublemaker." Nonunion nurses—still the vast majority in the United States—are employed "at will" and have little legal protection when they speak out, as individuals, about working conditions or patient care. Unless they form a union and come under the due process provisions of a collective bargaining agreement, management need not show "just cause" to terminate them. They have legal recourse, under state or federal laws, only if their firing is discriminatory: based on age, sex, race, religion, or national origin. Unfortunately, because the focus of nursing academics and associations has been on individual advocacy, most nurses have not been taught that they need to act in concert with others or to link their professional concerns about patient safety to employment conditions like forced overtime and understaffing. Joint action would give them protection under the National Labor Relations Act, which guarantees the right of even nonunion workers to engage in "protected concerted activity"—that is, to engage in efforts to improve wages, hours, and working conditions with one or more other people.

The unfair firing of vocal patient advocates, like Boston RN Barry Adams, has helped focus public attention on the need for a stronger collective voice among nurses, as well as on the need for stronger whistle-blower protection. Indeed, what happened to Adams is typical of the kind of management retaliation nurses can face when they try to advocate for better patient care. Adams's ordeal began in 1996, when the rehabilitation hospital where he worked—Youville Health Care Center in Cambridge—

cut staff and increased his patient load from six to twelve. He soon encountered mounting obstacles to delivering proper care. He took notes
on improper wound management and mistakes new nurses made because
they didn't have enough training, mentoring, and supervision. Adams
talked to two managers who agreed with him but could do little to help.
He tried to take his concerns to the director of nursing and the chief hospital administrator, also a nurse.

Neither Adams nor two coworkers, who lodged similar complaints, felt
they got a satisfactory response. Adams also took his concerns to the Massachusetts Board of Registration of Nursing (BORN). He filed a complaint of "unprofessional conduct," "unethical conduct," and "patient
neglect" with the BORN and also asked the regulatory body to clarify
nurses' responsibilities under the state's Nurse Practice Act. Adams
specifically wanted to know whether nurse administrators in charge of an
institution's finances could also be held responsible for care given at the
facility. Despite his excellent performance reviews, Adams received no response from Youville's administrators. Three days after he filed his
BORN complaint he got a dismissal notice. The other two nurses who
worked with him were assigned rotating shifts and soon resigned.[12]

Although Adams's facility was nonunion, he took his concerns to the
Massachusetts Nurses Association. With the union's help, he found a
lawyer who represented Adams at hearings with the National Labor Relations Board. Adams and the two nurses later won their complaints with
the NLRB, which found that the dismissal "was an illegal attempt to silence and retaliate against him." The judge in the case also ruled that the
hospital had to post a notice reassuring workers in the facility that they
wouldn't be harassed for joining together to protect themselves or their
patients.[13]

While Adams won his case with the NLRB, experiences like these convinced many RNs that when it comes to patient advocacy and professional
leadership, they are often on their own. Nurses increasingly feel isolated
and alienated from nurse executives and managers, and even from nurse
academics. They say they feel that academics often support nursing managers rather than working nurses. These tensions are often expressed in
debates about collective versus individual action that center on union activity.

The Union Conundrum

In the first part of this book, I described the enduring impact of nursing's
long apprenticeship in religious hierarchies. One of the talents nurses developed—a survival skill that many subordinate groups acquire—was the

294 ability to function without attracting unwanted notice or interference from ecclesiastical or secular authorities. Nurses no longer have to contend with potentially meddlesome bishops, cardinals, popes, or kings. Instead, they now have to deal with doctors and hospital administrators operating within the context of modern health care bureaucracies. To get things done for their patients and themselves, in a system of structured inequality, they constantly learn how to work the system quietly without drawing too much attention to how well they have, in fact, worked it. While remaining ever self-effacing, they become skilled in the art of indirect manipulation—polite wheedling, nudging, needling, and persuasion.

This pattern of conflict avoidance may be rooted in the nature of nursing work itself, as well as in the history of the profession. Nurses work with people—patients—who are already anxious about being in a hospital bed or on an examining table, particularly if that's due to a serious illness or sudden emergency. Calming people down, revealing bad news in stages, creating, as I've described before, order from the chaos of illness and its treatment—that's what nurses get really good at. Their job is to protect patients from risk without making them feel at risk. This is a task akin to that of parents faced with the challenge of warning their young children about "talking to strangers" without leaving them fearful of all unfamiliar adults.

Sick people don't need the additional worry that might be aroused by too much awareness of all the systemic problems swirling around them, sometimes quite visibly, in the modern hospital. When disagreements arise on the wards with doctors, nurses tend to avoid any direct confrontation, sometimes out of concern that the ire of medical colleagues might somehow have an adverse impact on the patient. Instead, when seeking a treatment option or adjustment, they may, through hint and suggestion, try to make the physician think that the nurse's idea was not only the right one but really his or her own idea as well.

As subordinates, this give nurses some measure of decision-making control and the ability to resolve what might otherwise become a worse patient care situation. But as the larger hospital system becomes ever more dysfunctional, such day-to-day coping mechanisms prove to be infeasible and ineffective. On crowded, understaffed wards, younger and less experienced nurses have too many patients and not enough mentoring or support for traditional strategies of accommodation to work. More RNs find themselves forced to choose between the strategies of exit and voice. The latter option inevitably requires shedding traditional reticence about ruffling feathers and, instead, engaging collectively and constructively in direct dealings with established authority.

Collective bargaining in most industrialized countries is well esta-

blished and rarely challenged. This means that RNs can fulfill their ethi- **295**
cal obligation to be forceful patient advocates, while also having a strong
collective voice that addresses workplace problems, professional issues,
and public policies related to health care. In Australia, for example, the
Victoria branch of the Australian Nursing Federation fought for and won
the first staffing legislation implemented anywhere in the world. In
Switzerland, the Swiss Nurses Association has negotiated pay equity in
some Swiss cantons, thus giving nurses equal pay with that of other civil
servants. In the canton of Zurich, nurses were awarded the equivalent of
$200 million in back pay.[14] Another powerful nurses' union is the Danish
Nurses Association, which represents everyone from staff nurses to the
vice president of nursing in a hospital. As a result, RNs in Denmark are
some of the most powerful and best treated hospital workers in the world.

Over the past decade, nurses in the United States have become increasingly restive about the deteriorating conditions of patient care work. One
expression of this trend has been a continuing series of shake-ups and
splits within nursing organizations themselves. In 1967 internal tensions
between nurse executives and fellow members of the American Nurses
Association (ANA) whom they supervised led to formation of a separate
group for managers—the American Association of Nurse Executives,
which is now a subsidiary of the American Hospital Association. In the
early 1990s, nurses in the California Nurses Association split off from the
ANA and formed their own independent union, because they felt the national organization was still not representing the interests of working
nurses as opposed to those of academics and advanced practice RNs. As
managed care continued to erode nurses' working conditions, the Massachusetts and Maine State Nurses Associations also voted to leave the
ANA. Since then, the collective bargaining wing of the ANA has sought
to bolster its union credentials and avert further defections by affiliating
with the AFL-CIO as the United American Nurses.

In the United States, health care unionization remains controversial
and limited (to 17 percent of the RN work force), in part because employer resistance is far greater here than elsewhere.[15] In addition, nursing
education rarely addresses the fact that legal protections in unionized
workplaces allow nurses to speak up about problematic practices or unsafe
working conditions and give them greater legal recourse against employer
retaliation. Nurses, like most workers, believe that everyone should have
due process rights on the job and the opportunity for a fair hearing when
their job performance is questioned or their continued employment is at
stake. What nurses usually don't know is that, without union representation and a negotiated procedure for appealing management actions, they
have no guarantee that their side of the story will ever be heard, and little

296   hope that an unfair personnel decision might be overturned. They're also rarely aware that unionized employers, as part of their legal obligation to engage in collective bargaining, must share large amounts of useful information related to their pay and benefit costs, staffing levels, training budgets, tuition reimbursement plans, and other personnel programs. Before altering existing personnel practices, hospitals must give affected RNs advance notice and the chance to bargain about proposed changes— an opportunity for input routinely denied in nonunion workplaces, where any such management consultation with employees is completely discretionary.

Despite such advantages, most nursing managers and academics—and even many working nurses—question the appropriateness of collective bargaining in health care settings. The harshest of these critics play on nurses' class and status anxieties and socialization in selflessness, according to Darlene and Paul Clark, Penn State University professors who've studied this phenomenon. Darlene teaches in the nursing school, where she tries to introduce her students to the subject of organized labor. RNs-in-training often equate unionism with being blue-collar and not really professional. "They go to nursing school to become professionals," Clark points out. "They are taught in most schools and in most organizations that they don't want to be seen as blue-collar, so if unions are blue-collar, then why would we want to do that?" In addition there is the concern that if you're in a union you might have to strike, an action that many nurses view as tantamount to abandoning their patients.

According to Clark, this feeds another worry, that labor-management conflict might erode public support for nursing. As the polls show, nurses are highly trusted, far more than lawyers, businessmen, and people in most other occupations. Many in nursing believe, however, that their profession's favorable rating is so rooted in an image of selflessness that any behavior contrary to that image would cost nurses dearly in terms of public esteem. Opponents of unionization play on such fears. They invariably depict nursing unions as strike-happy, as if some RNs were eager to spend their days shivering in the cold as they walk in front of hospitals with picket signs and no paychecks. In fact, such scenes are relatively rare and RN bargaining units have to be pushed to the brink before they walk out—in the United States at least. When they do go on strike, it's often because working conditions or management demands—related to overtime, scheduling, or staffing—are jeopardizing patient care. As Clark notes, when the issues involved are framed and explained in terms of their impact on patients, nurses' strikes often receive an impressive degree of public support.

The Clarks believe that antiunionism among nursing students or working nurses also reflects general ignorance about organized labor's contributions to society, as much as ideological opposition to the concept of collective bargaining. Most nursing professors, the Clarks say, tend to be as ill-informed as their students about basic employment law and labor relations. In Paul Clark's introductory classes for undergraduates on these subjects, he finds that most of his students, like their peers in the nursing program, are completely unaware of the "employment-at-will" doctrine, which deprives unrepresented employees of any due process in termination situations. Says Clark, "You tell them about that and they will say, 'That's not fair, you can't fire people because you don't like the way they look.' It may not be fair but it is perfectly legal and perfectly consistent with our economic system and the role that employers play in it." Meanwhile, at the nursing school, Darlene Clark reports that when she tries to "teach my nursing students about the role of unions, it may be the first thing they've ever heard" about them. "They don't read about it in the textbooks in school and they probably don't hear about it in most nursing programs. I have a three-hour window in their entire four-year education."

Interviews and conversations with deans or faculty members at many other nursing schools suggest that this is not an unintentional omission from the curriculum. When I talked with one New York State nursing school dean, she was irate over the presence of a nursing union in the hospitals of her local community. She criticized the RNs involved—many of them educated in her school—for being "unprofessional" even though their union displays a sophisticated understanding of public policy issues, has been an articulate advocate of health care reform, and has engaged in complex negotiations about the impact of hospital cost cutting and consolidation. Despite many such examples of union organization reflecting well on its RN members, the dean of another, more prestigious nursing school insisted that unions "were the worst thing that has happened to us." Harking back to the crudest of stereotypes, she exclaimed: "We don't want to look like truck drivers!"

Nurse managers universally deride the notion that nurses "need someone else speak for them"—even if that "someone" is a fellow RN acting as their union steward, not a burly Teamster business agent. (I first heard the "we're not truck drivers" refrain during a conversation with a manager who was attending a meeting of *her* group, the Organization of Nurse Executives in New York, which "speaks for" RN administrators in that state!) Whenever there's an RN organizing drive in the United States, hospital administrators mobilize all their nurse managers in an intensive campaign to convince staff nurses to vote No. When I was recently in Australia, an American nurse manager who had fled eroding working con-

298 ditions in California recalled a typical effort of this sort. He and his colleagues were forced to attend a series of closed-door meetings with lawyers from an outside firm specializing in union busting. They were supplied with antiunion scripts to be used (whether or not they agreed with them) in systematic workplace conversations with all the nurses they supervised.

It's hardly surprising, then, that new nurses and nursing students tend to be wary about collective action. Their attitudes reflect their socialization. Several years ago, for example, I interviewed a nurse who'd recently graduated from an elite four-year nursing program and then gone to work at a New York City teaching hospital, where nurses had never voted to join a union. This was her first job and she told the usual story—way too many patients, too little time, compromised care, no management support. "I asked the nurses on both the night and day shift was this normal for them, and they said, 'Yeah.' On the night shift they were working with two nurses for thirty patients and on the day shift they often had three. I asked them why they hadn't done anything or were they doing anything about it. They said their nurse manager was not someone they trusted or respected. They couldn't do anything about it because they were too scared for their jobs."

Although she understood the systemic nature of the problems she encountered on the job, this nurse had also been taught that members of her profession are supposed to be patient advocates. She believed that her colleagues had failed in their ethical obligations to their patients and were "pathetic." She finally left her position in New York City and went to work at a for-profit hospital in California. According to her, however, things were no better there, even though nurses were in a union and negotiated with management about salaries and working conditions. She considered such activity to be selfish and unprofessional. "I think [having a union] is an adolescent way to solve problems. It doesn't help the profession or add professionalism to our profession."

When I asked what "professionalism" meant to her, she responded that "what makes nursing a profession is an attitude, rather than a structure or organization. A professional nurse is one who is respected and respectful, who is able to handle problems and concerns in a mature manner. Which in my mind means going to the individual involved on one's own, rather than going to a union representative and meeting. It sounds like third grade, going to a union representative to arrange a meeting with a manager. It seems divisive. The leadership and the staff are separated by the union."

When I inquired whether this young woman understood that nurses were employees-at-will and could, without a union, be fired for no reason, she expressed surprise. "That can really happen?" she asked. "You mean **299** anywhere?" Yes, I said. "You mean like in a law firm?" she asked. Yes, I repeated.

She was dumbfounded. I asked her if she had ever been taught about the risks of speaking out, as an individual, in the workplace, under such circumstances. Or if her professors had ever explained the concept of "protected concerted activity" under the National Labor Relations Act, so that, if she ever raised any controversial issues about patient care, she would enlist one or more of her colleagues in the effort and link their complaint to workplace conditions or personnel practices, thereby making it easier to protest any management retaliation. No, she admitted. That wasn't anything they had covered in nursing school.

This lack of basic information about workplace legal rights—or the lack of them—represents a significant disconnect in nursing education and research, particularly in light of all the lessons that nursing students are taught about autonomy, professionalism, and patient advocacy responsibilities under the American Nurses Association Code of Ethics. That disconnect is reflected even in the one leading study—published in the *Journal of Nursing Administration*—which documents that when nurses are in unions their patients do better. This study found, for example, that there was a "significantly predicted lower-risk-adjusted AMI (acute myocardial infarction) mortality" rate in hospitals with unions.[16] Nevertheless, the authors of the study argue, union substitution schemes are better than unions: "Although further exploration of the relationship between unions and patient outcomes must be done, should nurse executives rush to embrace unionization as an organizational strategy? The answer of course is *no*. . . . As researchers work to scientifically explicate the mechanisms by which a union environment may be related to positive patient outcomes, nurse executives can try (in an operational setting) to identify organizational characteristics related to positive outcomes common to union environments that could be incorporated into their organizations."[17]

Similarly, high-ranking representatives of the nursing profession continue to oppose unions or wish them away rather than acknowledge the reality of workplace law and labor relations. For example, just before leaving to speak at a conference held by an ANA affiliate in the South, I received a phone call at home from the state association director, who said she wanted to remind me about something before I left. "What's that?" I asked. Her group operates in a "right-to-work" state, she explained, and therefore it was impossible for it to gain collective bargaining rights in any hospital. Because the state lacked legal protection for nurses' right to organize, she wanted me to be sure not to talk about unions, lest any of

300 her members get unrealistic ideas about how to deal with the workplace problems they face. "I always try to protect my nurses from thinking that collective bargaining is the answer in this state," she said.

Since my topic was how nurses could tell their stories to the media and public, I expressed curiosity about why she would call me to warn me away from the subject of unionization. "Well, you never know what's going to slip out of people's mouths," she said, seemingly oblivious to the fact that what had just slipped out of her mouth was a complete misrepresentation of the legal status of private sector nurses in her state, who have the same federally protected organizing rights as RNs anywhere else (if not the same ability to negotiate union contracts requiring payment of union dues).

Not surprisingly, given their frequent exposure to such paternalism and misinformation coming from some nursing elites, RN union activists reciprocate with their own hostile rhetoric, in which they accuse nurse academics and managers—"the pumps-and-pearls set"—of not being real nurses. They also remain deeply suspicious of nursing school faculty who are fighting to make four-year baccalaureate education a requirement for entry into practice in nursing. As one nursing union leader told me, this proposal is perceived as a direct attack on staff nurses and would, if implemented, give hospital managers an excuse to demote or get rid of anyone without a four-year degree. Since many nursing academics also promote an individualistic and (for management) voluntaristic approach to solving workplace problems, few support the more militant workplace agenda of union nurses. As we shall see in the concluding chapter, many academics oppose regulatory approaches to workplace problems and government restrictions on management prerogatives, yet favor government action when it establishes a four-year degree requirement for entry into practice, more authority and autonomy for advanced practice nurses, and better funding of nursing education and recruitment. This increasingly wide chasm separating the nurse in direct care from those in management and academia also makes it difficult for nurses to approach problems collectively when employees are powerless to solve them on their own.

Exacerbating Doctor-Nurse Relationships

If nurses feel they have little support from those within their own professional hierarchy, it is not surprising that they also feel unsupported by physicians and higher-level hospital administrators. Some doctors have spoken out to protest cutbacks in nursing. When cost cutting first began, John M. O'Donnell, director of the surgical intensive care unit and chairman of the

Department of Surgical Critical Care at the Lahey Clinic–Hitchcock Medical Center in Burlington, Massachusetts, became worried about the decline in nursing standards in his and other hospitals. As early as 1994, he tried to publish an article warning about the potential problems for patients, doctors, and nurses as a result of this trend. His article was rejected by all the prominent medical journals to which it was submitted.

O'Donnell then spoke at the conference on Abandonment of the Patient and his eyewitness account was reprinted in the book that collected the comments of patients, doctors, nurses, and other health care observers. O'Donnell described ICUs on which the sickest patients could no longer benefit from the continuous care of two nurses over a twenty-four-hour period—nurses who could "recognize subtle changes in vital signs," reliably administer risky sedatives, narcotics, and muscle relaxants, and act as the communications hub for doctors, families, and other personnel. Now, with the use of pool, float, and agency nurses, "four, five, or even six different nurses may be responsible for that patient over a twenty-four-hour period."[18]

In Massachusetts, a group of doctors and nurses joined together under the banner of the Ad Hoc Committee to Defend Health Care to protest the fate of clinicians and patients under managed care. But these alliances and supportive efforts have not been able to overcome the fact that interprofessional tensions will inevitably increase as clinicians in all settings and disciplines are under greater stress to be more "productive" and see more patients and sicker patients in shorter periods of time.

Clinicians who can barely catch their breath will have a difficult time catching up with one another, particularly when they have not systematically done so in the past. If scheduled deliberations that included doctors and nurses rarely happened in the best of times, they won't suddenly be put on the agenda when nurses can't even make it to the bathroom and doctors just want to turn off their beepers and take a break.

Doctors may become more curt and irritable with nurses, and nurses will become less able to communicate intelligently with doctors. Oncology nurse Erica Wilson feels that the good relationships she and her colleagues once enjoyed with physicians and with other clinicians have suffered. Physicians, nurses, and social workers, key members of the cancer treatment team, are under so much pressure that it's hard to communicate, much less collaborate. "We have the general feeling that the medical group is very stressed out too. There is a great deal of tension between the nurses and doctors, because we feel they don't understand how short-staffed we are."

Indeed, nurses who sometimes feel that the powerful players in health

302   care simply want to get rid of them may lump doctors and administrators together and feel scapegoated by both. In an article in the *New England Journal of Medicine*, Robert Steinbrook remarks that nurses' "perception is that physicians and hospital administrators often treat registered nurses as workers, not as clinicians and peers, and when possible seek to replace them with less skilled and cheaper personnel, such as licensed practical nurses and aides."[19]

In their dealings with physicians, nurses often claim they should be heard because they are closest to the patient and have, therefore, important knowledge about the patient's responses to illness, medication and other treatments. This argument, however, loses credibility when patients become increasingly unknowable as they're virtually catapulted through the system. Who does know the patient?

As one former hospital administrator who is sympathetic to the plight of RNs told me with frustration, nurses keep telling us they're the humanists in the hospital, but hospitals aren't hiring many humanists these days.

Dana Weinberg agrees. When she wrote her book *Code Green*, about the dismantling of the nursing service at the Beth Israel Deaconess Medical Center, she watched nurses stumbling to try to convince administrators and senior physicians of their worth. But, she says, "they couldn't move beyond traditional articulations of nursing" and that just helped bottom-line-oriented number crunchers to dismiss their complaints more readily.

RN Breakdown and Its Impact on Nurses' Health

The combination of heavy caseloads, lack of social and financial rewards, and often ineffective struggles against workplace restructuring has had a dramatic impact on nurses' health. According to the Bureau of Labor Statistics, 700,000 health care workers suffered injury or illness in 1996— twice as many problems as were reported in 1990. The rate of injuries surpassed that of manufacturing, construction, and mining—well-known high-hazard industries. In an earlier chapter we've seen the physical risks nurses incur on the job.

In 2001 the American Nurses Association questioned 4,826 nurses online to determine their exposure to workplace hazards. The association's report is alarming. Over the twelve months prior to being surveyed, 40 percent of nurses said they'd been injured on the job. Of nurses who reported an injury, the vast majority (74.7 percent) said they did not report their injuries, some because they didn't have time or feared retaliation from their employer. Many nurses were worried about potentially disabling back injuries (59.4 percent) and said they continued to work in **303** spite of having back pain (83 percent).[20] Interestingly, one Swedish literature review of the relationship between psychosocial factors and musculoskeletal disorders observed that "negative emotional states associated with low-status jobs, combined with a lack of economic resources, are also likely to reduce the individual's motivation to seek proper medical treatment and, thus, increase the risk that transient symptoms develop into chronic illness." The authors also suggest that stress induced by "psychosocial conditions at work" may shut down the individual's ability to recover from injury.[21]

Almost half of the RNs in the ANA study (45.3 percent) worried about contracting HIV or hepatitis from a needlestick.[22] The Service Employees International Union also reported a growing problem with needlestick injuries, which led the union to participate in a successful campaign to force hospitals to use safe needle technology.

Needlesticks can have catastrophic—indeed lethal—consequences for nurses who contract blood-borne illnesses like hepatitis B and C and HIV/AIDS. They lead to absenteeism due to illness, worker's compensation and disability costs, and huge costs for the nurse turned patient, as he or she deals with a chronic, life-threatening illness. Mandating hospitals to provide safe needle technology is a critical part of the solution. Improvements in nurse workload and staffing are the other part.

Hospital staffing and organizational climate correlate with needlestick injuries. A 2002 study analyzed retrospective data from 732 nurses and prospective data (describing incidents as they happened) from 960 nurses on needlestick injuries and near misses on forty units in twenty hospitals. When a nurse worked on a unit with poor staffing ratios and a poor organizational climate, he or she was twice as likely to get a needlestick injury than a nurse who was well supported on a well-staffed unit. Since the article revealed that only one in four needlestick injuries are actually reported to hospital officials, the results of this study are sobering indeed.[23] This study took place before hospitals introduced protective equipment—safety-engineered needles, in the jargon—that makes it harder to get injured. Using 1998 data in another article, the investigators found that nurses were still getting stuck and that staffing and work climate made a difference. "Poor organizational climate and high workloads were associated with 50% to twofold increases in the likelihood of needlestick injuries and near misses to hospital nurses." Although safe needle technology reduced the risk, the authors concluded, "nurse staffing and organizational climate are key determinants of needlestick risk and must be considered with the adoption of safety equipment to effectively reduce sharps injuries."[24]

Stress—the Perfect Storm

Given the realities outlined above, it shouldn't surprise us that the vast majority of nurses who responded to the ANA survey said they did not feel entirely safe from workplace-related injury and illness and 12.1 percent said they didn't feel safe at all. "Health and safety concerns have an impact on the kind of nursing work performed and on their continued practice in the field of nursing," 87.9 percent of the respondents confessed. The most prevalent concern these nurses voiced, and the greatest difficulty they said they had, was job stress. More than 70 percent said one of their three major health concerns was the acute and chronic impact of stress and overwork.[25]

Job stress and its Siamese twin, job burnout, are perhaps the most significant health problems that nurses face. Numerous studies document that nurses experience a great deal of job stress under even the best of circumstances. Nurses, Joel Hillhouse and Christine Adler tell us, "experience higher rates of mortality, suicide, stress-related disease, psychiatric admissions, and general physical illness than does the general population." The primary sources of nursing stress, the authors explain, "include work overload, death and separation experiences, poor communications and social support, emotional demands of patients and families, and a constantly changing work environment."[26]

Stress can lead to burnout, which can be understood to be "a psychological process in which chronic job stressors are translated into outward affective and physical symptomatology."[27] Burnout has also been described as "a prolonged response to chronic emotional and interpersonal stressors on the job, and is defined by the three dimensions of exhaustion, cynicism, and inefficiency."[28] RNs may perform poorly on the job, report to work late or not at all, and even abuse drugs or alcohol. Their resulting cynicism and exhaustion may make nurses appear to be discourteous or even callous toward their patients. It's easy, given the public's angelic template for the profession, to blame this behavior on the individual nurse's personality, character, or lack of vocation. Certainly some nurses probably should have chosen other work. When rude, callous behavior is, however, rampant in a hospital or unit, it's probably more realistic to look at job stress and burnout as the culprit, rather than the character or failings of the individual RN.

When we understand what job stress does to the worker, it's easier to understand its impact on nurses and thus on patients. In its booklet *Stress at Work*, the U.S. National Institute for Occupational Health and Safety (NIOSH) helps us understand why job stress is one of the most important predictors of health problems and behavior.[29] According to the St. Paul

Fire and Marine Insurance Company, "problems at work are more **305** strongly associated with health complaints than are any other life stressor—more so than even financial problems or family problems."[30]

Job stress should not be confused with a job challenge. A job challenge is good; job stress is always bad. A job that is challenging may stretch a worker's capabilities. When people successfully meet challenges, they get motivated, inspired, and energized. They feel powerful and gain a sense of mastery. Job stress depletes and enervates us. It can, under especially adverse circumstances, make us feel desperate and powerless. Another crucial caveat: job stress is not created by a worker's personal failings, flaws, or characteristics. It's a product of working conditions that produce harmful physical and emotional responses when "requirements of the job do not match the capabilities, resources, or needs of the worker."[31]

Why is job stress so harmful? At the risk of covering familiar ground, we need to go back to the African savanna and our ancestors to understand why. In *Homo sapiens*, the built-in stress response developed to protect us from threat and danger. When our ancestors encountered the famous saber-toothed tiger on the savanna, stress, or the fight-or-flight response, was a great boon. It allowed them to recognize danger instantly and to fight or scram. Within milliseconds of perceiving a threat, without having to think a thing or exercise conscious control, the brain goes into action.

When the modern equivalent of the saber-toothed tiger or another threat or danger emerges, the sympathetic nervous system—the body's fight-or-flight system—is jolted into action through a wondrously complex chemical chain reaction that releases hormones like adrenaline, producing the stress response: the heart pumps faster (it increases the flow of blood circulating through the body) and the blood pressure goes up (to pump the blood where it needs to go even faster), the stomach contracts or churns, bowel activity slows down, the level of blood sugar rises, and the extra energy thus produced is directed to our thigh muscles (rather than our arms) so we can run, if necessary. The body also produces cortisol, another stress hormone, which can help us recover from the effects of adrenaline.

This response is great at making sure a nurse bolts into a patient's room when she hears the sound of an alarm signaling a cardiac arrest. Her system races, so does she, and the crisis is addressed. Afterward, the body is programmed to begin to shut off the heightened state of arousal and return to normal, which doesn't happen instantaneously.

Herein lies the problem. If the stressors that confront a human being don't abate, the body is continually set on go and remains on hormonal overdrive. The heart won't stop pumping; the sense of being hyper-

306 aroused doesn't let up. You can't focus. You can get depressed. In humans, the stress response can be prolonged because people ruminate about the things that are stressing them out. Nurses can become just as stressed out by their thoughts about the patients they couldn't help or the fight they had with a nurse or physician colleague as they do when the incident is happening. Human beings can also launch the stress response by thinking about past or upcoming stressors. For better or worse, this is why, as Robert M. Sapolsky wrote, zebras don't get ulcers. Once they've gotten away from the lion, they don't worry about the encounter.

Constant contact with a stressful environment can turn acute stress into chronic stress. Constant contact with stressors and rumination about the stress they cause can create a state in which the sympathetic nervous system remains activated, which produces high levels of stress hormones like cortisol. In this way, the brain's biology begins to change, sometimes permanently, and the body can also be permanently damaged. When, NIOSH explains, workers are constantly confronted with "heavy workload, infrequent rest breaks, long work hours and shift work, hectic and routine tasks that have little inherent meaning, do not utilize a worker's skills and provide little sense of control," the body keeps up the pumping, churning, and heavy breathing and starts to use itself up.[32]

The negative health effects of chronic job stress can be severe. Long-term stress can produce anxiety, depression, hypertension, impaired immune system function, and an increased risk of recurrence of cancer and death from heart attacks. "Cortisol in the short term improves the immune system and makes it work better. Long-term exposure to cortisol has the opposite effect," Timothy McCall explains. "When you have high levels of cortisol in your system, you tend to do a couple of things that can be very disadvantageous for a number of diseases including diabetes. In addition to raising blood sugar, cortisol tends to lead people to put on intra-abdominal fat—fat between the viscera. Intra-abdominal fat has a very strong correlation with heart disease, metabolic syndrome (a precursor to diabetes), and other problems."

One study of overwork in Japan, for example, correlated extra hours at work with increases in heart disease due to long working hours.[33] And we know, McCall adds, that lack of job satisfaction is an independent risk factor for heart disease. "There's, in fact, a characteristic of the kind of job stress that really gets to people which is lack of recognition and no autonomy, precisely the kind of circumstances that describe the work of the modern nurse. While we think of heart disease as the major cause of death in men, it's also the major cause of death in women. Indeed, heart disease is such a major problem among women that the number of women who

die from it exceeds the number who die of the next seven causes com- **307**
bined."

Stress is also associated with obesity—which is a significant problem
among nurses, particularly in North America. "Rats that have high levels
of stress and high levels of cortisol tend to engage in what the researchers
call food-seeking behavior," says McCall. "Being stressed tends to make
you eat a lot. And people who are stressed and short on time often end up
eating junk food. The high levels of cortisol they produce make it much
more likely that they will turn that extra eating into intra-abdominal fat."

All of this is more bad news, because continuous high pressure pumping of the blood under stress can damage "branch points in arteries
throughout the body." When vessels begin to tear and scar, the substances
racing through the body because of the stress response begin to clog the
arteries. Through another series of complex processes, Sapolsky explains,
"chronic stress causes atherosclerosis."[34] Stress also exacerbates a whole
host of illnesses including colitis, asthma, diabetes, and high blood pressure. Stress may not cause all these problems, but if you have any of them,
it will surely exacerbate them.

People under stress are also more likely to develop depression, now
considered to be the single greatest cause of disease-related disability in
women worldwide. Some researchers have done studies that suggest that
"subordinacy" has an added impact in the damage stress can inflict.[35] If
someone of subordinate status is on hyper-alert all the time, they may develop problems associated with high anxiety. If they've given up, they may
develop problems with depression.

Stress can also cause sleep disturbances and sleep disturbances can
cause or heighten stress. In Anne Rogers's study, nurses reported getting
less sleep than they needed, being extremely tired at work, and even
falling asleep on the job. In earlier chapters, we've seen how resident
working hours have a negative impact on mood and workplace relationships. The same thing can happen to nurses.

To this mix of fatigue and overwork among nurses, add the stress of
conflict with physicians, who are themselves increasingly stressed because
of what cost cutting and managed care has done to their work lives. Combine high patient loads, conflicting demands, poor workplace relationships, conflict with stressed-out doctors, subordinate status, and many
other characteristics of the nursing workplace, and you have the perfect
storm of stress in the health care environment.

Hillhouse and Adler's study on nurses illuminates how this perfect
storm operates in the contemporary workplace. In their exploration of
the impact of job stress, they took account of hospital reengineering and

308 restructuring by moving from ward- or unit-based studies of different kinds of nurses—critical care versus general ward nurses—to a global hospital analysis. They sent out questionnaires to all the staff nurses (709) at a large university hospital and analyzed the reports of the 36.7 percent of nurses who responded to them. The authors then divided the nurses up into clusters. The first group, 31.5 percent of those who responded, was labeled "low stressor/low stress effect." The next two groups, however, illustrated some revealing problems. The second group, "high stressor and burnout/moderate symptom," included 43 percent of the respondents. These nurses said they had little social support, reported problems dealing with death and suffering, conflict with other nurses, and uncertainty. They also reported moderate caseloads and moderate conflict with physicians. The remaining 26 percent of the respondents were in the "high stressor/high stress effect" group. These nurses said they had low unit support and high patient numbers. They also added another important variable to the mix of stressors—poor relationships with physicians.

The nurses who had the most stress, and suffered the most from it, experienced "a combination of stressors, with particular emphasis on 'conflict with physicians,' and 'workload' stress, together with patient load," which resulted in these detrimental effects. It's worth quoting their comments at some length.

"High patient load or general nursing stress are not sufficient to create serious symptomatology," they concluded. "It seems that there is a two-stage process, whereby certain types of nursing stressors (specifically, 'death and suffering,' 'conflict with other nurses,' and 'uncertainty—lack of preparation') will typically result in feelings of burnout but fail to produce the high levels of affective and physical symptoms that are most personally and professionally damaging." To produce the most damaging personal and professional problems, the two essentials seem to be high caseloads combined with "greater levels of physician conflict."

Why is the issue of physician conflict so critical? the authors ask. "Intra-professional conflict is perhaps less threatening and offers more avenues for problem resolution than does conflict with individuals who have more power and status, and with whom one typically has less frequent contact," they speculate. Here the authors add a new twist to our understanding of excessive patient loads. Each additional patient the nurse cares for brings her into contact with an additional number of physicians. Some of these physicians may be a pleasure to work with. But we've seen the problems that arise in a medical system in which structured inequality and lack of interdisciplinary communication and collaboration is the rule. Today, the doctors nurses encounter are also under more stress and are experiencing less satisfaction on the job. In this way, a higher patient load and additional contact with doctors may magnify, to use the authors' words, the nurse's stress.[36]

Of course, not every nurse will suffer—and certainly will not suffer in the same way—from chronic workplace stress. Depending on their genetics, psychological coping mechanisms, personal risk factors, and so forth, people react to stress differently. Since no one knows in advance how well their genes, coping mechanisms, and risk factors will protect them, relying on human beings to adapt to a chronically stressful workplace (by, say, working smarter not harder, or mastering stress reduction techniques), rather than making the workplace less stressful, is a poor strategy. By asking nurses to take care of patients under such stressful conditions, we risk producing even more patients. By this I don't only mean patients who get sicker because nurses can't adequately care for them. We are definitely doing that. But we are also turning nurses into patients. Adding to the considerable burdens of caregiving, we are now asking them to take on an extra burden of illness—this time their own. This is a very poor way for health care systems that are supposedly strapped for cash to function.

Indeed, some nurses confess they are so stressed out they are in therapy, or on a plethora of medications, from cholesterol-reducing Lipitor to the antidepressant Prozac. They are as pessimistic about their personal prospects as their professional ones. What is so moving and ultimately so professionally and personally self-defeating is that many of them seem to blame themselves, because they believe they have somehow failed their patients and themselves. As members of Western industrialized society, we've all been told that we're responsible for our health and our health care decisions. So that doesn't help. Added to this, RNs probably shoulder an extra burden of self-flagellation. Nurses have been repeatedly told, "Nursing is the art of self." From the society, their administrators, journalists, children's book writers, and even their peers and professional organizations, they've been programmed to believe that altruism and empathy are an act of will. They're admonished to place their patients first, advocate for their patients no matter what, and continue giving and giving and giving. Sometimes, they're even congratulated for being particularly moral or ethical actors (all opinion polls confirm this image). But that's not how they feel when they work in bad systems, which they may actually help perpetuate through the very sacrifices they are called upon to make.

Loss of Efficacy and Empathy

When you ask working nurses who deliver direct care to fragile human beings what troubles them the most about their working conditions,

310   many will talk about the loss of their human connection to their patients. When Paul Duke complained about excessive patient loads to his nurse manager, she advised him to concentrate on getting five people through the emergency room alive and not worry about the rest. But one of the great psychological rewards of nursing—a reward that often made up for poor pay, physician disregard, and bad working conditions—lay in the positive consequences of this "worrying." Patients got better as a result. Or even if they didn't, the healing connections nurses forged were said to be part of the "difference" nurses make to quality patient care.

Today, many nurses say, the lowering of overall health care standards makes them feel that they are part of a machine that is actually doing the patient harm.

On the verge of quitting her own job, Maureen O'Keefe explained that "when you're determining how many nurses you need based on patients in the bed, this creates an environment where the nurse feels she's running around most of the time like a chicken with her head cut off. She can't focus on the essential things; she is frustrated with the system and feels like she doesn't make a difference. Most nurses in this institution don't feel like they're important or that they matter; they're a kind of commodity that is interchangeable."[37] One nurse was even more blunt. "We're being turned into people we don't even like."

Patients often complain about physicians who aren't empathetic, which is, of course, a serious problem. In spite of patients' complaints, physicians have an easy out that's not available to nurses. That's the oft-repeated rationalization that "he's a brilliant doctor who just happens to have no bedside manner." When people like David Nathan from the Dana Farber cancer hospital—or nurses themselves—fall into traditional angelic stereotypes, then how do we excuse their stress-related empathetic failings? Sometimes, we don't.

In 2002 the American Hospital Association recognized this important component of health care work. "Most health care workers entered their professions to 'make a difference' through personal interaction with people in need. Today, many in direct care feel tired and burned-out from a stressful, often understaffed environment, with little or no time to experience the one-on-one caring that should be the heart of hospital employment."[38] A nurse explained the problem particularly well: "Patients don't say, 'Oh, thank you for putting my plan together and making sure I have the right standards initiated and that my critical path is up to date.' They don't say that. When I do (direct) patient care (such as removing) the snarls out of their hair that hasn't been brushed since surgery, they're so appreciative."[39]

An ICU nurse talked about her despair because she no longer has time to deal with the emotional needs of her patients and their families. "As nurses, we pride ourselves on doing that. But it becomes harder and harder. If you have a patient in crisis, and you're running between them and a patient who's very sick, dealing with a patient's or a family's emotional needs is the first thing to go."

Some nurses have told me they almost don't want to find out that their patients or their families have emotional problems, because they won't have time to deal with them. For another ICU nurse in the Midwest, one particular patient symbolizes the plight of both patient and nurse. "This patient was dying. It was her last day on earth. I'm sure she knew she was dying, and I knew she was dying too. Even though nothing would have saved her life, I had to rush off. I literally had to peel her hand off mine to be able to leave the room."

12

No Nurse Left Behind

In the wake of the cost cutting and restructuring of the 1990s, and in the restructuring and cutting that continues today, no hospital, no area or group of nursing, no country—indeed no nurse—has been left behind. There are problems in almost every hospital in the United States. Nurses complain about the erosion of their work life and patient care, whether in home care and nursing home care, in rehabilitation hospitals and hospices, in schools and community clinics, or wherever else they work. Nurse executives and managers, who were asked to implement restructuring—and who often denied staff nurses' concerns about its impact—have been deeply affected, as have the nursing academics whom we count upon to educate all the nurses that hospitals and other institutions have suddenly rediscovered. And as the advocates of cost cutting and privatization of health care services travel the globe, the restructuring solution—with its cuts in length of stay, its excessive nurse workloads, overwork, and job stress, and its deprofessionalization and deskilling of nursing—is promoted in hospitals in every industrialized country and many developing ones.

Beth Israel

One of the most tragic stories is the demise of nursing at the Beth Israel Hospital in Boston.[1] During the merger mania of the mid-1990s, conventional wisdom held that a stand-alone hospital could not survive. To gain clout with insurers, hospitals needed to cut costs and merge into various integrated networks, so that they could reduce administrative overhead, save money on medications and supplies, cut labor costs, and also provide, **313** in one network, a vast array of patient care services. In Boston, two of the major Harvard teaching hospitals, the Brigham and Women's and the Massachusetts General Hospital, had merged into something called Partners HealthCare. The Beth Israel looked around for a partner of its own and found the New England Deaconess, located catercorner from the Beth Israel on Brookline Avenue in the Longwood medical area. The resulting merger created an entity called CareGroup that included the Deaconess and several other hospitals.

Both hospitals felt the merger would be financially advantageous. In fact, they would even try to out-merge Partners by engineering not just an alliance of convenience (a sort of health care equivalent of a civil union) but a real marriage that inextricably joined the two facilities. In forming Partners, the Brigham and Women's and the Massachusetts General merged administratively, but they did not try to consolidate their facilities and operations in a full integration. In fact, they duplicated services and even competed with each other. The Massachusetts General, for example, started an obstetrical service to compete with the Brigham's well-known service. The Beth Israel Deaconess was a full-scale merger. Departments were merged and financial operations were consolidated. Hospital staff and clinical units were joined and redistributed over what would now be two "campuses"—the east and west campuses that represented the old Beth Israel and old Deaconess respectively.

This marriage joined two hospitals with two very different reputations, cultures, and attitudes toward nursing and models of nursing care. The Beth Israel was a relatively small Jewish hospital that had originally been formed to give Jewish doctors and patients a hospital of their own. In the 1970s the Beth Israel began to develop its nursing department and to give nursing a much higher organizational profile. The New England Deaconess was started by Lutheran deaconesses during the great era of religious American hospital formation. The Deaconess evolved into a hospital that was surgeon and physician driven, and nurses were in a much more traditional relationship with physicians than were those at the Beth Israel.

The Beth Israel was world renowned for its "caring" and competence, and particularly famous for its nursing department and the advances nurses had made within the institution. Through primary nursing, Joyce Clifford, the hospital's chief nurse, had helped to establish a model for nurse empowerment that went from the top of the organization to the wards. The hospital had become a mecca for nursing worldwide. The management style at the Beth Israel was what Dana Beth Weinberg called "consensus driven." The Deaconess was known for a very caring staff but

314 was hardly in the forefront of innovation in nursing care delivery. Indeed, its former vice president of nursing, Judy Miller, was an early advocate of the kind of restructuring that many nurses at the Beth Israel and elsewhere felt was deskilling the profession. The Deaconess management style, Weinberg wrote, was "data driven."

It took only a few years of restructuring for a hospital noted for its satisfied nursing staff—and the innovations it pioneered in the delivery of nursing care—essentially to disappear. Two years after the merger, the *Boston Globe* was filled with stories about a "mangled merger" which was costing the hospital $1 million a week. Mitchell T. Rabkin, who had with his board led his hospital into the merger, soon left the helm, to be replaced by James Reinertsen. Like other hospital administrators frantic to cut the costs they could control, Reinertsen and the multiple consultants he would hire, as well as the hospital senior management team, began to cut nursing. Joyce Clifford remained as vice president of nursing for CareGroup. As the hospital continued to lose money, she was asked to watch as nurses lost many benefits they had won. The nurses' voice within the institution was muted. Patient loads increased, and educational resources disappeared.

Beth Israel's major innovation, primary nursing, became harder and harder to deploy as nurses worked with more patients and these patients were assembly-lined through the hospital. The hospital's nursing department tried to accommodate the new realities and still deliver high-quality care.

When our broader societal failure to understand the value of nursing was combined with an acute financial crisis, staff nurses and even nurse executives became sacrificial lambs. In 1997 Clifford was still chief nurse at the Beth Israel Deaconess, but then she was bumped up to a corporate position in CareGroup. In 1999 she resigned from her corporate responsibilities—some said because she could no longer bear to watch what had happened to the nursing department she had so carefully nurtured. She started the Institute for Nursing Healthcare Leadership, ironically at a time when the hospital she devoted her life to was systematically decimating its own.

After the merger of the Beth Israel and Deaconess was ostensibly complete, Trish Gibbons, who three decades earlier implemented primary nursing on the patient care units at the Beth Israel, was brought in to the hospital to be a vice president for inpatient care. When Clifford retired, Gibbons became vice president for patient care services. Her mandate was to cover nursing, social work, unit management, occupational, physical, and respiratory therapy, as well as chaplaincy and nutrition. Early one morning in September 2000, I received a call from a nurse at the hospital

informing me that just before she was supposed to go on vacation, Gib- **315**
bons was told that her services were no longer required.

Dozens of stars of the Beth Israel nursing department left for positions
in other hospitals or to work in academia, including Karen Dick, former
director of the home care department, and oncology nurse manager Ellen
Powers. After trying to adapt to the new nursing at the Beth Israel Deaconess for more than three years, Jean Chaisson said she was so frustrated
that she handed in her resignation before she'd even landed another job.
"I was so angry about what they'd done to nursing that I walked out."
Now she works in hospice and home care and her seventeen years of expertise are no longer available to newer, less experienced nurses. Even
nurses who remained at the Beth Israel Deaconess were deeply disheartened. At this writing, most of the old Beth Israel nurses have left the hospital. So have nurse managers and clinical specialists, many to go over to
the Massachusetts General. While the management team lead by Reinertsen has been replaced, the hospital has yet to recover fully, as the new director of nursing tries to regain a voice for nursing within the institution,
rehire clinical specialists, and rebuild confidence in the nursing staff.

Home and Community Care

Advocates of market medicine argued that nurses would find greater satisfaction in the home and community. Yet, nurses in home care are now
dealing with patients who have higher acuity and who are also raced
through the system. As the 2004 Institute of Medicine report points out,
"increase in severity of illness has had a ripple effect throughout all
health care settings." Reductions in length of stay also "transfer the risk
for adverse events from the hospital setting to the home, where such
events may be less readily detected and result in more serious consequences for the patient."[2] Patients sent out of the hospital more quickly
are sicker when they arrive at nursing homes, rehabilitation hospitals,
and home care settings. Nurses in those settings must deal with much
more complex patients who arrive on IV medications, ventilators, and
tracheotomy tubes. Their conditions could destabilize in a matter of
minutes. Even more stable patients at home have great difficulty moving,
dressing, going to the toilet, or feeding themselves. They may have difficulty mastering how to take their multiple medications safely. "No matter where you go, you're still dealing with the fallout of inadequate nursing staffing," says Jean Chaisson of her current work in home care and
hospice. "You leave the toxic environment of the hospital for home care
and spend eight months helping the patient heal the bedsores they got in
the hospital."

316   The reality is that in North America, insurers, and government payers don't want to incur higher costs for patients, whether they are cared for inside or outside the hospital. They thus have mandated shorter lengths of stays for patients in nursing homes and rehab hospitals and have reduced nursing services available in the home. In the United States, in an effort to cut the home health care program by $16 billion over five years, the Clinton administration and Congress slashed reimbursement rates to home care agencies in the Balanced Budget Act of 1997.

These cutbacks seriously compromised the care that home care nurses were able to give patients in the home. A number of home care agencies closed or cut back on admitting the sickest patients. Because of budget cuts, nursing home agencies also cut staff. After the Balanced Budget Act of 1997, Patricia Keliher of the Home Health Care Association of Massachusetts told me that virtually every home care agency in Massachusetts had cut staff, some by as much as 40 to 50 percent, but most by about 20 percent. In November 1999, members of the Massachusetts Nurses Association who worked at the Visiting Nurses Association of Boston (VNAB) voted to walk off their jobs because of pay and working conditions. Three days before the strike was scheduled, the two sides reached an agreement. In January 2000, when I interviewed Joe-Anne Fergus, a nurse who had worked as an intravenous specialist for four years, she outlined conditions that were not dissimilar to those that hospital nurses were experiencing.

Fergus's trajectory is typical of that of many RNs today. She was majoring in biology in college and wanted to be a doctor, but she switched to nursing when she shadowed a physician and realized that nurses had more patient contact and did critical work with patients.[3] Fergus worked at the Medical College of Virginia Hospitals in Richmond when she graduated in the early 1990s and loved it. In 1995, at the height of restructuring, she went to work at the Massachusetts General Hospital in the transplant unit. "But things were beginning to change in health care," she says. "We were beginning to feel the strain of increasing patient loads. We didn't have enough time with patients."

Trying to find a safe haven for patient care, Fergus moved again, because in home care she thought you would "have more control over your time with patients." She did, for a while. But starting in 1997 or 1998, she said, managers at the VNAB started talking about nurses' "productivity per day." By that measure, her patient load was increased from 5 patients per nurse to 7.5. "When you add that to the fact that patients are now being discharged from the hospital sicker than ever before, our caseloads are even more arduous," she said.

"We recently had a patient discharged from the hospital after complications following a mastectomy," she told me. "She had a gaping wound in her chest . . . and the nurses had to pack the gauze into the wound it-self. . . . Just changing the dressing can take anywhere from a half hour to an hour. She had no family or outside support and was totally dependent on nursing and home health aides."

She was also frightened and anxious and wanted to talk about her fears. The nurses who took care of her, Fergus said, had to organize community support and teach her how to take care of her wound when they weren't around. Not to mention talking about her disfigurement and future sur-vival. "But when home care nurses deliver that kind of care to seven pa-tients a day," Fergus said, "they're under tremendous stress because the system is telling them they're providing too much care. . . . We call it drive-by nursing. And for this, nurses were, before the threat of a strike, being paid $45,000 a year to live in one of the most expensive cities in America."

In 2004, the story hadn't changed. Patricia Keliher reported that Medicare cuts in home care were ongoing. "In the last two Medicare re-form acts, home health was further cut," she said. "In October 2003, we took a cut of around 4 percent to our Medicare reimbursement. The Medicare Modernization and Improvement Act of 2003, which gave us a prescription drug benefit, actually included a provision to eliminate what would have been an inflation update on home health rates that was due this spring."

Keliher says that all of these cuts have produced a shortage in home health care nursing because cash-strapped agencies just can't compete with the salaries and benefits given by hospitals and can't hire enough nurses. This shortage, however, isn't manifested in nursing vacancies. In-stead, it means that home care agencies turn away clients who need serv-ices because there's no one available to provide them.

"The financial squeeze is on every agency or facility you work for," says Jean Chaisson. "From the point of view of the individual nurse you don't have a sense of efficacy anywhere you work," she says. "It's hard to be a hospital nurse and not provide adequate care and know you haven't, and then discharge the patient before you can rectify that. And it's hard to be a home care nurse and have to send them back to the hospital or, even worse, have them ill and home and saying, 'I will never go back to the hospital.'"

Chaisson insists that "this is psychotic. Basically, we're fracturing the health care experience and pressuring our health care institutions to try to pass the buck so they won't go under. And the buck is both the patient and the nurse."

Nursing Executives

The army of restructurers, consultants, and market advocates who helped to change hospital nursing aimed many of their arguments at nurse executives and managers, who would be putting their theories into practice. These nurse executives and managers would be some of the hardest hit by the policies they implemented. "Nurse executives and nurse managers were squeezed the hardest and were the first eliminated," argues Leah Curtin, current editor of the *Journal of Clinical Systems Management* and former editor the *Journal of Nursing Management.*

Until the 1980s, most chief nursing officers (CNOs) did not hold executive-level positions. They weren't involved in hospital strategic planning and didn't even control or develop the budget of the nursing department.[4] Joyce Clifford at the Beth Israel Hospital was a notable exception. This situation changed in the 1980s, and in many hospitals chief nurses were to gain more power and voice for themselves and for their nurses and nursing departments. But according to Clifford's 1998 study of nursing leadership, the hard-won victories of nursing in the 1980s were turned back in the 1990s.[5] One of the first things that happened during restructuring was that the chief nurse executive position in the hospital—which was changed from vice president of nursing to vice president of patient care services—became a staff rather than a line position. With this move, says Leah Curtin, "chief nurses lost line authority in a critical mass of hospitals."

For those uninitiated in management jargon, what this means is that the position of nurse executive, which used to give the administrator "line authority" (i.e., control over budgets, people, and departments), was transformed into to a staff position, where, Curtin explains, CNOs moved from top management to middle management.

Restructurers, Curtin believes, would have eliminated vice presidents of nursing if they could have. "In fact," she recounts, "I heard the president of American Practice Management (APM) say there was no need for any nurse manager in any hospital above the level of the head nurse. But because of legal and regulatory requirements, they had to keep them, so they made them staff under a chief operating officer. If they were lucky, they might be put in charge of quality assurance, which gave them influence. They could influence, but could not exercise authority."

The change in title from vice president of nursing to vice president of patient care services was also a significant one. Like nurses who were told that restructuring would take them to a higher level of power, responsibility, and authority, nurse executives were promised that they would gain more power by moving from exclusive responsibility for the nursing department to overseeing a variety of other disciplines. Along with nursing, these might include social work, behavioral sciences, respiratory, occupational, and physical therapy, transport, nutritional services, case management, housekeeping, dietary services, or any variation on this theme. It never included medicine or pharmacy. In addition, they would manage nursing services.[6]

This move generated a fair amount of controversy. Some in nursing management believed it gave nurses more power. Leah Curtin, for example, believes that nurse administrators gained greater impact and greater reach within their organizations. But some nurse executives worried that this expansion of the nurse executive's portfolio would dilute the executive's efficacy and rob nurses of representation at the management table.

Joanne Disch argued that nursing executives, because of their holistic view of patient care, could best represent both nursing and other service disciplines. This move would be problematic, she said, only if the nurse executive who became director of patient care services forgot nursing as she diffused her span of control. "In a lot of institutions," she said, "people worried about speaking up for one particular discipline now that they were everybody's boss. If an issue warrants support, it should be supported no matter what it relates to. Some people went too far the other way and supported nothing related to nursing."

Whatever their view of the wisdom of this move, more nurses were forced, or volunteered, to make it. A survey by VHA Inc., a nationwide network of community-owned hospitals, found that nurse executives across the country had expanded roles and duties and that those "holding the position whose title included 'nursing' declined from 55 to 24 percent." A 1997–98 study found that in 97 percent of teaching hospitals surveyed, the chief nurse was now a "patient care" nurse. Surveys show that many hospital redesigns have eliminated the department of nursing and others report that formerly strong chief nurses have lost power and authority in relationship to other top hospital officials.[7]

It's no wonder. Nurse executives would quickly see their workload and portfolios expand. Just as staff nurses have had more responsibility heaped upon them with less authority and control over their work, chief nurses have experienced a simultaneous increase in responsibility and decrease in control. In the late 1990s, a nurse executive in a New York hospital told me she no longer had as much time to listen to and work with her own nurse managers because her portfolio had significantly expanded. She was busy administering a nursing council made up of executives from more than six hospitals. The nurse managers directly under her complained that they felt lost in the shuffle. On the units, nurse managers, she said,

320 echoed their complaints: nurse executives no longer have time to hear their concerns.

Many nurse executives said they also felt they were working in an increasingly hostile environment. The traditional tension between the nurse executive's mandate to protect the profession and her job description—to protect hospital priorities—clashed with increasing intensity as consultants and top executives presented them with benchmarks they were ordered to achieve. Joanne Disch explained that because of the push to contain costs in the 1990s, "There was a failure to recognize that you could actually support the institution by developing strong professional practice. Nurses would bring forward legitimate concerns. A staff nurse might complain about a piece of equipment that wasn't functioning. In fact, it was a patient safety hazard. Yet there was rigmarole that a nurse had to go through to provide unbelievable data that indeed this was a problem."

If a nurse executive insisted that staff were being pushed too far, Disch said, the response was " 'Well, you just don't want to make changes; you just want to keep things the way they are.' There was such a resolute pursuit of financial savings that we lost sight of 'Wait a minute, let's get some balance.' Institutions would say, 'Well, we are balancing,' but the whole industry was taken up by this rush to cut costs."

Nurses' concerns weren't the only things to be dismissed. Many nurse executives were dismissed as well—literally.

Jennifer Hawkins* is a case in point. Hawkins had been director of nursing at a children's hospital for nine years when restructuring hit. During her tenure, several CEOs had come and gone. So had the administrators to whom she directly reported. Although her hospital was not in any imminent or even future financial difficulty, consultants had made a pitch to the CEO and board promising that they could save the hospital some $4 million a year on staffing costs. With that lure, they reeled the hospital in. Hawkins and another manager and upper administrators began meeting with consultants—both of them nurses, with no current clinical experience or experience in pediatrics. Although the consultants wanted their deliberations to include as few people as possible, Hawkins insisted that staff nurses and managers had to be involved. But it soon became clear that the involvement of managers and staff was merely sugarcoating an increasingly bitter pill.

The consultants told Hawkins that nursing was their target. When Hawkins protested that the work of other departments, like the OR and physical therapy, affected the efficiency and productivity of nurses, they reiterated that their goal was to reduce the number of nurses, to replace

RNs with nursing assistants, and to teach the remaining RNs to multi- **321** skill.

The consultants also wanted to eliminate what was known as the line team. These nurses were expert at inserting what are called central venous lines that are often inserted in the veins of children with cancer or who are patients on ICUs. For these patients the use of peripheral IVs—placed in the arm or back of the hand—is not recommended because the patient needs drugs or nutrition that may scar smaller veins or because the patient has had so many peripheral lines inserted that their veins have been damaged and no longer allow access. So lines are placed in larger veins, like the subclavian vein, a big vein under the clavicle. It takes special skill to insert theses lines and the risks of doing so are greater. For example, it's possible to puncture the lung when inserting a central line into the subclavian vein. Risk of infection is greater with such lines because bacteria can get right into the heart. In fact, research studies have shown that on ICUs infections of these lines are the most common causes of hospital-acquired bloodstream infections. These lead to between 2,400 and 20,000 deaths and cost between $296 million and $2.3 billion annually.[8] In spite of the risks, the team was cut and a smaller group of staff nurses was asked to manage these catheters themselves.

As meetings went on, Hawkins says, she tried to fight some of the consultants' proposals, to no avail. They not only ignored nurses' concerns, they urged higher management to fire the people who voiced them. "Some managers disagreed with the consultants during meetings. After the meeting, the consultants would go tell the administration that they weren't on board. One of the things I'm not proud of at all," she confided, "was that my boss told me that I had to terminate my managers."

Hawkins said that her boss's philosophy was that "if things weren't going well, it was the manager's fault." She offered several managers a severance package and they were gone. "You weren't really free to talk about your concerns in front of the consultants because you were concerned about your own job. With the new administration, staff started disappearing. Not just nursing staff. They were there one day and they weren't there the next day. They were just gone."

Hawkins also complained about the pace of the changes being implemented in the institution. The hospital staff, she said, had to adapt to the consultant's timetable. Because of the haste of the enterprise, Hawkins said, she had to quickly replace the nurse managers she'd fired and cut more staff. She did. Her boss was delighted, took her to celebratory dinner, gave her a large bonus, and the highest possible performance evaluation: she had substantially exceeded expectations.

322   By this time, the hospital was on its second consultant and things were not going well on the floors. Nurses who had more work and less time with patients began to complain to physician colleagues, who in turn took their concerns to higher-level management. Neither her boss nor the CEO was pleased with this turn of events. She was called into her boss's office and told that she would have to fire the manager she'd just hired. He said he would sit in on the meeting when she fired the manager and she summoned the woman to his office. With him at her side, she offered the manager a severance package. "She was really upset. I felt horrible," Hawkins said. But she had to go.

After the distraught manager left the room, she says, a man whom she'd never met came in. "You know what happened?" she asked me. "My boss turned around and fired me. . . . They wouldn't let me go back to my office. I'd been there for years. I'm the most trustworthy person. I would never do anything to hurt any hospital where I'd worked. They had someone go get my purse and escort me out of the building. . . . They let me come in the next Saturday with the head of the security forces, to let me get my things out of my office. My secretary was afraid to call me. She didn't know what was going on."

Hawkins went to a lawyer. The hospital had offered her a six-months severance package. She'd asked for eighteen months, and they split the difference at twelve.

With nurse executives overburdened and overwhelmed by their own insecurities, nursing lost more power. One study revealed that hospitals whose directors of nursing were "highly visible and accessible to staff" fell from 89 to 41 percent. When Linda Aiken and her colleagues looked at Pennsylvania hospitals, they found that 58.3 percent of nurses surveyed said they had fewer nurse managers and 16.8 percent had lost a chief nurse officer who had not been replaced.[9]

Nurse executives who have lived through—and are still dealing with—restructuring have told me that their lives have become a nightmare of coping with consultants and managing or trying to fend off cuts in services, in staff, in equipment, and in resources. "We're on the sixth or is it seventh restructuring," a New York State nurse executive told me. "Now we have Cap Gemini at the hospital, which makes the Hunter Group, which we had a couple of years ago, look like a day at the beach. Most of my time is spent managing consultants. And believe me, this is a full-time job. Their view of managing care is that it's about managing supply and demand. They want us to have a just-in-time float pool, which can dispatch nurses anywhere, like a taxi dispatcher. My view is that nurses create relationships with patients that save lives and bring comfort and healing." That does not seem to be a view many consultant share.

For Trish Gibbons, the job became as demoralizing as it was for the **323** staff nurses who worked under her. As her enthusiasm for cost cutting waned, the hospital CEO, she said, withdrew from her. "He stopped rounding with me. He canceled meetings. I felt alienated from the work of the organization. There was no place to talk about patient care. I felt very alone. I felt like I wasn't in health care. I felt like someone had dropped me on this corporate island far from civilization. I kept thinking maybe they won't last forever and I'll hunker down and build some tunnels of clinical quality and wait for new leadership."

Mid-Level Management

Trouble at the top of the nursing management hierarchy quickly percolated to those mid-level nurse managers who are supposed to be in charge of the day-to-day management of patient care. "Nurse managers, like vice presidents of nursing," Curtin says, "are caught in the middle. The nurse manager's job is to translate the decisions made in upper administration into reality on the units. That's your job and that's what you're hired to do. . . . That's what it comes down to. They are also there," she adds, "to communicate the concerns of clinical staff to administration in order to assure that adequate and safe patient care is delivered, and so they are the folks in the middle."

These mostly middle-aged women, however, were radically reduced in number during restructuring. According to Curtin, about half of nurse managers lost their jobs or were replaced, if they were replaced at all, with people who had little or no experience. A manager who had a great deal of clinical and management experience in, say, oncology would be laid off. A staff nurse might be promoted to head nurse and her duties would be to manage scheduling, budgets, and evaluations, as well as respond to staff concerns and do staff development. Then she would be rotated out of that position after a few months and another staff nurse would be made charge nurse. Given this paradigm, it's not surprising that Carol Lincoln was offered the position of nurse manager only a year after graduation from nursing school.

"When I began, the manager of each unit was a specialist in that field and could actually do the nursing involved," Susan Davis says. Davis, a nurse manager in a West Coast teaching hospital, began her career in nursing management almost two decades ago. "They could understand what the patients needed and the nurses needed in order to be able to do their job. Now you'll find managers who really don't know anything clinically about the unit they're managing. When things get tough and busy, they don't know how to operate the IV pumps."

324   Davis said that the position of nurse manager has always been problematic because many nurse managers got their jobs not because they had management experience but because they were good clinicians. Obviously, not every excellent clinician made an excellent manager. What is needed, she says, is someone with good clinical and managerial skills. Or a good manager can be coupled with a clinical specialist who takes over staff education and development. Today, clinical specialists have been fired and, Davis says, people with good management and clinical skills feel the pressure is too intense to do a good job in either area. "So we have managers leaving the field right and left. The newer managers who come in and who tend to stick it out have very little understanding of what it takes to be a clinician. We're getting very young nurses going into management who don't understand the stresses and strains of nursing work. Or experienced managers have simply thrown up their hands and said, 'I'll do what I can do and that's the best that I can do.' We're in a real nursing frontline management crisis," she insists.

Nurse managers' frustrations stem from an increased workload. Executives interviewed by the VHA said that along with nursing directors, nurse manager positions have been reduced and the work of the remaining managers has been consolidated, with most managers having responsibility for two units. Another study of teaching hospitals found that the number of nurse manager positions fell in 91 percent of the hospitals surveyed. In fact, the researchers reported that nearly half of the nurse managers were also given additional responsibility for supervising personnel other than nursing staff (e.g., housekeepers, transportation staff, dietary aides).[10]

All the nurse managers I spoke to told me that their job has totally changed during the past decade. "When I started out as an assistant head nurse I was very involved with the clinical component of the job," Susan Davis said. She worked at least once a month to maintain her clinical skills and, with her head nurse, did all the staff evaluations. "We had very little to do with the budget at the time. There wasn't this heavy emphasis on justifying everything that we did. The assumption was that we did what we did because it needed to be done. If we had that many nurses it was because we needed that many nurses."

That was then, and this is now, Davis says. "The job has become impossible. Most managers have two units, which means they can have eighty to a hundred employees or more. The manager is responsible for doing the budget and filling out an unbelievable number of forms to justify it, and yet has no control over it. You just can't effectively manage like this."

Maureen O'Keefe recently left a hospital where she had worked for over a decade because she simply couldn't handle the strain of endless cutbacks and her inability to support her staff. Before cost cutting, O'Keefe **325** says, nursing had an identity, a voice. When her hospital began to restructure, all that changed. Neither the rotating crews of consultants nor the administration, she says, were interested in hearing the views of mid-level nurse managers or staff nurses. When objections were made to proposed changes, top-level administrators "accused nurses of being obstructionist and just afraid of change."

Indeed, as she describes it, high-level nursing administrators used patient acuity calculations as an excuse to coercively ration nursing care. In one meeting with a high-level administrator, she relates, "We were looking at budgets and hours and she said, 'You have to sign off on these numbers. You have to sign off on this; you have no choice.'" But the hours per patient day were budgeted on the unit's midnight census which, O'Keefe said, "kills you, because that's your lowest census. You really don't have the capacity to handle the patients as they come in during the day."

Her objection was overcome by the new logic of the system. "You need to see so many patients and have so many operations. They benchmark and tell you that this is how long patients stay, this is how much nursing they get in another hospital. And then you ask them, 'Well, does that hospital do bone marrow transplants?' And they pause and say, 'Well no, it's a community hospital.'" In fact, she says, speaking almost in disbelief, at one point things got so bad that upper-level administrators actually directed the nurses to skimp on how much bed linen they gave patients. "They told us that each bed will have one top sheet, one bottom sheet, no pull sheet, one blanket. They were trying to control how much linen we use."

When I have asked nurse executives if there was any alternative to restructuring or if they felt they had too readily acquiesced to the consultants' demands, their responses have been ambiguous and ambivalent. What were our options? one director of nursing asked. We tried to fight within our institutions and we lost. When I asked if nurse managers and executives could have moved their protest outside their institutions, she seemed puzzled by the question. Talking to the press? Making private knowledge public to state legislatures? Although she is deeply distressed—and that is an understatement—about what has happened to nursing nationwide, such action did not fall within her repertoire of behavior. "Maybe I see things in too many shades of gray," she said, after painting a black-and-white picture for me.

Jennifer Hawkins was very distressed about what had happened to her and pretty shamefaced about the way she complied with executive directives to lay off managerial and nursing staff. I asked her if she felt that managers had too readily cooperated with consultants. Not at all, she replied. "We all wanted to do the right thing. No matter what we did we

326 were going to have trouble getting all the staff on board and have them understand why we had to do things differently."

As we talked it became clear that to her the problem was not the premise—get rid of RNs—but the schedule—do it quick. "What I believe happened," she said, "was that there wasn't enough help in getting the whole organization on board." She was distressed that change was rapid rather than incremental, that managers were blamed for inevitable problems, that the consultants took the money and ran, and that she was poorly treated. "If the change is difficult to implement and you have a lot of turnover of staff as a result, you don't blame the manager, you provide resources to support that manager."

Hawkins had pointed with pride to her great accomplishment during the process of restructuring—bringing staff into the process. Wasn't it just window dressing? I asked. She thought for a moment and admitted that yes, probably it was. She nonetheless insisted that there was a way to reconcile downsizing with efficiency, a good work environment, and nurses' control over their practice. Whenever I questioned the premises of restructuring, rather than the behavior of the restructurers, she replied that the hospital had suffered from inefficiencies.

"But you told me that your hospital faced no financial difficulties," I countered. Why then, was restructuring such an urgent matter? "Well, they didn't want to be wasting money," she said almost petulantly.

Hawkins's response is an interesting one. She said that her hospital was financially sound but was convinced it had to restructure anyway. Her comment also indicates the paradoxical position of the nurse manager, who serves two masters. She is supposed to represent and lead nurses, but she is also hired to implement the decisions of the hospital board and executive team, even when they compromise nursing care. This divided loyalty was evident in all her comments and in those of many other nurse managers.

In the balancing act between these two contradictory imperatives, Norrish and Rundall write, "the nurse executive's role on the executive management team and the need to demonstrate sensitivity to cost pressures may, at times, take precedence over the commitment to the profession of nursing. Can the nurse executive refuse to participate in redesign efforts or to implement changes in the skill mix? Not only would such refusal place his or her job at risk, but the nurse executive may also see little choice in the matter, thinking that 'If I don't do this, someone else will.'"[11] If this is the logic and the predicament, then it is difficult to give credence to nurse executives' claim to professional leadership. Indeed, in my conversations with many of nurse executives, they seem to have bought the rope with which they were eventually hung.

A number of top-level nurse administrators told me they felt that nursing executives failed because, early on, they didn't become chief operating officers of their institutions when they had the chance. "If I had to recast the 1990s or 1980s and do things differently, nursing should have taken over chief operating positions and run these organizations as nursing organizations. Many nurses wanted to go that route. The discussion at that time was that it was a reasonable thing to do but people feared that you're leaving nursing. It's a different career track."

"That's a flaw," she continued. "Physicians are CEOs of hospitals. Nurses should have taken over day-to-day operations of the organization, because bringing in business types doesn't work." She insisted that clinicians wouldn't squeeze out more than the fat and would have refused to cut into the muscle of patient care. "If you had a nurse and physician running an organization they would not have turned to twenty-five-year-old MBAs from these companies who had to come in to learn the business in order to give you some goddamn formula to tell you you could do it with five fewer people."

While her passion and belief in clinical loyalty is perhaps admirable, is it also naïve? It was, after all, physician Mitchell T. Rabkin, who under immense pressure, decided he had to merge his hospital into CareGroup. James Reinertsen, who took over from Rabkin and implemented the merger, is also a physician. In fact, he was as disliked by MDs as he was by RNs.

Physicians—much to the chagrin and ire of many of their colleagues—have been key, as a nurse executive pointed out, in promoting HMOs and managed care. Many now run hospitals like businesses and seem to view patients as guests who will fare better if they get a chocolate on their pillow and turn-down service at night. Why would nurses be any different? In fact, the experience of restructuring demonstrates that they aren't. As we saw in Chapter 9, many nurses themselves became management consultants who advocated downsizing and deskilling.

When this fact is raised, a number of managers respond that these nurse consultants don't really have the "heart of a nurse" or that they don't remember where they came from. Sadly it is one's job definition rather than one's former job that usually determines behavior. A nursing license, after all, is a professional credential, not a moral shield. Most people, no matter the letters after their name, usually do what they are told and act to save their jobs.

Which leads us to perhaps the saddest part of this story. Nurse managers and executives were not only asked to cut positions inside their institutions. They were also asked to publicly defend actions that they pri-

328 vately bemoaned and to denounce the concerns of those staff nurses who tried to alert politicians and journalists to the problems brewing in re-structured hospitals. Throughout the 1990s and continuing today, staff nurses have publicly protested cutbacks in nursing care and the declining quality of care, and have predicted a future nursing shortage. Nurse exec-utives and nurse managers, far more than physician CEOs or other non-nurse hospital administrators, were the ones who disputed these claims. In legislative hearings, in testimony before groups like the Institute of Medicine and other investigative bodies, or in discussions with journal-ists, nurse executives were the first to claim that staff nurses were alarmist and driven by a desire to protect their jobs, not their patients, or that they were benightedly impeding the march of progress. While many of these nurses were privately complaining about the same problems their staff nurses were publicly parading, they became guardians of a process about which many had serious reservations and which would eventually turn on them.

Their situation, at least in the United States, was further compli-cated by antiunion and anticollective biases and definitions of profes-sionalism that preclude collective action, and anything that smacks of militant political protest. Their actions were also colored by the kind of antigovernment biases that have become almost obsessive in post-Reagan America.

Although I'll explore these issues at some length in my conclusion, one brief example illustrates how these attitudes hurt both managers and the nurses they are supposed to represent. In the spring of 2003, a number of nurses from the Beth Israel came to a book launch party for Dana Wein-berg's *Code Green*. None of these nurses worked at the Beth Israel Dea-coness anymore. As they gathered with nurses from other hospitals to talk about the book, a rare rapprochement occurred between these former Beth Israel nurses, many of whom had been hostile to union organizing and activities and some of the union nurses in the room. With tears in her eyes, one of the nurses told the group that she felt the Beth Israel nurses hadn't fought hard enough. "We should have picketed, protested," she said. "We shouldn't have let it happen without a much more public fight."

One former nurse manager who has left nursing altogether continued to muse about their mutual loss. "We didn't do enough. You know, we could have gotten together as managers and written a letter to manage-ment and all signed it. But we didn't. You know why? Because putting ten signatures on a letter would have seemed too unionlike."

"What did you have to lose?" I asked her.

Well, it turns out, nothing, she said, We lost it all. Thirty years of work gone, for us and for nursing.

Nursing Academia

If nurse managers have experienced problems because of cost cutting, problems are no less serious for nurse academics, and tensions are similarly heightened. During the cost cutting of the 1990s, as many nurses lost their jobs or were increasingly dissatisfied with the ones they had, it became clear to those considering a career in the field that nursing, which had never paid enough, no longer seemed to offer its two traditional enticements, job stability and mobility. If nurses were to be rewarded with a pink slip every decade or so, that certainly undercut any promise of job security. And how could you move up into management, academia, research, or any other field if you couldn't even get a job at the so-called bottom of the ladder in bedside nursing.

When hospitals began to offer higher salaries and better benefits to resolve the nursing shortage of the late 1980s, these produced a steady increase in nursing school enrollments. In 1994, the American Association of Colleges of Nursing (AACN) issued an optimistic press release. When the association—which represents schools of nursing that offer bachelor's, master's, and doctoral programs—calculated enrollments, they found a "steady climb" in master's degree programs and a "modest increase" in enrollments in bachelor's programs.[12] By 1999, the releases the organization was issuing had a distinctly pessimistic tone. A March 1999 press release carried the bleak title "While Demand for RNs Climbs, Undergraduate Nursing Enrollments Decline." It reported that "enrollments of entry level bachelor's degree students at U.S. nursing schools fell by 5.5 percent in fall 1998, the fourth consecutive decline in as many years."[13]

The same was true in two-year associate degree programs in community colleges. "According to the National Council of State Boards of Nursing, the number of first-time, U.S.-educated nursing school graduates who sat for the NCLEX-RN, the national licensure examination for registered nurses, decreased by 20 percent from 1995 to 2003. A total of 19,820 fewer students in this category of test takers sat for the exam in 2003 as compared with 1995."[14]

As hospitals began searching for nurses in the late 1990s and the early twenty-first century, enrollments have increased. The AACN stated in May 2003 that enrollments in entry-level programs to nursing increased by almost 17 percent since 2002. But, sadly, in the same year 5,283 qualified applicants to various programs had to be turned away because there were not enough faculty.[15]

The AACN has also found promising increases in what are called "accelerated programs." These are programs designed to attract people who have four-year or graduate degrees in another field—say, music, or his-

330 tory, or biology—but who are interested in changing careers and disciplines. These programs allow potential students to complete a nursing school course in perhaps twelve or eighteen months and "provide the quickest route to becoming a registered nurse." These include programs that give people with a degree in another field a BSN in nursing. Accelerated programs also educate students in "generic master's degree programs" intended to appeal to second-degree students as "the natural step in their higher education." People who have four-year degrees in another field can be fast-tracked into advanced practice or nurse practitioner roles after completing three—or in some cases two—years of school. They can sit for their RN exam after only one year of course work. These are increasingly popular programs in the United States, and American nursing schools are trying to export them to other countries.[16]

Increased enrollments in bachelor's programs, accelerated programs, and master's and doctoral programs have been applauded for a variety of reasons. Nurses, as we've seen, have traditionally lacked the educational preparation of the other clinicians they work with. Some professors and deans of nursing schools believe that when some nurses have advanced degrees, doctors will at least show this group of nurses more respect. One prominent dean of a school of nursing explained that a lot of bedside nurses really didn't deserve to be treated collegially by physicians because they lacked the appropriate educational credentials. Why should doctors treat nurses with respect, this woman asked, since most of them don't have the educational preparation to think critically, problem-solve, and make important clinical decisions?

If bedside nurses have more knowledge, others argue, they will be able to provide higher-quality care to patients. That's the conclusion reached by at least one recent study, in which Aiken and researchers at the University of Pennsylvania School of Nursing found a correlation between educational preparation and lower mortality rates in hospitals.[17] Nurse educators also believe that nurse practitioners and advanced practice programs will also attract the kind of ambitious, intelligent woman—or man—that the profession needs, and provide nurses with opportunities for advancement and job mobility.

Unfortunately, it's not at all clear whether these future nurses will want to practice in shortage-plagued areas like hospitals. But even if they do, these increases in enrollments in nursing schools will not produce the nurses needed by the year 2010 and 2020. The Bureau of Labor Statistics has predicted that as a result of combined job growth and net replacements there will be over one million job vacancies by 2010.[18]

In order to meet the huge demand for nurses over the next decades, the AACN estimates that enrollments will have to increase by at least 40 per-

cent, but this may be an underestimation. To produce both nurses and **331**
nursing faculty, however, a society has to produce enough nurses who will
do both clinical and academic work. If there aren't enough nurses who
want to construct a long-term career in the clinical setting, particularly in
hospitals, home care, clinics, and other areas of direct care, then adding
more nursing students to nursing schools may not necessarily address future direct care nursing shortages. Indeed, if nurses leave the clinical setting to go into academia, it may actually exacerbate, not resolve, the nursing shortage in direct care. Similarly, if there aren't enough nurses who
want to teach in nursing schools, that will also worsen the shortage of
nurses in direct care, because there will be no one to teach new recruits, if
they're enlisted. To resolve future shortages, both the clinical and academic setting have to retain sufficient numbers of clinicians *and* faculty,
and recruit new replacements.

This project is hampered by a severe a shortage of nursing school faculty, which mirrors the shortage of bedside nurses. Nursing faculty, like
bedside nurses, are getting older, and younger recruits aren't nipping at
their heels. Many nursing faculty, particularly younger and junior faculty,
feel burnt out and report high levels of job dissatisfaction because of excessive student loads, escalating job-related demands and student need,
and salaries that fail to make their efforts at least financially worthwhile.

According to a 2002 survey from the AACN, the average age of a nursing faculty member with a master's degree is forty-nine, and fifty-three
with a doctoral degree. Many faculty with master's degrees will soon be
eligible to retire at age sixty-two. In 1993, the median age of nursing
school faculty was fifty years old (that is, those over fifty and under fifty
were equal in number). By 2002, things had changed dramatically, with
those over fifty increasing by 20 percent. New people just aren't entering
the pipeline, yet older faculty are inexorably moving on and out. Between
2004 and 2012, more faculty will become eligible for retirement each
year.[19]

While enrollments in masters programs have been rising, the number
of people graduating from them has been declining. This is particularly
significant because future nursing school professors and instructors are
taken from this pool of masters and doctoral students. Moreover, there
has been a decline in numbers of faculty in the 36–45 age group with a
PhD. "Advancement to the next age category accounts for some of the
decline, but egression from academic life is the major reason for the loss
of younger faculty members."[20]

The shortage of nursing faculty is making it difficult for schools to accept more applicants in a field in which education is very labor intensive.
Most faculty members who teach a lecture course will also be taking stu-

332   dents into a clinical setting off campus for at least one day of the week. Although the students will be paired with an RN and will accompany that nurse as he or she takes care of patients, the professor or lecturer will oversee their clinical learning experience and must be with them in the clinical setting. Since there may be thirty or forty students in a class, there must be enough faculty members to take students onto the units. This means that the ratio of faculty to students is much higher in nursing than it is in, say, sociology or French literature.

Nursing faculty are expected to take care of an increasing number of students, conduct research, and write a steady stream of grant proposals to finance their work. They must produce scholarship, which then must be published; if it isn't published, the faculty member might perish. They must advise, supervise, and mentor students, and offer service to the university community. "Time," faculty members said, "is becoming their most precious commodity," so much so that 73 percent of faculty respondents expressed frustration at "never having time to complete a piece of work."[21]

Like floor nurses, faculty also have to deal with increasing student "acuity." Nursing students were never the typical college or graduate students. A nurse may begin by going to community college, and then work for a while. She may then decide to get her bachelor's degree in a program designed to accelerate the process. Since most nurses continue working while studying, these programs are designed to accommodate full-time work and school. Then she may work some more. She may then go to get a master's or doctorate. But she may still be working either part-time or even full-time. (This is why almost half of all graduates of doctoral programs in nursing are between forty-five and fifty-four, which means the number of their "productive teaching and research years" is far fewer than other similarly credentialed academics.)[22]

Students who spend so much time working may have difficulty keeping up with their studies. Moreover, they no longer come from homogeneous cultural or national backgrounds. In public universities and schools of nursing, students may come from poor communities and need a lot of remedial help in reading, writing, and study skills. As more foreign nurses are recruited to the United States and are lured by the promise of continuing education, nursing professors have to deal with a huge ethnic and cultural mix in their classrooms.

Since students in accelerated programs may come from other academic disciplines, integrating them into nursing school culture—or in classes with students who are RNs (typical in generic master's programs) may prove a challenge. "It's not so easy to teach forty students—twenty of whom come out of a grab bag of different disciplines and twenty of whom were registered nurses for twenty years," one lecturer in a nurse practitioner program said. "The RNs have great clinical skills but aren't that assertive. The other students are more assertive but have no clinical skills. Sure, these students can learn a lot from each other. But facilitating that exchange and learning process is not easy," he commented.

"Faculty presence in the hospital and other health settings," says Victoria Palmer Erbs, a professor at University of Massachusetts in Boston, "is even more important today because staff nurses have less time to answer the student's questions." But establishing this presence may be difficult for several reasons. Although nursing is a clinical discipline, there is an increasing divide—or some say mismatch—between, on the one hand, lecturers who have a great deal of experience with the contemporary practice of nursing and are prepared to devote their careers to teaching students in clinical settings and, on the other, university-based academics with doctorate degrees who are pursuing tenure and are expected to engage in scholarly research. In contrast, most doctors who teach continue to practice medicine, because they have permanent appointments in teaching hospitals and an independent patient base. Neither nursing teachers nor their students have a permanent place in the hospitals in which their teaching and learning occurs. It is difficult for them to get advanced education and do research while remaining at the bedside. This problem is aggravated by the structure of academia. As nursing has moved into the university, more nursing academics are expected to have PhDs. But with the PhD, which is the only academic track that gives faculty the guarantee of tenure and thus job security, professors, whether junior or senior, must spend their time doing the kind of research that often takes them away from nursing practice. Yet, if a school has a faculty shortage and needs someone to accompany students into the clinical setting, faculty members who've spent years doing research or scholarly work may be asked to take groups of students onto a hospital ward and to be informed about clinical issues they may not have dealt with for years. "Because these are rapidly evolving complex systems, someone who worked there twenty years ago will be at sea today," a frustrated professor at a university school of nursing in the Northeast said.

Moreover, just like their students, faculty members have to deal with resentful floor nurses who are annoyed at the students'—or the faculty members'—questions. "Hospitals or other agencies invite groups of students for things like medical surgical rotations or in other specialty areas because they think it will be good for their recruiting—some of these nurses will be candidates for future employment. But they may be unaware of how staff nurses feel about teaching students and juggling heavy patient loads," one professor commented tersely.

334   One possible solution is the use of more lecturers—nurses with master's degrees and a clinical track record—who are comfortable and knowledgeable clinical teachers. In nursing academia, these people have neither job security nor job mobility. At the University of Toronto, for example, a lecturer is on a three-year contract and has no assurance that the time and money she puts into teaching will help her move higher on the academic career ladder. The same is true in the United States. This helps explain why there is a shortage of people graduating from master's programs and moving on to teaching. Why should they do it? What's in it for them, particularly since they can earn far more in the clinical setting?

Money is also a significant problem for nursing faculty. Nursing schools, like hospitals and other health care institutions, are not paying their faculty enough. The AACN white paper compared faculty salaries with those in nonacademic settings. The median salary of an associate professor of nursing with a master's degree was $60,556, while a nurse anesthetist earned $105,890. Associate professors with a PhD had a median income $74,556, while a chief nurse anesthetist had a median income of $128,879.[23] As one nursing faculty member explained, a professor with fifteen years experience and a doctorate can earn $57,000 a year. But she can go over to the Massachusetts General Hospital and earn as much as $90,000.

Nurses, particularly those in public universities, cannot expect any financial relief anytime soon. That's because cutbacks in education have affected them dramatically. The University of California at San Francisco cited permanent budget reductions of $18 million in 2002–3 and $11.6 million for 2003–4, and indicates a similar budget reduction is proposed for 2004–5. The university is trying to preserve its educational mission through increased student and professional fees.[24]

At the five campuses of the University of Massachusetts, all of which have nursing programs, nursing has been affected by the same systemwide budget cuts as all other programs. Each campus of the University of Massachusetts system has lost millions in state funds over the last five years. Faculty and staff morale is low because salary increases have not kept pace with private sector salaries and opportunities. The University of Massachusetts has many students interested in attending the School of Nursing but can't admit them because it doesn't have enough nursing faculty to teach them, says associate professor Genevieve Chandler. The school's faculty shortage has been exacerbated as the university urges more experienced and expensive workers to take early retirement. Using this typical business strategy, the idea is to winnow out the most expensive professors and replace them with new and cheaper blood. The problem is that in nursing there is little blood available for the transfusion. Try as they might, the school, like many others, simply can't find cheaper, or even more expensive replacements. "It a moral struggle for me," Chandler reports, "because I teach so many freshman and I think they'd make great nurses. Because of layoffs in other areas, we're seeing more diversity, more men, yet it's not clear how many will get into the school, so we have to refer them out to community colleges, which we've fought against doing for years."

The dean of the School of Nursing at the University of Virginia, Jeanette Lancaster, reports that because of funding cutbacks in the state, she lost about 10 percent of her budget for two straight years. "We had no ability to take in more students, and it stretched our ability to do the best possible job with students we had. We're at fixed enrollment right now," she reports. There have been no further cuts in the school's budget, and there have been no increases. "This year," she says, "we will take about one out of every ten applicants. But we could take many more. Last fall (2003) we had 284 applications from students coming from high school and we took 48. We know that 50 more fully met University of Virginia requirements. This year we have 310 applicants. We accepted 20 through early decision and we have 28 more spots, but again we could take more. If, between the fall of 2004 and the fall of 2009, we increase our enrollment of high school students entering BSN programs from 200 to 288, we will need $1,148,939 to support faculty and facilities. If we look at demographics in Virginia we know that by 2010 only two out of three of us will have a nurse, the others will just have to do without. Unless we do something about the supply and demand ratio."

What she needs in order to fulfill that requirement is not only more students but also more faculty and a place to put both. "What it would take for us to increase enrollment would be an addition to our building. We don't have a place to put extra students, or the faculty we'd have to hire to teach them." She says she's hoping for funding from the legislature and the university. Until she gets it, Lancaster, like many deans and faculty in nursing schools, is being asked to live on the usual mix of hope, altruism, and self-sacrifice. It's a cocktail that nursing faculty, like the nurses themselves, are swallowing with increased bitterness.

Other Countries

When I was in France in the summer of 2002, my husband and I sat in the usual crush of cars lining the Autoroute du Soleil, the major toll highway going from Paris to the South of France. Cars with license plates from all over Europe were idling in the usual August thousand-kilometer traffic jam. There was, however, something unusual going on this summer. At

336 the tollbooths, home care nurses were standing holding picket signs, begging the French government for a raise and better treatment. They, like nurses who had recently gone on strike in Poland, were among thousands of European nurses complaining about wages and working conditions which were fueling shortages of nurses throughout the European Union.

In a study published in *Health Affairs* in May/June 2001, researchers from the United States, Canada, the United Kingdom, Spain, and Germany analyzed reports from forty-three thousand nurses from more than seven hundred hospitals in those countries and documented serious complaints about eroding working conditions and quality of patient care. Nurses reported job dissatisfaction, burnout, and desire to leave nursing. The United States leads the pack: 41 percent are dissatisfied with their present jobs and 43 percent feel burnt out. In Canada, the numbers for dissatisfaction and burnout, which are two distinct categories, are 33 and 36 percent respectively; in England, 36 and 36 percent; in Scotland, 38 and 29 percent; and in Germany, 17 and 15 percent.[25]

Many nurses say their workloads have increased: in the United States 83 percent say the number of patients assigned to them has risen; in Canada it's 64 percent, and in Germany 44 percent. They report a reduction in number of nurse managers (58 percent make this report in the United States, 40 percent in Canada, 14 percent in Germany). Many also report the loss of a chief nursing officer without replacement (17 percent make this report in the United States, 25 percent in Canada, and 23 percent in Germany). An alarming number also report declining quality of care and an increase in adverse events. In all countries (again the situation in the United States is especially worrisome) only between 29 and 36 percent reported that quality of care on their unit was excellent. In Germany, a startling 11.7 percent of nurses said that their unit delivered excellent care. Nurses also reported that patients were "not infrequently" receiving the wrong medication or dose, getting hospital-acquired infections, and experiencing more falls with injuries, and that there were more complaints from patients and more verbal abuse directed at nurses. The authors conclude that "nurses feel that they are under siege and hospitals cannot find enough nurses willing to work under current conditions in in-patient settings."[26]

Canada

Nurses all over the world echo these sentiments. Canada has also experienced a decade of restructuring, often initiated by U.S. consultants and promoted by those who have long tried to privatize the Canadian health care system and introduce a more U.S.-style profit orientation. With variations in each province, Canadian nurses have experienced similar problems. According to Kathleen Connors, who was president of the National Federation of Nurses Unions in Canada until 2003, provincial governments across Canada began to lay off nurses because of debt and deficits, and to convert full-time positions to part-time and casual ones. Nurses who worked part-time would be guaranteed a predictable schedule of part-time work, while nurses who worked as "casuals" would have no guarantee of a predictable schedule. They would be called in to work as hospitals felt they were needed. Canada, like other countries, closed or consolidated hospitals, reduced the number of beds, shortened lengths of stay, and restructured the work of nurses, sometimes with the help of U.S. consultants.

"Among all Canadian provinces, Ontario was the hardest hit," explains Pat Armstrong, professor of sociology at York University, where she is a professor of sociology and women's studies and CHSRF/CIHR Chair in Health Services. In 1995, for example, the then finance minister Paul Martin (who became prime minister of Canada in 2004) cut an estimated $6 billion from the health care funding the federal government transferred to Ontario over a four-year period. The premier of Ontario, Mike Harris, then followed suit by cutting $1.3 billion from hospitals. He also cut taxes in the province, which added further financial pressure on the health care system.[27] Almost immediately, nurses began to feel the results. "Ontario cut back the number of nurses by ten thousand," Armstrong explains. "Other provinces cut less drastically and there was not quite as much damage."

Casualization, Armstrong says, made nurses' jobs precarious by reducing the number of people who have full-time, full-year jobs. This trend was reinforced by the government's encouraging the use of temporary nurses, who were rented out on a per diem, per week, or monthly basis by a growing number of temporary nurse agencies that sprang up during the 1990s. In contrast to the U.S. experience, Canadian nurses are 85 percent unionized throughout the country. Since most hospitals in Ontario were unionized, even part-time nurses had good salaries and benefits and some guarantee of schedules. Hiring temporary nurses allowed governments to avoid paying benefits and better salaries to nurses and protected them from any commitment to their working nurses. "If hospitals hire from temporary help agencies, they don't have the same kind of obligations to them. All the union contract provisions don't apply," Armstrong explains.

"I have only worked full-time in the United States, where there is plenty of full-time work in many areas of nursing," one Ontario nurse said, expressing the feelings of many. "Canada is very limiting to nurses. Casual positions are available where you can work a lot with no benefits.

338 With all the distress occurring, nurses are in conflict with other nurses, friends are competing for the same jobs, nurses are being bumped as seniority rules are in effect, and there is a lot of negativity while nurses are struggling to provide excellent, compassionate care."[28]

In an effort to cut the nursing work force, the Quebec government limited enrollment to nursing schools by 50 percent, froze wages and positions in hospitals, and closed seven hospitals in Montreal, says Ro Licata, who is president of the union of nurses at the McGill University Health Center's Royal Victorian Hospital, which is affiliated with the Fédération des infirmiers et infirmières du Quebec (FIIQ). Largely in response to those hospital closures, the government offered retirement packages to three thousand nurses, so it could avoid placing nurses from the closed hospitals into other facilities. Karen Lee, a nurse in Montreal graduated during this period and was unable to get permanent work for almost five years. In order to work at all, she had to be essentially on call, available to come in and work different shifts at a moment's notice. If she said no to a shift, she felt she risked not getting any work in the future. After this introduction to nursing, she finally got full-time work. But patient loads were so high she eventually went to work in Switzerland.

During the 1990s and into the twenty-first century, nurses across Canada protested and picketed, and some—in Saskatchewan, Quebec, Newfoundland, and Nova Scotia—went on strike. Nurses in British Columbia struggled to attain wage parity with RNs in the United States, so they could stem the tide of nurses leaving the province. Nurses consistently warned the government that its policies would produce problems for patients and a shortage of nurses. Yet Canadian policy makers and politicians, like those in the United States, did not heed those warnings. Ontario and other provinces are trying to woo back nurses who have left the work force—or the country. Indeed, Armstrong says, the Ontario government has finally realized that hiring temporary nurses is far more expensive, and money has been allocated to hire nurses for full-time, full-year positions. But, as we shall see in a moment, they have still failed to alter some of the main problems in the system.

In Quebec, the FIIC has fought for years to gain pay equity and pay comparability for nurses. According to Licata, pay equity in Switzerland and other countries addresses gender inequality by comparing nurses' work to occupations with a similar level of workload and responsibility—for example, police and firefighters. Pay comparability would compare nurses' work to that of other people in health care, like social workers. Since nurses in Quebec have lagged behind in both areas, equity and comparability, the government's recent promise to implement and even combine the two categories was hailed by nurses in the province. Unfortunately, Licata says, the government is not moving forward to implement its promise. In fact, the government has just informed nurses that if they want pay equity, they will face salary freezes. "That wasn't the idea," Licata says. "The idea was to equalize salaries not freeze them."

In other provinces, cutbacks in health care expenditures threaten nurse retention and recruitment. The Canadian Association of Schools of Nursing reports that government promises to increase funding for nursing education and thus the number of nursing school slots available to new students have not materialized.[29] Canada faces a shortage of one hundred thousand RNs by 2007, and the Canadian Nursing Advisory Council called for a 10 percent increase in the number of slots in nursing school programs in all provinces in both 2000 and 2001. Instead of increasing, the number of seats for nursing students has declined since 1997. Although clinical education costs have escalated, funding for those costs has stagnated or even been reduced. As in the United States, there is a shortage of nursing faculty in Canada.

In 2004, the government of British Columbia once again announced cutbacks in home health care, long-term care, and hospital nursing care. Debra McPherson, president of the British Columbia Nurses Union, told me that the nursing shortage in British Columbia includes both a shortage of bodies and a shortage of nursing care provided to patients. "We have the second lowest nurse-to-population ratio in Canada, and I would suspect that the amount of nursing hours per patient day that a patient can get is among the lowest, about twenty-four minutes a day, which is a paltry amount of hours."

Although McPherson says there is no decline in nursing school enrollments, there are not enough funded places in nursing schools to accommodate those who want to enter the profession. Moreover, nurses in hospitals are so busy that nursing schools are having a difficult time placing students on wards for the clinical rotations that are essential to their apprenticeship. U.S.-style privatization of nursing education in British Columbia has, according to many academics, complicated matters. The Conservative government in British Columbia has deregulated nursing education at the community college level and there are now several U.S.-based private colleges offering training to Licensed Practical Nurses. These trainees need clinical experience and supervision on the wards to finish their training. To get this needed clinical training, private colleges offer to pay cash-strapped hospitals to place LPN students on hospital wards, and financially troubled hospitals are accepting these payments. At the same time, however, they are turning away students from the public university system because the private colleges have bought all the nursing time that hospitals—with fewer nurses in them—can afford to provide.

340   The government in British Columbia insists that it doesn't have a shortage of nurses. McPherson believes that optimistic estimate is not based on a sober assessment of patient needs but on the fact that the provincial government has cut services and cut jobs. If there are no job openings, obviously from the classical labor market point of view, there is no shortage of nurses. But as we have seen, when nurses are cut in a country with an aging population and rising levels of chronic illness, patient acuity goes up and the remaining nurses suffer escalating job strain and stress. They may choose to leave their posts, which eventually produces not only a shortage of nursing care but of the nurses who can deliver it. When governments do not facilitate the appropriate education for nursing students, the future is assured: there won't be enough nurses when governments or hospitals acknowledge that demand has increased or when the public insists that legislators provide them with adequate levels of nursing care.

McPherson says she feels that the seeds of ongoing shortage have been planted and are being well fertilized. One-third of the British Columbia nursing work force is nearing retirement age. Under different circumstances, they might postpone retirement for a few years. Now, she says, they are calling the union to ask about the intricacies of their retirement plan and benefits. What can we expect to get if we leave now? they are asking.

SARS in Toronto

In 2003 health care cost cutting, combined with traditional physician disregard, created its own fatal synergy when Toronto was hard hit by the international epidemic of severe acute respiratory syndrome, what has become known as SARS. Thousands of patients and health care workers were immediately affected. When health officials made their calculations in June 2003, 6,800 people were in quarantine and 5,200 health care workers were placed on what is called "working quarantine." In other words, these health care workers were not totally segregated from the Toronto public. Instead, they were allowed to report to work in hospitals and other facilities. After work, however, they had to return home, being careful to make no contact with anyone en route. Once at home, they would voluntarily remove themselves from their families, friends, or roommates, using separate bathrooms, cooking and eating with different utensils, wearing masks, and above all else, having no physical contact at all with loved ones.

From the initial weeks of the first outbreak of SARS, nurses feared that health care cost cutting was hurting patients, jeopardizing the public, and endangering nurses. Because of the lack of full-time work and increased casualization, many nurses worked in several hospitals and moved from **341** one facility to another. Doris Grinspun, executive director of the Registered Nurses Association of Ontario (RNAO), explains that because of the fear of cross-contamination, the government issued a directive prohibiting nurses from working in more than one facility. "This aggravated the nursing shortage that some organizations were experiencing since they couldn't rely on their pool of casual or part-time nurses. It also meant that nurses who were working multiple employers could not rely on that income."

Nurses, says Barb Wahl, then president of the Ontario Nurses Union, also began to worry that hospitals were skimping on protective gear and failing to educate nurses about the need to wear gowns, gloves, and masks when they were in contact with patients suspected of having SARS. In March, Wahl recounts, several patients at the Grace Hospital were not isolated and the nurses treating them were not gloved, gowned, and masked. Nurses became ill with SARS. The Ontario Nurses Union told government officials that this hospital and its sister hospital, Scarborough General, should have been quarantined and that visitors should be restricted. The government did not issue the quarantine until a few days later. Since minutes count when trying to prevent the spread of a disease like SARS, the nurses felt the government's failure to heed their warnings put more people in jeopardy.

Minutes aren't the only things that count in containing an epidemic. Equipment also matters, particularly for bedside caregivers. But hospitals, Wahl says, did not give nurses appropriate equipment and did not alert them in a timely fashion, so they could don whatever equipment was available. To protect themselves against SARS, Grinspun explains, nurses needed to double-gown, double-glove, and use a face shield. They needed masks that had appropriate filtration material. Moreover, these masks had to be specially fitted so they formed a close, protective seal around the mouth and nose. But the province didn't provide nurses with enough masks that actually fit.

"Right from day one we were concerned that the masks were not adequate," Wahl says. Nurses insisted that hospitals were telling them to reuse their masks. The union had requested that the government initiate a serious mask-testing program. But with cutbacks in public health personnel, there weren't enough people to test the masks. "We had ten thousand nurses in Toronto, and six people to test the masks, and it takes a half an hour to fit a mask," Wahl explains.

Nor were there enough Stryker suits, high-tech gear with a large face shield, hood, and full gown that protects nurses, physicians and respiratory therapists from the respiratory droplets that are the main route of SARS transmission. These suits were particularly critical for nurses who

342   worked with patients who have to be intubated. Whenever a tube is put down a patient's throat, the patient will cough, which adds even more risk for the transmission of SARS.

"At some hospitals," Wahl adds, "there were policies that said doctors and respiratory therapists had to wear Stryker suits but not nurses." A month later at North York at a SARS unit, a patient required intubation. Nurses were not wearing these suits, and two of them contracted SARS. "Our position," Wahl stated adamantly, "is that nurses on SARS units should be wearing Strykers or equivalent gear all the time with the sickest patients." If a patient suddenly goes into respiratory arrest, it takes too long to put on this complicated gear and respond to an urgent situation. "Patients don't come up to you and tell you they're going to get into trouble in a couple of hours so you should be dressed and ready," says Wahl. But the government and hospitals balked because of the expense.

The most egregious and devastating result of cost cutting and disregard of nurses' expertise occurred, however, in late May, when nurses at North York Hospital told their managers, physicians, and administrators that they suspected a patient had SARS. While the doctors they worked with didn't dismiss their concerns, the heads of infection control and of the SARS committee—neither of whom had any relationship with these nurses and apparently distrusted the warnings of people who were "just nurses"—did so. Unfortunately, it turned out that the nurses were right, and Toronto experienced a second outbreak after the first one had abated.

"It's the old tradition that nurses get respected for clinical knowledge only after they have developed a trusting and knowledge relationship with the physician partner," explains Grinspun. "They are not respected by all physicians who understand that nurses have the education and training and know their patients." Because of this debacle, the RNAO has called for a full public inquiry, and both the Ontario Nurses Association and the RNAO have called for whistle-blower legislation to protect nurses who report unsafe practices. Because of the hue and cry raised by nurses and their organizations, the government was forced to institute a full independent inquiry known as the Justice Campbell Commission. Nurses testifying at this inquiry will have full protection from employer retaliation.

The United Kingdom

In the United Kingdom, lack of time, lack of money, and lack of respect are all fueling a serious nursing shortage. Throughout the late 1980s and 1990s, the British National Health Service faced a great deal of restructuring. In her testimony at the Bristol Inquiry, Patricia Dorothy Fields and other nurses described the chaos that they experienced as a result. "The structure became very fragmented. Everyone had their own budg-

ets, all the way through the structure. . . . Units no longer worked together as closely and cooperatively as they had before, always being concerned about the implications for their own budgets, which were jealously
guarded."[30]

The Royal College of Nursing reports that "although progress in
bringing new nurses into the NHS [National Health Service] is welcome,
retention of staff has become the critical issue facing the NHS. An ageing
nursing work force means almost a quarter of registered nurses (24 percent) will be eligible to retire in the next five years." The RCN also warns
that despite more nurses entering the profession, nursing shortages continue. The "demand for nurses in the NHS is projected to rise, yet the
number of registered nurses is diminishing. . . . The UK nursing population—the overall population of registered nurses—is declining. Between
1990 and 2000, 170,000 nurses left the register, with over 21,000 going in
1999/2000 alone. . . . In the NHS in England, there were nearly 9,200
whole time equivalent (wte) long term vacancies at 31 March 2001. The
number of these 'hard to fill' posts has reduced slightly from the previous
year, but remains higher than in 1999."[31] By the year 2008, the Department of Health says it will need 35,000 more nurses in England alone.[32]

Tom Keighley, former editor of *Nursing Management* in the United
Kingdom, contends that these shortages are due to a combination of demographic changes and the failure to provide decent wages and working
conditions for RNs. "Since the 1970s and 1980s there just aren't enough
people born to fill the exploding number of jobs in the health care sector,"
Keighley says. "With increased sophistication of health care delivery,
nurses need to have a serious educational background to do their work.
But a nurse leaving university to take an entry-level job will make £17,500,
while someone going into the law or accounting will get a starting salary
of £21,000 or £22,000."

Add to this the erosion of working conditions, and the picture is hardly
reassuring. Nurses in hospitals in the United Kingdom now take care of
anywhere from six to twelve patients. Since the average length of stay in
the United Kingdom is down to 4.1 days, these patients, like those in the
United States, are acutely ill when they are in the hospital. Working conditions seem to have pushed nurses out of the work force in the United
Kingdom just as they have in the United States. There are currently
110,000 qualified RNs who don't work in nursing, out of a work force of
650,000. Anecdotal evidence suggests that many nurses are leaving the
profession to work in another job. After a period away from nursing, they
may or may not return.

The current Labour government has tried to address the nursing
shortage by raising salaries and increasing the number of places in nursing
schools, but these initiatives, while well intentioned, may not be effective.

344   Raises are not given across the board, based on level of education or experience. Instead, to qualify for raises, nurses are asked to go through a complex process in which they submit forms that describe the content and nature of their roles. A senior team of nurses and managers then reviews these applications. If the managers approve the application, nurses are given a raise. But, says Keighley, many nurses feel the raises aren't commensurate either with their education or their experience and are excessively difficult to obtain.

As in the United States, increasing the number of nursing students—while a fine idea—may also be stymied by staffing shortages and the aging of the nursing faculty work force. Nursing faculty in the United Kingdom are getting older, but more worrisome, says Keighley, is the fact that there simply aren't enough working nurses on the floor to educate students and mentor new graduates. "So," Keighley concludes, "while the UK government has increased the number of students it has put in schools of nursing, it's not possible to give them a sufficiently wide range of clinical experience."

The combination of inexperienced nurses, overworked veteran nurses, and an emphasis on throughput and doing just the minimum to make sure patients survive, has also affected the care of patients in the United Kingdom. Like many nurses, Keighley has experienced the results of these problems personally as well as professionally. His eighty-year-old mother with advancing dementia has had several recent hospitalizations, and he has observed the nursing care she has received with distress. "My mother was recently sent to the emergency ward, where she waited for seventy-four hours, rather than what should have been eight," Keighley told me. "The nurses went about their jobs exactly as the procedures dictated. If my mother was in bed, she got her tablets and her meals. If she wasn't, she didn't. The unit just didn't have enough staff to properly supervise and monitor her whereabouts, so she wandered around the unit."

Australia

Australian nurses have experienced similar problems. As they became more militant and better organized in the 1970s and 1980s, they won a number of important gains, such as improved salaries and benefits and political recognition. Mary Chiarella, former chief nurse in New South Wales, explains that in the early 1990s, as Australian federal and state governments began to worry about containing costs and increasing productivity in their national health system, "the need for 'productivity savings' became the call. Nurses and other health care professionals were asked to do 'more with less,' 'work smarter, not harder,' and comply with other

similar euphemisms." Australian government leaders began to adopt the
same economic rationalism as their business and political counterparts in
the United States and Canada and were intrigued by the development of
diagnostic related groups in the American Medicare and private insurance
system.[33]

Hospitals began to develop spending cut targets. To cite only one example, in 1991–92 one New South Wales hospital was told it had to cut $7
million (Australian), with $3.5 million coming from cuts in nursing jobs.
"By 1994, the 'productivity savings' had been so effective," Chiarella
writes, "that there was a declared shortage of specialist nurses." Without
job prospects, nurses were looking for work outside the hospital, and even
in other fields. Over six years, the New South Wales nursing work force
lost one thousand positions.[34]

Nurse managers and directors of nursing (DONs) also lost line authority and control over the nursing budget. "Bed usage drives costs, but it is
not controlled by nurses," one NSW report stated bluntly. "Because
nurses are kept right out of budgeting (especially in private hospitals) they
cannot even see what income they are generating."[35]

The same kinds of cuts were going on throughout Australia. The result
was enormous disaffection and even despair among working nurses.
Chiarella quotes one nurse in Western Australia:

"I stand by the bedside of a patient with cancer, who I know wants my
time; she wants to talk to me about her fears and her feelings. She wants
to ask me questions, what can I do?

"I have someone to pick up from theatre (the operating room), someone else in pain; I have the 'obs' (observations) to do, the 'meds' (medications) to do. I am already behind because someone is vomiting. I have to
go; maybe if I 'skimp' on other patients' care I can get back to talk to her
and the moment will not have passed.

"I don't get back to her. Someone's chemotherapy leaks onto them and
the bed, that takes a lot of time. A few days later she dies. I go to bed that
night (I was late off duty as usual) and now I can't sleep. I hope someone
had time to listen to her, because I failed her. . .

"These things go on day after day, week after week. I feel ashamed and
guilty, maybe it's me. I'm not up to this, I can't cope, but I look around,
very few people are doing any better. I move from that ward because it
tears the heart and soul out of me."[36]

In Victoria, a conservative government was elected in 1992 and cut
funding to the health care sector, eliminating three thousand nursing positions. The government offered these nurses huge buyouts—so-called
redundancy pay. Belinda Morieson, secretary of the Victoria branch of
the Australian Nursing Federation between 1989 and 2002, explained that

346   nurses took advantage of the offer because they could get the buyout and then leave the public sector to work in private-sector hospitals. Because of the strain of their workload, other nurses also began leaving hospitals, leaving nursing, or working part-time. "A lot of nurses who stayed in hospitals deliberately moved from full-time to part-time work because they couldn't cope with the strain of working full-time. So some began to work four days a week rather than five. Because hospitals were having trouble getting nurses to work for them, temporary agencies stepped in to fill the gap. But this simply exacerbated the shortage. . . . Agencies were paying their nurses three times the amount of money permanent staff were getting," Morieson explains. "So more and more nurses left permanent work in the hospital and went and worked agency."

Philip Della, the chief nurse of the state of Western Australia, explains that the culture of nursing management changed because of restructuring. "Instead of rewarding permanent nurses to fill in schedule deficits, nurse managers were going to agency nurses and offering these nurses their schedules six weeks in advance. The agency nurse received a greater hourly rate than permanent members, and they could pick their shifts and their hospitals, their ward location. That caused a movement out of the hospital from the permanent staff to agency staff. The permanent staff saw that the agency nurse was getting flexibility, shifts they wanted to work, and also more pay. So they left permanent work for agency work." Costs of agency nurses rose from $30 million to $55 million a year.

According to a report by the University of Sydney, 60 percent of "Acute Ward nurses reported that inadequate nurse-patient ratios were the single biggest source of clinical workload problems and the greatest source of stress."[37] Of those surveyed, 87.5 percent of nurses reported that the use of agency nurses in Victoria was a concern. Because some temporary nurses were "unfamiliar with the working environment," this increased their workload.[38] Although the nurses' union, which is strong in public-sector acute care hospitals, was able to block use of unlicensed personnel as RN replacements, nurses were replaced by assistants with minimal training throughout the aged care sector. These cuts to the nursing work force, when combined with the fact that nurses caring for the elderly may receive up to 20 percent less than nurses in the acute sector, created a major shortage of RNs in aged care in Victoria. Because of funding cuts and poor pay, Australia has suffered a particularly severe crisis in the care of the elderly. Throughout the 1990s, nurses abandoned work with the elderly because they could earn more working in the public sector. These disparities in funding meant that nurses in aged care were run even more ragged than their colleagues in acute care hospitals.[39]

Nurses say that patients in Australia have begun to suffer from nursing **347** understaffing just as they have in the United States. Anne Marie Scully, a Victoria nurse who worked for the Department of Health and Human Services as well as the Victoria branch of the Australian Nursing Federation, has done research on the fifty-five deaths that triggered coroners' inquiries in Victoria between 1990 and 2000. Scully found that a number of these deaths were produced by a complex constellation of factors that included changes in nurses' working life.

"Management and organizations failed to provide appropriate numbers of nurses to deliver safe nursing care," she told me. Nurses, she said, didn't have enough information and education to do their job, particularly when it concerned new medical equipment, medications, or treatments. In one case, physical restraints were placed on a patient, but neither nurses nor doctors were taught the basics of safe use, and the patient died.

Cuts in staffing and scarcity of time, Scully said, led nurses to cut corners when caring for patients. When I asked her to elaborate on the issue of time, she reflected for a moment. "How do you describe time? Time comes from having the extra hands at the bedside. It's time to read the notes of the previous shift. Time to listen to what the nurses from the previous shift are telling you. It's time for the less experienced nurses to come up to a more experienced nurse and say, 'This is what I've got; how do I deal with it?' Or to find out what the norm is when you're caring for particular patients. This time to teach also allows the experienced nurse to see what's happening on the unit."

Finally, said Scully, "it's time to spend with the patient. It's time to stand at the end of the bed and say, 'My name is Anne Marie Scully and I'm the registered nurse who's looking after you this shift.' It's time to find out exactly how the patient feels before you move on. This is critical because when you're taking that time, you're assessing how they cope with their illness. They tell you all sorts of things in that five minutes."

The problem is, Scully says, nurses no longer have those five minutes.

Norway

In Norway, to cite one more example, nurses for decades were proud of the fact that every Norwegian hospital was run by an administrative team made up of a chief nurse and chief physician. At the Rikshospitalet in Oslo, for example, Inger Margrethe Holter was the chief nurse alongside a chief physician. At least she was until August 2003. In 2001 the Norwegian government began to introduce market mechanisms into the health care system and divided the country into five health regions. The dual

348 hospital leadership by a chief nurse and a chief physician was ended. Now in most hospitals there is only one hospital leader, usually a physician. Under this administrator, and reporting to him, is the director of daily operations, a Norwegian version of the head of patient care services. Sometimes this job is filled by a nurse but often it is not. The position of nursing director at the department level—in pediatrics, cardiology, general medicine, and orthopedics—was also cut. The only specifically nursing management position remaining is the unit nurse manager.

In early 2000 Holter gave me a guided tour of the newly rebuilt Rikshospitalet, the biggest and most important public hospital in Norway. Holter had given nursing input throughout its design and construction, and she and her nurses were pleased with the result. The building was a magnificent architectural achievement, filled with original sculptures and paintings, linoleum mosaics decorating the floors of unit corridors, and clean, elegant Scandinavian furnishings. Only two years after the hospital was opened, the content of Holter's chief nurse position was changed and she was sidelined and given less significant assignments. Her authority over nursing and patient care was thus significantly reduced. Most of her staff support was removed. Because she felt that her situation had become impossible, she left her job in August 2003.

Holter feels that nursing management has lost much of its power in Norway. What is worse, she says, nurses on the wards are dealing with the same difficulties as their counterparts in the United States. "We were able to maintain much of the great staff development we built at the Rikshospitalet, but that has not been true in other hospitals," she says. She worries that the programs in the major hospital are in jeopardy. "It is taken away little by little. First they cut one nurse, then another. And who can say what the end result will be if no one is responsible for nursing at the top level of the institution?"

Although these cuts are new and their impact on patients has not yet been analyzed, Holter fears that patients will suffer the same problems that are being documented in other countries. Like an epidemic of an infectious illness, Holter says that restructuring, cost cutting, and dismantling of nursing are spreading through Europe. "There is no longer a chief nurse at the biggest hospital in Sweden," Holter says. "Pretty soon nursing management as a force will be gone in most hospitals around the world."

The World Health Organization

The power of nursing has diminished not only in hospitals in a variety of countries but also within governmental health departments, ministries of health, and even in international organizations like the World Health Or- **349** ganization. Nurses have lost chief nurse positions in some ministries of health, says Mireille Kingma, who works on nursing and health policy at the International Council of Nurses (ICN). Chief nurses were eliminated most recently in Costa Rica and El Salvador. There was an attempt to do away with the position in Nicaragua but the effort failed, only because legislation establishing the Ministry of Health mandated that such a position exist. It wasn't eliminated, says Kingma, because the government didn't want to undergo the arduous process of changing the legislation.

Within the World Health Organization nursing has been losing ground over the past ten years. According to a statement Kingma prepared for the ICN on nursing in the WHO, "Nursing is considered an essential service and should therefore be mainstreamed and included in policy-making throughout the WHO structure. . . . [Yet], the overall number of filled WHO nursing/midwifery posts had decreased 43 percent since the 1992 nursing/midwifery resolution. In 1992 the secretariat reported that nurses represented approximately 3.2 percent of the professional positions throughout WHO. In 1996, the percentage had fallen to 1.6."[40]

The justification that the WHO gave to nurses who complained about this move was that in its restructuring, it wanted to move away from a "corporatist" approach to health issues and planning to a more interdisciplinary one. If each discipline continued to have its chief and worked in its own silo, the new management theory held, disciplines would look out for themselves and their own profession or occupation, rather than dealing with critical issues holistically. So the organization had developed a matrix system in which people would participate in what are known as crosscutting projects. For example, an HIV-focused campaign about safe injections would include members of the human resources, infection control, and accident and injury prevention sections, and this would supposedly provide a way for nurses to give their input into health initiatives and decisions.

While this theory may make sense in the abstract, it often hurts marginalized groups like nursing. Unlike physicians who are represented on every level within the WHO, nurses have had only limited representation. There simply aren't enough nurses, Kingma explains, to participate on those overlapping teams. This means that nurses are disempowered by the matrix, while physicians maintain their dominance within the organization, even as they ostensibly dismantle their individual silos and work in interdisciplinary teams.

In 2001 Kingma prepared a statement about the ongoing problem. WHO statistics continued to show the underrepresentation of nursing—

350   "only 2.9 percent of the category 'Dental, nutrition, medical, nursing and veterinary specialists' are nurses—and this includes regional and national as well as headquarters staff. When considering *all* professional staff, this percentage is reduced to 1.2 percent—in complete dissonance with the needs and realities of health systems worldwide." The organization also said that, considering health needs and their cost-effectiveness, it believed nursing and midwifery services were not amply utilized within the WHO.

Kingma's comments concluded with a sobering assessment: "There have been calls to strengthen nursing and midwifery from the 42nd, 45th, 47th, 48th and 49th Assemblies. This year there is once again a resolution that recognizes the importance of nursing as an essential service for health promotion as well as health care delivery. The resolution urges Member States to increase the participation of nurses and midwives in policy-making positions and ensure the involvement of nursing experts in the integrated planning of human resources for health. Yet, nurses worldwide must face the fact that these recommendations are not being applied within WHO. This double message harms efforts to address the acknowledged global critical shortage of nurses."[41]

The issue of nursing representation in the WHO is indeed significant, not just because nurses are the largest profession in health care worldwide, but because nursing is also a predominantly female profession. Its absence in the highest policy-making councils suggests not only that health policy making will be influenced primarily by physicians—who present only part of the health care picture—but that women's voices will also be underrepresented in global policy making. "They are constantly whittling away at the visibility of any nursing position at the policy-making level of the WHO. And that means that women's voices are not being heard," Kingma says.

The problems nurses are experiencing in these different settings sets the stage for local, regional, national, and international quests, in which nurses move from hospital to hospital, from state to state or province to province, and from country to country looking for a workplace in which pay is decent and working conditions are at least tolerable. The problem is that nonnegotiable conditions for a stable work force seem nowhere to be found.

13

Management by Churn

hen Philip Wilson took his first job in a hospital after graduating
from a four-year nursing program in 2001, it didn't take him more
than a few days to understand what it would be like to be a registered nurse at the turn of the twenty-first century. As a junior
nurse, he had to work a lot of night shifts and holidays. The pay wasn't
great. More distressing was the patient acuity—pretty much off the
charts—and the understaffing. As a new nurse, he'd find himself on a busy
neurology floor with as many as twenty-eight patients having seizures and
just one other nurse. Some nurses had called in sick. No one could be sent
over from another unit. The float nurses were drowning not floating. He
was in way over his head way too often. He'd already left a career in
teaching to go into nursing. He'd invested too much in his education to
switch careers again. He wanted to stay in nursing but not on these terms.
A couple of his friends were doing travel nursing so he looked into the option and decided to try it.

So after a year in the hospital, Wilson stopped working as a permanent
staff nurse and, at the age of thirty-two, joined the expanding corps of
traveling nurses, who move from hospital to hospital or work on a semi-
permanent basis for hospitals after contracting with what are known as
travel nurse agencies. These nurses sign on with companies like InteliStaf
Healthcare Travel and Cross Country TravCorps, to name only two of
the many agencies, and work on thirteen-week contracts with hospitals
across North America and around the world. The enticements are almost
irresistible. Wilson, who works in a major Boston teaching hospital,
makes a couple of more dollars per hour than the permanent RNs on his

352 neurology floor. He works three twelve-hour shifts. And he names his conditions. Day shifts. No weekends. He'll sometimes agree to come in and work extra, but he says no to nights. He can leave a hospital if he finds that the conditions are not to his liking. The travel nurse agency, he says, owes the hospital a body for thirteen weeks, but if he opts out, it doesn't have to be his body. He can take that and work elsewhere.

The travel agency gives him health care benefits and a 401K retirement plan. As a permanent employee, he might have a better pension plan and medical benefits. But nurses in the United States have read the headlines. Many companies agree to provide workers with good pension plans and retiree health benefits. Then, decades later, when the company is sold or is hungry for more profit, it reneges on those commitments after the worker actually retires. If you can't bank on the future, some American nurses feel, at least you can make some short term gains.

As a travel nurse, Wilson says, he can avoid getting involved in hospital politics—no committee meetings or discussions about how to improve care, unless he wants them. He can check out a place. If it's really awful. If, for example, he thinks his license is on the line because of unsafe conditions, he can leave and the agency will furnish the hospital with another RN. If he just finds the usual dose of stress—too few nurses, too many too sick patients, not enough support—he can grin and bear it. "By the time you figure out you don't like the place, you probably have only six more weeks to go. That's eighteen three-hour shifts, or eighteen days." If he likes it, he can sign on for an extra thirteen-week stint. In fact, given the nursing shortage, hospitals no longer limit travelers to a year's work in their institution. He's worked at his hospital for going on two years now and, if the nursing shortage continues, he thinks he could probably work there longer.

But the best thing about the job is you get either free housing or a living allowance. If he decides to take a job in another city, he gets high-quality accommodations for nothing. But you don't even have to travel to be a traveling nurse. Subsidized by his employer, and indirectly by the hospital he works for, Philip Wilson has spent the last two years in his own apartment in Boston. In Boston, he tells me, travel nurses can get between $1,500 and $1,700 a month for their living allowance. A couple he knows who work in town get $3,000 between them. Do the math, he suggests. If your apartment costs $2,500, well, you can't beat that. True, he doesn't get paid for sick days and personal days and doesn't get any vacation. That doesn't worry him in the least. Each year he works for the company, he gets a bonus—maybe $1,000 a year. That can go to sick pay. And if he wants to take a week or two off between contracts to take a vacation, that's hardly much of a loss. Particularly when you consider what he doesn't have to put up with on the floors. Needless to say, hospitals are paying enormous sums to hire travel nurses, since the hospital is paying the agency enough money to offer this level of benefit and salaries. Plus, the hospital is also paying the agency enough to make this a profitable business.

Wilson occasionally works for a temporary nursing agency when he isn't doing his "travel" work. There he makes $36 an hour. Some agency nurses make up to $50 an hour. Most permanent new staff nurses in Boston make between $21 and $26 an hour. Sure, the agency can call and cancel a shift if the hospital doesn't need him at the last moment. But given the nursing shortage, that doesn't happen all that much. So here he is, after just three years out of nursing school, working only the shifts he wants and making as much as—or more than—a nurse with fifteen years of experience. He tells me that it would take a lot to convince him to work as a permanent staff nurse at a hospital. He'd be giving up $20,000 to $25,000 a year, and for what? To take care of too many patients with too few resources. This way, when he gets bored, he just travels on. Maybe he won't like the next place as much as he likes this one. That's no big deal, he says, "You can take anything for thirteen weeks."

Philip Wilson is part of a small army of what are known as contingent nurses. The working conditions that have exacerbated nursing's long-standing problems are increasing their numbers. Those conditions are also leading to increased reliance on immigrant nurses, many of them from developing countries. And then there's another, less well publicized—and certainly less studied—kind of "migrant" worker in nursing. That's the nurse who gets fed up with the bedside and decides to migrate to a nursing job with more status and better conditions and pay. These transitory nurses will temporarily ease the shortage of nursing bodies at the bedside. Depending on their status within the institution, their personal commitments or fears and anxieties, they may also inadvertently exacerbate the very conditions that produced the need for their services.

Travelers and Temps

In the late twentieth century, both agency nursing and travel nursing have appealed to a small group of nurses seeking adventure or constant change. Because recent cost cutting has eroded working conditions, many nurses who would never have thought of working for travel or temporary agencies now tell their unions and organizations that their hospitals are filling up with agency and traveling nurses, and some of them are becoming contingent nurses themselves.

The growing use of contingent nurses is part of a broader corporate

354   trend to use temporary employees who may be churned over—that is, turned over—rapidly as they move in and out of a particular workplace and on to the next.

Many traveling and agency nurses, says Sean P. Clarke, a nursing work force researcher at the University of Pennsylvania School of Nursing, used to be thought of as the bottom of the barrel—people who couldn't get along with their colleagues, who had a "past," who didn't quite have what it takes. Although that may have been an unfair representation of temporary and travel nurses, the image is now changing. Now the administrators he talks with, Clarke says, are often very pleased with their traveler and agency nurses.

Stories about the increased use of contingent nurses are borne out by the data. Although only 2 percent of nurses "working in their principal nursing position" worked as temporary workers in 2000, this was a 36 percent increase over figures documented in 1996, and was a departure from declines in the use of temporary nurses that occurred between 1988 and 1996—that is, between the last nursing shortage, when conditions began to improve for RNs, and the beginning of the current shortage. Moreover, 71,490 nurses said they worked with temporary agencies in 2000 to supplement their permanent jobs. "Taken together, the total number of nurses employed through a temporary employment service was 110,994— a 65.6 percent increase over 1996 and considerably higher than 1988 and 1992 estimates," the Institute of Medicine reports.[1] A 1997 study of 736 hospital-based nurses found that RNs were much more likely to leave their jobs if they saw little opportunity for promotion, had to do highly routinized work, had little ability to make decisions, and felt there was poor communication in their workplace. Nurses who were most likely to leave were those who'd been there for the shortest periods of time, "expressed an intent to leave," or didn't have "enough time to do the job well."[2]

Just as hospital and health care restructuring has been transplanted to health care from other sectors of the economy, so too the use of contingent nurses is part of the much larger trend toward the use of part-time and temporary workers. As early as 1988, workplace researchers were recording an increase in the use of contingent workers. Lonnie Golden and Eileen Appelbaum noted a $2\frac{1}{2}$ fold increase in temporary help in the U.S. economy between 1982 and 1988.[3] These authors argued that temporary workers were part of a move to cut labor costs, diminish the bargaining power of labor unions, and hire an increasingly overworked "core" of permanent employees. One sees this kind of temporary outsourcing in every area of the new global economy. High-status attorneys as well as low-status secretaries and clerical workers were the subject of Jackie Krasas Rogers's book *Temps: The Many Faces of the Changing Workplace.*[4]

Some of the workers whom Rogers studied did scut work, some didn't. Some of them were poorly paid, some weren't. As we've seen in the war in Iraq, even the military is using contingent workers—civilian soldiers to fight and employees of outside companies to gather intelligence.

Although temporary workers are costly to employ, they are irresistible to managers, whether in the military, the law firm, the corporation that needs a quick clerical fix, or the hospital. Temps offer something no permanent worker can promise: relief from the cumbersome obligations an employer incurs when he takes on a permanent worker. In a global economy where flexibility and curtailing obligations to one's workers is the name of the game, this is a huge plus.

Some health care managers these days, says Sean Clarke, are obsessed with flexibility. "All some of them talk about is the ability to change units and beds and rooms from one purpose to another. The upside of temporary workers for the hospital is that they allow managers to be flexible. They can bring in people when they want. They can bring them in for two weeks, four weeks, six weeks. You don't have the inflexibility of bringing someone in full time and being obligated to them potentially for years on end. The reason hospitals are using so much temporary assistance is because on one level it works for them."

Yes, employers have probably read the studies documenting the obvious—"that," as Clarke explains it, "nurses only get good at their jobs when they're doing the same thing and are allowed to develop in a role for months and years. That's when you get the real proficiency." The problem, says Clarke, is that too many people are looking for "the quick hit." But can proficiency and expertise compete against flexibility? Not unless nurses and patients make flexibility too expensive. Here, of course, the question is, too expensive *to whom*? While it's beyond the scope of this book to consider the economic rationality of many corporate practices today, it's clear that they have not been working in health care. In spite of all the talk of efficiency and cost saving, which we certainly need more of (so long as savings are recycled into effective and compassionate care), health care costs are mounting. The United States spends more per capita on health care than any other industrialized country. In 2004, that's about $6,000 per person, yet its health outcomes—such as the number of uninsured, and infant mortality rates—are very poor.[5] Similarly, many have argued that even in other industries where restructuring has created a flexible, temporary work force, promised savings have not materialized.[6]

Like a handsome young man fleeing from a "committed relationship," today's hospital administrators seem to be fearful of commitment when it comes to their employees. If employers won't make the long-term investment required to improve the workplace, nurses will control what they

356 can—their working hours and salary. "In a free economy, people can move with their feet," says Alan Sager. "This isn't like the emperor Diocletian in the late Roman empire chaining people to their ploughs, where if your father was a farmer, you're a farmer. In a free economy people move when working conditions aren't offset by higher pay." For better or worse, staffing companies are successfully appealing to the material interests that nurses have hidden under their angel's wings.

When appealing to nurses, travel agencies hit all the high spots. InteliStaf Healthcare Travel, with its seventy offices in fifty-five major markets,[7] offers nurses "a higher rate of pay than most full-time staff positions, cash bonuses on every assignment, travel reimbursement, free private housing or housing subsidy, and an array of other benefits including health, dental and life insurance or a cash bonus and recruit a friend bonuses." We're not going to put you up in a shack, InteliStaf assures. The agency promises nurses "generously furnished apartment homes located in safe neighborhoods and convenient to the facilities where they work. Our experienced and professional housing staff work diligently to ensure your new home is customized to fit your needs and to make you comfortable. . . . Unlike many of our competitors, we offer private housing as a first option. That way you don't have to deal with the 'unknown' of sharing your living quarters with someone you have never met. We take care of the details, so all you have to do is unpack and begin exploring and enjoying the sights and sounds of your new community."

A recent article in *U.S. News and World Report* featuring InteliStaf said the agency pays contract nurses between $23 and $35 an hour, or $43,000 to $66,000 a year depending on skill level and benefits package. In San Francisco, a nurse right out of college can earn $75,000 a year as a contract nurse. A contract nurse must have one year of experience and two references from an employer.[8]

Cross Country TravCorps, another large agency, regales nurses with offers of shift differentials and bonuses for the completion of every assignment. Nurses can look forward to cash bonuses of up to $5,000, free housing or generous housing allowances, travel reimbursement, emergency twenty-four-hour on-call support, and dental and medical coverage. To sweeten the appeal further, annual bonuses may be applied tax-free to education, BSN and MSN programs, and licensure reimbursement.[9]

Nurses in temporary agencies also earn much more than staff nurses at the hospital in which they work. Like Philip Wilson, they can earn $15 or $20 an hour more than staff nurses. While they may lose out on benefits, they can choose their hours. A nurse who had worked at a Catholic Health Care West hospital in Sacramento told me that CHW pays agency nurses between $32 and $35 an hour, while a nurse who's worked for the hospital for sixteen years "maxes out" at $27.82. Some nurses, he says, have quit their jobs at CHW (a increasingly common practice) and then later come back to the hospital to work on a shift-by-shift temporary basis at salaries higher than colleagues who have worked there for years. "Can you imagine how many nurses would come back to work for the system permanently, if they made that kind of money," he said, barely able to contain his ire.

Meredith Jenkins* gave me a pretty distressing picture of the neurology floor in her Boston teaching hospital, where she works as a clinical nurse specialist with Philip Wilson. Many travel nurses are employed on the service. During one period, Wilson himself estimates that there were nine travelers among the approximately fifty nurses who staff the unit. Jenkins said it didn't take some nurses much time to figure out that traveling was a better deal than working in the hospital. While some travel nurses decided they liked working at the hospital and stayed on after their contracts expired, some decided to quit and become travelers.

"This is a real Catch-22 for nurses and for the unions who represent them," says Diane Sosne, president of the Service Employees International Union district 1199NW in Seattle and cochair of the SEIU Nurse Alliance. "It can be demoralizing for nurses to work side by side with someone who is making more money than they are, who has less commitment to the institution, and who may be making more mistakes. At the same time, if you have to work short, or the hospital asks you to do overtime, or you can't get a vacation request, that's upsetting to people too."

The agency/travel nurse phenomenon certainly offers nurses a way out of the dilemmas of working permanently for a flexible and, therefore, often unpredictable hospital. But it raises as many problems as it solves, the most critical of which is patient safety. Travelers and agency nurses may be smart, ambitious, infinitely elastic, well intentioned, and highly qualified. But how many times do administrators have to hear it? Expertise is not just something you pack up in your bag, or your brain, and unpack in a new setting. It's context dependent, says nursing researcher Patricia Benner, an expert on expertise. "Hospitals are very complex. To navigate your way around in them you need not only general but local and specific knowledge." If we remember James C. Scott's description of the role of the harbor pilot (in the introduction), that helps here. The pilot knows the context-dependent local conditions of a particular port, which is why the captain depends on the pilot to get his ship to harbor.

"Hospitals are so complex, the array of pharmaceutical delivery devices, IV lines, equipment is so varied, and then you have all the local specific knowledge of specific styles of practice, and you have travelers or

358 agency nurses, to whom the institution can't afford to give much orientation to the local setting. It's just created accidents waiting to happen because there are so many gaps in knowledge that people don't even know they have. There are so many expectations they come with from a former institution that can lead them down the wrong path. They're rendered incompetent by that local knowledge in the way care is delivered in practice." And will the traveler or temporary nurse know what she doesn't know?

I ask Benner for an example. She tells me she was just observing a nurse in an ICU who was, in fact, a traveler. "She was trying to deal with a new IV delivery system and she was very confused about how to deliver medication in the system. It was purely a design and mechanical problem. But she'd never encountered this style of equipment before." Or consider, Benner suggests, the way surgical patients are treated after they get out of the OR. That too varies from hospital to hospital. "One institution may do a lot of invasive electrical monitoring of cardiac output, and so the nurse comes to rely on the machines to provide her with a lot of information. She needs to know how to read those machines. Then she goes to another hospital where less invasive means of monitoring are used. In this facility, nurses get very skilled at checking peripheral vital signs: they stay on top of shifts in fluids, blood pressure trends, and urinary output. It changes the focus on the meaning of the vital signs if you have a different array of vital signs."

Then there's the people problem. When you come into an institution, you don't know whom you're working with. You don't know who's the less experienced attending physician and who's the more experienced one. You don't know which physician will be helpful and how to deal with a physician who might be curt and dismissive. You don't know when to call the intensivist (the doctor who works the intensive care unit) in on a consult. It's called working the system, and the new folks on the block won't know how to work it because each system is different. "Even getting lab work done in a timely way varies from institution to institution," Benner adds. If you look at all the system savvy someone amasses when they work somewhere overtime, how can someone who parachutes in, even for thirteen weeks, figure it all out so the patient gets what he needs?

As a the first step on the road to system savvy, a nurse would have to get a very thorough orientation indeed. But what kind of orientation or training do travel or agency nurses get?

Philip Wilson, almost fresh out of nursing school, got two days orientation at a very prestigious high-tech hospital. Had he been a new nurse taking a permanent position in this particular hospital, he would have had six weeks of orientation. He would have been given a much lighter patient assignment and been accompanied by a more experienced nurse who also had—it is hoped—a lighter patient load, so that she could introduce him to the unit, its patients and particularities. So here's the question. Why was Wilson, the traveler who was also a fairly new nurse, considered safe to practice after only two days of orientation when Wilson, had he been hired as a permanent employee, would have been considered unsafe at the same educational speed and then been given six weeks of orientation?

"The traveling nurses get a one-day orientation to the hospital—things like fire safety and so forth," says Meredith Jenkins, who is, in fact, assigned the job of educating these travelers. "And then they have one or two days with a nurse and then they're expected to function with a full assignment. They could be working nights with no one but a bunch of new grads, and they don't know how to work a mechanical ventilator. We have patients who are on special epilepsy monitoring units where we make them seize, so we can tape their brain activity. These nurses are expected to function at a very high level in a very short time. And it's my job to train them and my challenge to pull them away and give them specialized training in a very short time." In twenty-four to forty-eight hours, by the way.

"Yes, these nurses," Jenkins said, "are good and smart, but can anyone get up to speed in this kind of high-tech environment in two days?" What about traveling nurses who work in hospitals where there are no clinical specialists to give them a quick tour, or where travelers work with more new grads than experienced RNs?

We've seen that many hospitals have been skimping on their orientation of new staff. Most hospitals do give staff some orientation, and there certainly needs to be action taken to make sure there is a standard period of orientation for new nurses in hospitals (with adjustments made for what "new" means—whether freshly graduated, new to the hospital, or new to the unit). But patients can't afford a dubious double standard in which a temporary or traveling nurse is deemed to be safe with a cut-rate orientation while a new hire has a longer orientation.

Wilson and his employers, however, argue that this double standard is what makes travelers cost-effective even though they cost millions of dollars more. (In Western Australia, the use of agency nurses cost public hospitals $20 million extra a year at the turn of the century). "If they had to hire a new nurse they'd have to orient her for six weeks," Wilson says. "So for six weeks they're paying a more experienced nurse to train a new nurse. So pretty much they're paying for two nurses for six weeks. Then there's no guarantee that after six weeks of orientation the permanent hire will stay. While I've been there, six nurses left after four weeks of orientation. With the traveling agency, the hospital is guaranteed a body for thir-

360 teen weeks. It might not be this body. They'll bring someone else in at a flat rate of pay. If you have a traveler you just bring them on, give them two days of orientation, and then they're on their own." That's precisely the point. They're on their own, but are they safe?

Travel nurses may get a couple of days of orientation. Temporary nurses may get none at all. When Philip Wilson calls up the temp agency he occasionally works for, he tells them what shifts he'd like to pick up and where he would like to work. The agency then calls him and sends him over to a hospital. With not a second of orientation, he will work on a medical surgical unit, an orthopedic unit, or maybe a cardiac unit. This, in spite of the fact that he usually works on a neuro unit. The only place they won't send you, he explained, is someplace where you need special knowledge, like a cardiac telemetry unit.

Philip Wilson is a very appealing fellow. He's spunky and is probably a very good nurse and a pleasure to have around. Again, this issue is not whether temp and travel nurses should exist, but how they are used and how often. Are there agencies with better and worse training programs for temps and travelers? Are there hospitals that use temps and travelers well or badly? Are there ways of structuring nursing staffs that make it easier to apportion care among permanent nurses and temp and traveling nurses? Are there units that are more or less appropriate for staffing by travelers and temps? Is equipment being standardized or designed in a way that makes it easier to use for everyone, and especially for temp nurses? Right now, the answers to these questions aren't reassuring. It seems that hospitals use travel and temp nurses to plug an increasing number of holes without much concern about who plugs them and how well, or about the possibility that unplugged holes might line up and lead to medical errors, as in the Swiss cheese analogy we saw earlier.

Katherine Harris, the labor and delivery nurse in western Massachusetts, was, for example, very concerned about her experiences as a temp nurse. Harris got her first job at Bay State Medical Center. There, she says, she felt she was adequately trained, particularly since she'd done an internship in the hospital before going to work there permanently. The problem was that after about a year, Bay State started cutting back on her hours. She'd be scheduled to come into work and someone would call her and tell her, sorry, they didn't need her that day. Since nursing was not a vocation but the way she made her living, she had to find supplemental work. While continuing to work at Bay State when she was needed, she signed up to work with a local agency that provided temporary nurses to hospitals, particularly to long-term care facilities.

Most of the people who entered the agency with Harris were also new nurses. Before the nurses went out for their first job, the agency was supposed to give them an orientation. The orientation consisted of a four-hour video presentation given in the basement of the agency's headquarters. Harris says it seemed like the video was produced in the 1970s. It showed nurses how to move patients safely and gave some instructions in medication administration. After four hours, the instructors laughingly reassured their students that they wouldn't have to carry the code beeper, which meant they would not be in charge of running rescue missions on patients who'd had cardiac arrests until they'd worked in the facility for some time.

Harris was shocked. She'd never learned to run a code, she'd never even seen a code, and here they were talking about code beepers. She was even more shocked to find, a month later, that she was given the code beeper to carry with her, even though no one had given her any instruction in running codes. She was also told that she should follow the rules governing how the facility delivered care, even though no one at her first assignment ever told her what those rules were or how to find out about them.

When Harris reported to work at that long-term care facility, she was assigned to a floor that was devoted to long-term ventilator-dependent patients—patients who were paralyzed or in a coma and stayed on breathing machines, sometimes for years. When Harris got to the floor, she found patients lying in bed in what seemed to her to be a limbo between life and death. No one guided her through the maze of human suffering to explain who was in a coma or who was paralyzed but mentally alert. At the sight of all these patients, she says she experienced wave after wave of sadness. She wanted to be compassionate and kind as well as competent. But she could be neither. "They weren't concerned about me knowing how to talk to the patients or being comfortable with this kind of patient, with whom I had never had any experience. All they wanted me to do was to put medications into the feeding tubes that were permanently inserted into their stomachs."

No one taught Harris how to master what turned out to be a complex skill. "I had to figure out which meds I could mix together in their G tube. I had to look it all up because no one told me, and then people would get upset because I was so slow. No one helped me. Not the managers or the other nurses. It seemed like because they'd been doing it for so long, they assumed everybody knew how to do it."

Harris found the experience frightening and depressing. "There was no time for me to ask the most basic questions. When I asked a question, as one would have to do when you don't know what you're doing, people were very short with me." Harris says that after only a few hours she felt utterly defeated by the whole experience. "I felt really sad and scared for

362 everyone—for me and for the patients I was supposed to care for. When I went in there, I thought I could learn how to communicate with these patients and be kind. It was something I would have liked to learn how to do, but the place didn't allow me to do that. I was surrounded by fences of mean people and so after a few shifts I said 'forget it.'"

Harris, by now reduced to tears, told her agency managers that she refused to work on that floor again. They did not offer to help her attain a level of competence with this group of patients. Nor did they offer to discuss the lack of orientation with the hospital nursing management of the institution. Instead, they simply said, "Well, no one ever wants to work there."

No wonder, Harris comments.

Fatigue is another critical safety issue involved in the use of travel and agency nurses. If hospital administrators are truly concerned about patient safety, they can easily monitor how many hours their permanent staff are working in their institution. They can verify when the nurse arrives at work and leaves. Hospitals obviously can't control what a nurse does when she's off the job, but if nurses are well paid and well treated, they have less incentive to moonlight elsewhere. Hospitals have no control over travel or agency nurses. They don't know how many extra twelve-hour shifts a nurse like Greg Wilson is working. They don't know how many extra hours they're putting in for a temporary agency. "It's like the Wild West, where people can work where they want," says Sean Clarke. "You basically have to trust individuals to be responsible about only taking assignments that they are really in a position to take, and you have to be confident they're going to work a reasonable number of hours and are not going to run themselves into the ground and take their patients with them."

In fact, some studies find a correlation between an increase in patient complications, medical errors, and deaths and the use of travel or agency nurses. The Institute of Medicine report on patient safety states, "Medication errors have been shown to increase with the number of shifts worked by temporary nursing staff and to decrease when permanent staff work overtime to ensure adequate staffing." Similarly, infections from intravenous lines that may snake close to patients' hearts, known as central lines, have increased when nurses are floated onto units.[10]

In 1996 a nurse from a temporary agency was assigned to work on the burn and trauma intensive care unit at the Brigham and Women's Hospital in Boston, even though she had little experience with an intensive care unit. She was taking care of a sixty-seven-year-old surgical patient who was receiving an IV infusion of potassium chloride. Although potassium is necessary to help the heart function, giving too much potassium to a patient too rapidly is a perfect way to stop the heart. Unfamiliar with the IV **363** that delivered the drug, the nurse inadvertently gave a dose in thirty minutes that was supposed to drip into the patient's vein over two hours. The patient died. Who was responsible for checking the nurse's ability to function on the unit, the hospital or the employment agency? As the *Boston Globe* reported, "the credentials of agency nurses aren't usually checked."[11] The case of nurse Charles Cullen, who admitted to murdering as many as forty patients, raises another concern. Given a hospital's lax attitudes toward those rare nurses whose peculiar behavior signals serious emotional problems, will the use of contingent nurses make it more difficult to protect patients from mentally unstable caregivers?

There is now a movement of sorts to assure the safety of temporary nurses by credentialing staffing agencies that are themselves unregulated and uncredentialed. The Joint Commission on the Accreditation of Healthcare Organizations (JCAHO) has recently announced that it will offer a new service to hospitals and certify health care staffing agencies. Speaking for many in the industry, Frank Shaffer, of CrossCountry Health Care, lauds the move, saying that it will bring standardization to the industry and "level the playing field . . . help[ing] the health care industry differentiate among high quality staffing companies and those who are less concerned about quality."[12] Diane Sosne and many other leaders of nurses' unions disagree. They believe it will simply legitimate the use of contingent nurses as a solution to the nursing crisis and channel energy away from the real issues that drive nurses out of the workplace and necessitate greater use of staffing agencies.

More than this, JCAHO's long and controversial history makes this move very problematic. Although JCAHO is in the business of accrediting hospitals and other health care facilities, business may be the operative word here. JCAHO isn't a government agency; it's a private company that, thanks to the U.S. Congress, has been given near-monopoly power to accredit the quality and safety of hospitals. Some HMOs won't use non-JCAHO-accredited facilities, and Medicare demands a JCAHO or, alternatively, a state government inspection, before it will reimburse a hospital for its services to Medicare beneficiaries. To receive Medicare reimbursement, which amounts to almost half of their revenue, hospitals and other health facilities must pay JCAHO a great deal of money to inspect and accredit them.

Observers have criticized the ethical problems embedded in this arrangement. "They are bought and paid for by the people they investigate, which is an absolute conflict of interest," Representative Fortney "Pete" Stark (D-CA) commented when he spoke to *Chicago Tribune* reporters Michael J. Berens and Bruce Japsen. In November 2002, the two

364 journalists published a major investigative report documenting numerous flaws in the JCAHO inspection process. "Less than 1 percent of hospitals failed to receive accreditation from the commission in the past 17 years and some hospitals received high accreditation scores even in the midst of a public health crisis," they wrote. Thus a Florida hospital retained its high JCAHO accreditation after federal public health investigators warned that "patients were in 'immediate jeopardy' of harm because of infection-control deficiencies."[13] Hospital inspections, the reporters said, are almost a sham, since hospitals know they're going to be inspected three months in advance. Imagine if a health department inspector called a restaurant on April 1 to tell the owner he'd be over on June 1. When the inspector arrived, the place would be spotless—and if he stopped to grab a bite, the cuisine would be divine, and the service impeccable. The next week the roaches could safely return. That's what the reporters say happens after a JCAHO inspection. "In some instances," the authors say, "medical centers have temporarily hired more nurses and transferred patients to ease overcrowded and unsafe conditions."

Berens and Japsen also insist that JCAHO's voluntary reporting system "vastly underestimates the number of avoidable patient deaths. The organization, for instance, documents just 12 cases of preventable hospital-borne infections. . . . The *Tribune* found about 75,000 such deaths in just one year, a figure supported by state and government files."[14] These problems and many more that the authors catalogue stem from the fact that members of major medical associations—the American Medical Association, American Hospital Association, American College of Surgeons, American College of Physicians, American Society of Internal Medicine, and American Dental Association—exactly the people JCAHO is inspecting, make up three-quarters of the association's board.

JCAHO's proposed accreditation of staffing agencies seems to parallel its hospital operations. An advisory council made up of members of staffing agencies explored the issue of certification and okayed the idea. An expert panel, made up of representatives of staffing agencies, is developing the Standards and Application Process and will determine the qualifications of surveyors. Will this new service replicate the same problems that have plagued JCAHO's hospital accreditation programs? Will JCAHO insist that staffing agencies risk alienating hospitals by asking where a nurse will be assigned, what kinds of—and how many—patients she'll be caring for, what equipment she'll be using, and which staff she'll be working with? Will they know what kind of orientation hospitals provide nurses of different levels of experience? Will large agencies that work with tens of thousands of nurses be able to follow each and every one and make sure their work records are stellar? How deeply will they be forced to check a nurse's background and work record? If hospitals assume **365** JCAHO-accredited agencies have checked up on nurses, they certainly won't have any incentive to do so themselves. We've learned that it takes nurses years to obtain expertise. Yet travel agencies advertise that they will accept applicants with only a year of bedside experience. Will expertise even be a part of the calculation that agencies and the hospitals make when they hire traveling or agency nurses to staff the wards?

In March 2004 an incident occurred that raises further questions about whether JCAHO sides with the industry or with patients. At the end of January of that year a group called Joint Commission Resources, which is a subsidiary of JCAHO, called the sociologist Dana Beth Weinberg to invite her to do a by-phone audio conference on her book *Code Green: Money-Driven Hospitals and the Dismantling of Nursing.* Although Weinberg takes a stand for staffing ratios, her book is not a polemic against the hospital industry, and it was favorably received by journals like *Health Affairs* and *JAMA*, whose reviewers complimented her on her evenhandedness. (In the interests of full disclosure, the book is part of this series at ILR Press and I had significant editorial input.) The conference, scheduled for April 15, 2004, was advertised on JCAHO's website on March 18. The notice announced that Weinberg would offer a "stinging indictment" of hospital practices.

Weinberg was looking forward to presenting her research and engaging in a reasoned discussion about the issues of hospital restructuring and the nursing shortage. This was, however, not to be. On March 19—the announcement wasn't even up for twenty-four hours—it suddenly disappeared. Then Weinberg got a phone message from a representative of the Joint Commission Resources informing her that the conference was canceled. Why? "There had been a great deal of concern voiced to the Joint Commission. . . . We posted the audio-conference on our website yesterday, in the afternoon, and I have been barraged with phone calls. And so we just wanted to make sure that you knew our sentiments and kind of what was happening," the woman said. Weinberg didn't. When she called the Joint Commission Resources to find out more, she was told, "It was pulled by our leadership. They felt there was a lot of negativeness going on. We accredit hospitals and they thought we were pushing the envelope a little too much. It was a board decision. We didn't want to show the hospital industry in a negative light against the nurses. . . . We felt we needed to be more sensitive to issues with our hospital associations." When Weinberg asked if people had expressed concern about her research methods or findings, she said no, not in the least.

When reporter Scott Allen decided to write a brief story on the cancellation, he called JCAHO's Charlene Hill, who told the *Boston Globe* that

366 callers didn't like the book's title because it "cast a kind of disparaging light on hospitals."[15]

"JCAHO is supposed to be the watchdog for the hospital industry, not its lapdog," Weinberg commented. "The information about what is happening to nursing really needs to get out to hospitals. Hospital directors hold the key to solving the nursing shortage. But they don't seem to want to open the door and take the necessary action and responsibility, or sadly, even to talk about the working conditions in hospitals. This stifling of intellectual discussion and debate is a chilling reminder of the power of industry over research that can't be ignored."

If JCAHO cancels a serious discussion about the issues confronting hospital nursing because a few people don't like the title of a book, this hardly bodes well for any process in which the organization is involved. What is more troubling is that the cancellation of this event is part of a larger pattern. Other researchers have had similar experiences as they try to collect, discuss, or present data on the impact of hospital restructuring on nurses' work. In 2001 Senator Edward Kennedy's office asked Boston College School of Nursing professor and researcher Judith Shindul-Rothschild to present findings from her research on nurses' views of their changing working conditions to a hearing of the Senate Health, Education, Labor and Pensions Committee. The committee would hear from only one representative of the nursing community. In the opinion of many groups that were polled, Shindul-Rothschild should represent research documenting the claims of staff nurses. Over the years, as both a professor and former president of the Massachusetts Nurses Association, Shindul-Rothschild had spoken about—and researched—the eroding working conditions of nurses.

Shindul-Rothschild said that a day or two before she was scheduled to present, she received a call from Kennedy's office telling her the hospital industry had threatened not to send a representative to the hearing if she appeared. Since the hearing could not be held without the participation of the hospital industry, the chair of the committee, a pro-industry Rebublican, told Kennedy's office to replace her, and they did. "I was told," she says, "that the industry felt I was too radical. This was an affront because I was presenting well-documented scholarly research."

Sean Clarke says the group of researchers working at the University of Pennsylvania School of Nursing have had difficulty gathering data from the hospital industry. When it comes to the use of temp and travel nurses, Clarke says, it's very difficult for researchers to get a clear picture of the extent of the problem and the money hospitals really spend on contingent nurses. "This is one of these political hot potatoes that everybody would

love to have some good data on, and people are either finding it too difficult to study or don't want to wade into the political morass. It's like the
staffing issue and patient outcomes. Hospitals don't want their freedom
restricted to make their decisions as they see fit. They don't want bad
public relations around this particular issue. So the bottom line is that
they don't want to make data available."

It's the same issue with nurse staffing, Clarke says. "It's very hard to
get unit-level staffing data on representative groups of hospitals. You
have to go to hospitals individually. The data that are available in these
national data sets are very crude because human resources and nursing
represent such a large proportion of a hospital budget. Frankly, the way
they choose to manage their nursing work force is part of a competitive
advantage of a hospital. They don't want to make that open to their competitors in the same market or even in the broader world. The researchers find the research too difficult to do because the research is too
hard to get a hold of."

Follow the Money

Hospitals' use of contingent nurses raises another serious problem: the
way in which supposedly scarce health care resources are used. Travel and
agency nursing appeal to RNs because they are promised more money,
benefits, and perks than the people they are working with. When nurses,
either on their own or through their unions, ask hospitals to pay them
more and give them better benefits, hospitals usually claim they are cash
strapped and can't do it. But how is it that hospitals find the money to hire
travel and agency nurses and undergo the expense of sending recruiters
abroad? According to one travel/temp agency, hospitals pay hourly rates
plus 50 percent more for the company's overhead for a travel nurse, and
the hourly rate plus 20 percent more in overhead for the agency nurse. In
the United States, when the American Hospital Association surveyed its
accredited organizations, 56 percent spent $71 million a year for supple-
mental staffing. Is this the real figure? Who knows?

In the United States, nursing unions waged long strikes to address understaffing, mandatory overtime, and stagnating pay. During those
strikes, hospitals used temporary nurses to replace striking workers. Ted
Iorio is the attorney for the nurses represented by the Teamsters Union at
Northern Michigan Hospital, in Petoskey, Michigan. Iorio explains that
in just the first six weeks of an almost two-year strike, the hospital spent
$5 million on traveling nurses used to replace those on strike for better
benefits and greater voice in patient care.

368   During its 103-day strike against Brockton Hospital in 2001, the Massachusetts Nurses Association (MNA) found a pay stub for one of the traveling nurses hired to replace striking RNs. For one week's worth of work, the nurse was paid $5,000. She worked eighty-four hours in one week and was paid $45 an hour for straight time and $60 an hour for overtime. This didn't include the cost of a stay at the Marriott, her meals, and living and travel expenses, or the fee the agency charged the hospital.[16]

Is this use of patients' and the public's money (Medicare dollars, after all, supply almost 50 percent of a hospital's revenue) cost-effective? In the calendar year 2002, total hospital spending was $487 billion, and of that Medicare provided $149 billion, or less than a third. But it's the second largest source of hospital income after private health insurance.[17] What are hospitals really paying for? If hospitals have this much money and can work out scheduling for nurses who have demonstrated no loyalty to the institution, why can't they pay permanent nurses more and treat them better?

Not surprisingly, the disparity in salary and perks between temporary and full-time workers does not endear agency and travel nurses to the permanent staff with whom they work. Indeed, nurses express the same feelings of resentment and disillusionment when hospitals try to recruit new staff with sign-on bonuses, while they fail to pay loyal workers in the very same facility as much as they pay new recruits.

Hospitals insist they are forced to use temporary nurses if they have vacancies or if nurses are on strike. Unfortunately, the travel/temp solution to a shortage breeds an even greater shortage of its own. If working conditions are pretty much the same in different hospitals, why not bail out and sign up with a temporary agency and go to work at another facility— or even the same one—for more money? If nurses see that agency and travel nursing is more lucrative and less stressful, it makes sense to join up.

In Mississippi, the number of RNs who sought license verification in other states spiked dramatically—from 1,338 to 5,359—between 1998 and 2001. Some nurses I spoke with speculated that Mississippi RNs were signing on with travel agencies and replacing nurses who were on strike or seeking better pay elsewhere. Since 2002, perhaps because of efforts to increase retention and recruitment, the number of Mississippi nurses seeking out of state "endorsements" has decreased.

This pattern may help explain some statistics. The Institute of Medicine reported that "high rates of turnover characterize the nursing staff of both hospital and long-term care facilities. . . . [O]n average 21.3 percent of all full-time registered hospital nurses had resigned or been terminated during the preceding year. While most hospitals reported turnover rates **369** of 10–30 percent, some cited much higher rates."[18] Turnover rates of 50 percent and more were even noted.

Internal Migration

All sorts of migratory patterns may be observed in the new nursing universe. One little-discussed pattern is migration away from hospital and bedside into higher-status roles. Nurses have always found it difficult to advance while staying at the bedside. When they wanted a raise, higher status, or a different set of challenges, they usually went into management or academia. But today they have another option—advanced practice.

Dave Latham is one of these internal migrants. Latham began his nursing career in 1994 at a Southern teaching hospital. He enjoyed his work, first on the emergency unit and then on neurology, cardiac, and burn intensive care units. But it didn't take long for him to get worn down working so many nights, hassling with the bureaucracy, and coping with physicians. After moving to Illinois, he began to work at a smaller hospital. But the hospital started losing money during the cost cutting of the 1990s and brought in the Hunter Group, a consulting firm known for its slash-and-burn, cut-no-matter-what mentality. Cut they did. In the ER, instead of covering three or four beds, nurses had to deal with five or six. "So you have potentially high acuity in all beds. You have a tech to help out but you're drawing your own blood, doing a lot more running," said Latham. Then he went to the orthopedic floor, where staffing was better until the cuts followed him. Suddenly nurses were told, "We're going to cost-contain you," and they'd be sent home where they were supposed to be on call for the rest of their shift. Alternately, they could stay in the on-call room in the hospital but wouldn't get paid.

"Staffing was cut and acuity increased. We had people with fractured hips who were old and frail—and sometimes big—and you had to help them out of bed and get them their meds, and they needed bedpans and they were on pain pumps." Latham almost breathlessly catalogues the problems. "There were thirty-two patients and one tech for the whole floor. So you had to prioritize. And how did you do that?" he asked. "Based on patient need? Not at all. Based on how likely it was that the patient would sue. So people weren't getting a bed bath or changed or fed because you weren't going to get your license jerked. That's when it became a moral issue for me. If people can't get well, that's when I got disgusted at what happened here."

So Latham decided to become a nurse practitioner. "With the staffing cuts going on, I wanted to have the ability to do something else."

370   While the opportunity to move into a different kind of work is one of the good things about nursing, many of the nurses I have talked to over the past decade are not making what can be considered to be voluntary career moves. Like nurses who feel their stagnating wages force them to accept overtime work, many nurses feel eroding working conditions are forcing them to abandon bedside nursing.

This internal migration is not only affecting frustrated veteran nurses. When I recently spoke to fourth-year classes at five different university nursing schools around the United States, I asked students where they wanted to work after graduation. Most of the students said they wanted to work for a year or two in direct care nursing of some kind—in the hospital or home, or a rehab facility or clinic. When I asked how many saw themselves working in direct care in ten years, I'd see one or two hands flutter up in a class of sixty or more students. In one class, not a single hand was raised. These students said they wanted to work in hospitals for maybe a year or two, get some skills, and then move on and away. The hospital was too stifling, conditions were deplorable, and nurses were telling them to leave. Why should they stay? Nursing students I interviewed at the University of Toronto School of Nursing echoed these sentiments.

This should give us pause. Restructurers' predictions of the demise of the hospital are clearly premature. People are still getting sick, still need care, and still depend on expertise at the bedside—in the hospital, clinic, and home. Even if the number of nurses working in the hospital setting were to drop to 45 or 50 percent, which it probably won't, nursing schools should be producing enough students to fill a significant need. If they aren't, then why should taxpayers support legislation allocating funds to recruit new nurses and educate them?

When I asked students in these classes if they were worried about the fate of hospitalized patients when so many of them were eschewing hospital work, most assured me that there would be plenty of students who would fill their shoes and work on the wards for a year or two. Since so many nurses are reaching retirement age, I asked them if they thought that hospital units staffed predominantly with new grads would be safe. "Oh, no," they groaned in unison. Well, think about it, I suggested, how are patients going to get expert hands-on care if no one wants to stay at the bedside for more than a year or two?

Worldchurn

On a dreary February day in 2002 nursing students attending a conference of the Canadian Student Nurses Association held in Victoria, British

Columbia, strolled through a hotel lobby where hospitals exhibited their desperate need for nurses. Canadian hospital recruiters weren't the only ones trying to corner interested new prospects. Recruiters, mostly from the southern part of the United States, were aggressively snagging students and trying to lure them away from Canada. "We hear they're disgruntled because of unions and socialized medicine, and not being paid enough," a recruiter from a North Carolina hospital told me. To try to sweeten the pot, she said her institution offered them a union-free environment, no national health care hassles, and a $5,000 relocation allowance, living expenses, and $2,000 for a friend.

A Kentucky hospital would pony up a $5,000 recruitment bonus, as much as sixty days' free housing, and an intense eight- to twelve-week orientation. A hospital in Texas dangled the promise of relocation money, tuition rebates to cover expenses left over from nursing school, a $1,500 signing bonus, and tuition reimbursement should the nurse want to continue his or her education while in Texas. A recruiter from a hospital in Dallas didn't believe in relocation bonuses. Nurses wouldn't stay if you just give them money, she said. Her hospital had devised another enticement, a three-month internship for new graduates in medical surgical nursing, critical care, or six months in the ER. "Nursing is a calling," this particular recruiter said. When I wondered then why there was such a shortage of nurses across the United States, she told me that the new generation seems to lack the necessary spiritual receptors to heed the call. Conveniently, this interpretation absolves health care employers—no matter which country they're in—of any responsibility for the nursing shortage. In fact, this game of musical nurses responding to the siren song of hospital recruiters traveling from country to country has little to do with the failings of nurses and everything to do with the failings of the health care systems or institutions that employ them.

Nursing has always been a profession that offered opportunities for national and international mobility. Think of all those nineteenth-century nuns who packed onto steamers traveling from Europe to the New World. What was unique about this migration, as Sioban Nelson points out, was the new economic and social opportunities it provided to women, who often moved alone. Apart from the opportunity to be a maid or nanny, no other occupation gave women a legitimate reason to travel far from home and earn their own keep or become a breadwinner for their family. Nelson argues that this was, in fact, one of the attractions of work that often had many unattractive characteristics.

Nurses move from country to country for a variety of reasons. Some want an opportunity to advance their education and move up an occupational ladder they cannot find in their home country. Some can't find sat-

372 isfactory paid employment at home. Some are escaping deteriorating working conditions. Some go abroad to earn money they can send home. Among countries that produce nurses for export, the Philippines are perhaps the best known.

For decades, the Philippines have actually mass-produced nurses for export. Because of the country's colonization by the United States, Filipino nurses speak English and were trained in American nursing practice. They are thus perfect products for export in an economy that depends on the money that Filipino nurses working in industrialized countries send home. The Philippines owe some $46 billion to the World Bank, the International Monetary Fund, and other North American lending institutions. "Overseas workers' remittances have been the country's largest source of foreign exchange," writes Catherine Ceniza Choy in her excellent study of Filipino nurse migration. "According to the Central Bank of the Philippines, between 1975 and 1994, Filipino overseas contract workers sent remittances totaling $18.196 billion."[19] Choy found that migration was such a common phenomenon that stores sell an entire line of greeting cards devoted to the overseas worker. Go into a shop and there they are, Choy told me, cards for all sorts of special occasions with the message "missing you across the ocean."

Lesleyanne Hawthorne, an international expert on the migration of skilled workers, adds that 25 percent of Philippine gross domestic product (GDP) is dependent on money sent back to the Philippines by migrant workers. Hawthorne explains that in some Asian countries like Indonesia, the Philippines are considered a successful pioneering model of the production of workers for export. "A major goal of Ministry of Health in Indonesia is now to train people to work internationally in nursing so they can be exported to Western and Middle Eastern nations." Whether in Indonesia or the Philippines, nurses, Hawthorne elaborates, are valued as loyal producers of remittances because, as women, they can be counted upon to actually send money home rather than spending it on themselves in their new host country.

Between 1950 and 1970, entrepreneurs opened scores of private nursing schools in the Philippines.[20] A number of private universities grant Filipino nurses what they claim is the equivalent of a baccalaureate degree in the United States or Canada. These schools deliberately overproduce nurses and make it difficult for them to get entry-level jobs at home. Although the Philippines have registered a shortage of thirty-one thousand nurses, most of these positions seem to be in rural areas—some of them the scene of armed conflict. A new graduate of a Philippine nursing school usually has to work for a year as a volunteer in a hospital if she wants to keep her skills up so that she is a candidate for emigration or for a job at home. If she does find a job at home, her wages and working conditions are so low and so poor that she won't be able to help support her family. These conditions are constructed to push Filipino nurses offshore so they can work and send money home. A World Health Organization Study on International Nurse Mobility reported that in 2001, eleven thousand nurses left the Philippines for jobs primarily in the United Kingdom, Saudi Arabia, and Ireland.[21] UK and Singaporean recruiters, among others, have targeted the Philippines and are quite explicit about the critical role that foreign nurses play in keeping their health systems afloat. Many nurses who migrate do so not only for economic but physical survival. Their countries are wracked by war, ethnic violence, or crime born of poverty. Some nurses—they are probably the minority—travel for adventure. All of these motives, which economists call push factors, propel a nurse to leave her home country and relocate, sometimes in a very alien culture.[22]

No matter how hard they are pushed, nurses can't migrate easily unless push factors are complemented by pull factors. Today, Hawthorne and others explain, one of the major pull factors is a shortage of nurses in the host country. The shortage is due to all the factors described here—as well as the fact that, with the exception of the United States, where Hispanic and other immigrant populations have more children, most industrialized countries have such low birthrates that they rely on mostly Asian nurses to provide nursing care to increasingly needy populations. Host countries provide the pull by helping nurses find the job, obtain the visas, pass the licensing exams, and get the work permits. The nurse will have to pass licensing exams in the host country. If they continue their education, schools in the host country have to offer them courses, which may require special services. They have to have help with relocating and with buffing their language skills. Nursing migration doesn't just happen. Someone—government and health care institutions—must turn on the faucet of demand.

Today that faucet is wide open. In the year 2000, for example, the U.S. Department of Health and Human Services reported that there were about a hundred thousand overseas-trained nurses in the country.[23] "Between 1998 and 1999," Choy writes, "the number of foreign-trained nurses in the United Kingdom increased by 25 percent. According to Singapore Minister of Health Yeo Chow Tong, without foreign nurses 'some of our services would be decimated.' "[24]

Hundreds of recruiters are scouring the globe, and individual recruitment agencies, hospitals, and even educational institutions are cutting deals with governments willing to supply nurses. Governments are facilitating the entry of nurses into their countries just as others encourage the

374   exit of nurses from theirs. What's unprecedented about this period of nurse migration is not only the sheer numbers but also the commercial potential unleashed by mass nurse migration. Today, almost every industrialized nation is experiencing a nursing shortage and is using immigration as a solution of choice.

It's hard to pinpoint exactly how many nurses are actually migrating around the world, Mireille Kingma of the ICN explains, because each country has different qualifications and descriptions of what a nurse is and does. Kingma does point out that contemporary migration patterns differ from those in the past. "We used to see more migration between developed and other developed countries. Now we are seeing more migration from developing countries to developed countries." She likens it to a carousel. "People are migrating and eventually finding their way to the United States, as the endpoint. Nurses will go from Nigeria to South Africa or from the Philippines to the Middle East to get training in more high-tech work. Then they go for a year to the United Kingdom and then from the United Kingdom to Canada, and from Canada to the United States. That's the flow we're seeing." Nothing seems to stand in the way of this migratory flow. After terrorist attacks hit Saudi Arabia, European, and American nurses left that country, but Indian and South African women took their place.

While globalization is a fact of life and migration impossible to halt, this new nurse migration is different, Kingma explains, because "now we're seeing aggressive and massive recruitment by agencies. These recruitment campaigns are taking such numbers at the same time that it's becoming a real problem."

While nurse migration certainly affords women greater opportunities for advancement, it also offers entrepreneurs and large companies enormous opportunities for profit. To take advantage of those opportunities, agencies have sprung up all over the globe. I open the pages of the *Australian Journal of Nursing* and find ads from Worldwide Healthcare Exchange: "Working in Scotland will put a smile on your face";[25] from Nightingale Nursing: "Itchy feet? We can get you walking in the right direction"; from Austra Health International: "Launch your nursing career in beautiful British Columbia [with its] snow-capped mountains, fertile valleys, lush green forests and one of the world's most spectacular coastlines." Not a mention, you will notice, of what it's like to work in the hospitals of any of these countries.

Recruitment has not only become a big business, it is a very lucrative business. Most agencies in the United States don't make their money off nurses; their big fees are paid by the hospitals. Expenses alone can be significant. One agency I spoke with told me that for an Australian nurse looking to work in the United States, they will pay airfare and a week's worth of hotel expenses to take the NCLEX, the U.S. licensing exam for nurses. The nurse will then have to go back to Australia to wait and see if she passed. Then the agency will pay the fees associated with getting the potential recruit an American green card—or work permit—and they will pay the nurse's airfare back to the United States when she comes to work in the hospital where she's been placed. She'll be given three months free lodging, if she agrees to share with another nurse, or if she comes with her family and wants to live with them on her own, she will pay one-third of her lodging expenses and the agency will pay the rest for three months.

Because nurses are in such short supply in the United States, the agency told me, the nurse, her or his spouse, and any child under twenty-one will get a green card, which means they can stay in the United States for as long as they want and ultimately apply for citizenship. The U.S. nursing shortage thus allows RNs to be fast-tracked toward work or citizenship because, as a representative of this agency told me, there are not enough qualified nurses in the United States, and foreign nurses aren't therefore taking the jobs of U.S. nurses.

But consider the facts. Hospitals are paying thousands of dollars in fees and expenses for every foreign nurse they recruit (this doesn't include the money they spend training the nurse once he or she arrives in the United States). If hospitals were to put this kind of money into retaining nurses, they might be able to keep nurses on their floors and recruit new ones into the profession. Indirectly, then, the expenditures for fees to recruitment agencies (or even to pay the hospital's own recruiters to go overseas) is money that is taken out of the pockets of American nurses and potential candidates into the profession.

Many recruitment agencies are legitimate and deliver—or at least try to deliver—what they promise to the nurses who sign on with them. But some are not so scrupulous, and as nurse recruitment agencies mushroom, so do the opportunities for exploitation. Because there is no regulatory framework governing recruitment or recruitment agencies, groups like the International Council of Nurses have received complaints that suggest the possibilities for exploitation as nurses move from country to country. Some nurses, says Mireille Kingma, are misled by recruitment agencies. A nurse signs a contract to work in a hospital on an intensive care unit, but when she arrives in the United Kingdom or the United States, her passport is confiscated and she's forced to sign a new contract to work in a nursing home. Or an agency brings nurses to a particular country and they can't pass the registration exams. The nurse has to take job in a nursing home, which means the nursing home benefits and the nurse suffers. In the United Kingdom, says Kingma, the Nursing and

376 Midwifery Council is supposed to scrutinize a candidate's CV and degrees and decide whether someone needs to go through an orientation period. If the immigrant nurse has to go through this orientation period, some facilities pay her salary, some pay reduced salaries, and some pay no salary at all. A recent report by the Public Services International detailed problems with the recruitment and abuse of migrant nurses in Ghana, Fiji, Ecuador, and many other countries.[26]

The Royal College of Nursing in the United Kingdom also recently released disturbing findings about some of the hidden costs of recruitment. "Over one in three internationally recruited nurses have had to pay fees to their employer or a recruitment agency to work in the UK. Over a third (37 percent) of Filipino nurses had to pay a commission after securing their job and for half of them this was between £500 and £2,000."[27] Some nurses have faced so many problems and are so fearful that one nursing union in England, UNISON, has set up safe houses to offer nurses some protection. In January 1998 a group of American recruiters pleaded guilty to charges of "illegally bringing hundreds of registered nurses from the Philippines into the United States to work in convalescent homes and other medical facilities. Expecting wages of $13 to $15 an hour, these nurses earned as little as $5 per hour as nursing assistants."[28] "There is no standardization in the global marketplace," Kingma says, "and people working in a system that has no standardization are a target of exploitation."

Hospitals, nursing homes, and commercial recruitment agencies are not the only ones that may benefit from the increased use of migrant nurses. Nursing schools may also profit from the new commercial opportunities migration affords. One of the lures used to draw nurses from Canada and other countries to the United States has been the promise that hospitals will reimburse their tuition if they continue their education in the United States. When hospitals offer foreign nurses money for education, that money is going to a nursing school in the United States. So nursing schools that suffered during the cutbacks of the 1990s, when many hospitals stopped providing U.S. nurses with tuition reimbursement, are now recouping their losses and then some.

Marcia Martin, a nurse and union representative of the United American Nurses at St. Mary's Medical Center/Duluth Clinic told me that the director of her hospital and of the graduate program of the local nursing school, the College of St. Scholastica, journeyed to the Philippines to find recruits for both the hospital and the school of nursing. The hospital was looking for experienced nurses with a baccalaureate education, and the school was looking for candidates for its master's program. Filipino nurses were told that if they worked a few days at the hospital, their master's education would be paid for. They were thus brought into the United States on a student visa, which permits them to work for only a few days a week.

Without informing the nurses in the hospital about this new program and offering them the opportunity to pursue their studies, Martin says, the two directors returned and enthusiastically reported that they were going to bring over twenty nurses. The number was eventually whittled down to ten. These nurses were working and studying while coping with life in a new country. A year later only two remained.

Of course, some might argue that the benefits to foreign nurses, particularly those from underdeveloped countries, far outweigh the risks that they incur. Nurses who migrate to industrialized countries and advance their education and skills have the opportunity to bring back many innovations and use their newly acquired knowledge to help patients and other nurses in their home countries. Tom Keighley in the United Kingdom has done a great deal of international work, including a study of the integration of Eastern European nurses into the European Union. Unfortunately, he says, there is little evidence that migrant nurses are returning home after they receive their advanced education and learn new skills. They will return only if things change for the better in their home countries. When nurses stay in their new home, Mireille Kingma says, this represents a significant drain on taxpayer investment in nursing education in those countries that fully or partially fund nursing education.

While many nurses who migrate end up working well alongside their new colleagues, nursing migration also has the potential to fragment the nursing work force. While migrant nurses may be forceful advocates for positive change in the workplace once they have established themselves in their new land, new arrivals may passively accept the kind of working conditions that have led to shortages. They may agree to work longer hours and more overtime, and might be reluctant to complain about just-in-time staffing. They may not speak up about unsafe patient loads or other problems that threaten quality patient care. They may be hostile to or frightened of joining unions. And depending on their country of origin, they may be more deferential to physicians. Their understandable acquiescence to employer demands may make them far more attractive to hospital administrators than the cranky, demanding, homegrown nurses who are fighting for improved working conditions.

A recent article in the *New York Times* profiling Filipino nurses sketched out some of the problems and benefits of migrant nurses who are fortunate enough to get good jobs in their new country. Nurses from the Philippines, the article explained, are well educated and, with enough overtime, can earn up to $80,000 a year in New York. While the article painted a rosy picture of their life in the United States, the subtext was

378   less than reassuring. Many of these women leave families and children behind and work very long hours. While their salaries of $80,000 or more sound like a lot, we have to remember that New York is one of the most expensive cities in the world, and migrant nurses aren't pocketing their entire salaries. Unlike American nurses, they're worried about more than paying the rent and putting food on the table. They have to set aside money to send to their families back home. That's why some may be willing to be workhorses for their hospitals. This may endear them to hospital administrators like Diane Aroh, the chief nurse executive of Montefiore Hospital, who lauded her Filipino nurses not only because they are so caring but because "they're very flexible, willing to take new assignments on the spur of the moment, willing to work extra-long hours."[29]

While these extra-long hours may be good for hospital executives who need to put a body at the bedside, how alert will that body working those extra-long hours be? And how do American nurses fighting against these extra-long hours feel about Filipino nurses who accept them? An illustrative case of the problems that can arise between homegrown and foreign nurses took place in British Columbia. In 2000 the British Columbia Nurses Union (BCNU) launched an ongoing campaign to increase the salaries of nurses in the province. Concerned about the exodus of nurses to the United States, the nursing union was asking for a significant raise to make salaries competitive with those south of the border. The conservative government was not eager to comply. That's when Filipino nurses in Vancouver entered the debate and an even more dramatic and heartwrenching battle between foreign and Canadian nurses started.

During nursing shortages of the 1960s and 1970s, Canada began heavily recruiting Filipino nurses, and the country became one of the destinations of choice for this group of immigrants. Because nurses were in short supply, Immigration Canada gave Filipino nurses extra "points" or more favorable immigration status. In fact, they didn't even have to sit for the Canadian nursing exam and their education was given equivalent status to that received by Canadians. In the 1990s, as the government laid off nurses, foreign nurses were no longer such valuable commodities, and the government withdrew its favorable immigration status for Filipino nurses. Nurses coming from the Philippines were also told that, like all Canadian nurses, they would have to write the Canadian nursing exam and they would also have to pass an English competency test. But the push pressures in their home country didn't disappear merely because the pull pressures from Canada had evaporated. To survive, Filipino nurses still had to move and they found a way to do it.

Through Human Resources Development Canada, a new program of "live-in caregivers" began to recruit Filipino nurses who wanted to get to

Canada but couldn't do it through the normal route. If they signed on for **379** two years to be domestic servants, agreeing to care of the children or eld-erly parents of well-to-do Canadians, they could work; whether they could stay was another issue altogether. And sign on they did. Recruited by brokers in the Philippines, nurses signed two-year contracts, thinking that they had been informed about who they would work for, what they would be paid, and what their duties would be. Their contracts stipulated that they could not study for Canadian nursing exams while working as domestics and couldn't leave their jobs without fear of deportation.

When they came to British Columbia, many received an unwelcome surprise, says Debra McPherson, president of the BCNU. "We've just met with a group of these women," McPherson said in the spring of 2004. "Many find out, once they get here, that they are not just looking after a couple of children from 9:00 to 5:00. One of them told us she was work-ing for a Japanese businessman in West Vancouver, which is a very rich part of town. She thought she was only going to look after two children. Well, she's certainly doing that. But she's also looking after the man's aged father and mother. The father has had a stroke and is bedridden. The woman takes care of him and the kids and does the housekeeping, and is expected to do some gardening, and wash the car. These women become indentured servants. If they leave the program, they must find another domestic service position in order to maintain immigration status. So they endure terrible circumstances and, in some cases, even report physi-cal and sexual abuse."

The union is very concerned about the abuse these nurses endure. The BCNU has lobbied the Canadian government to regulate or end the pro-gram and to allow nurses in it to study while they work. Since the union has tried to ease the nursing shortage by fighting for better salaries and working conditions for its members, the efforts of Filipino nurses to lib-erate themselves from servitude have created serious ethical and political dilemmas for Canadian RNs. Groups representing the Filipino nurses have asked the BC government to allow nurses to leave their domestic employment and take nursing jobs. "These nurses are saying, Look, you have a nursing shortage, we're qualified to be nurses," McPherson ex-plains. "They want two things, which is where the rubber hits the road."

Some Filipino nurses say they will take nursing jobs at current salaries, but they want to be allowed to study. They also want their credentials to receive reciprocal status and be treated as equivalent to those of Canadian nurses. They don't want to have to sit for the Canadian nursing exam, as all Canadian nurses are required to do. Their argument to the govern-ment is that if they can work in British Columbia, there won't be a nurs-ing shortage. So, McPherson says, they are effectively undercutting the

380 union's argument that there is a shortage of nurses that can be corrected by giving better wages and working conditions to Canadian nurses.

This puts the BCNU members in a terrible moral position, McPherson says. "We don't support the exploitation of these women and want it to end. But we also have to protect our members and our patients from the kind of exploitation that results when hospitals don't pay nurses enough and don't treat them with respect." In fact, the Canadian government has now recognized the seriousness of the nursing shortage and has set up a federal task force that will look at national credentialing of nurses with a specific focus on how foreign nurses are credentialed. McPherson and others worry that Canada will continue to poach from other countries rather than addressing the causes of the shortage and that the government will lower standards in order to obtain a quick supply of nurses.

The debate illustrates the complexities and tensions created by nurse migration. These tensions may arise wherever migrant nurses work. When nurses were wooed from the Philippines to Minnesota, says Marcia Martin, none of the nurses working for the St. Mary's Medical Center/Duluth Clinic was offered the kinds of opportunities for study offered to nurses from thousands of miles away. "They never came to our staff and said, If you're willing to pick up hours and sign contracts that say you'll work here for x amount of time, we'll help you get to grad school. None of that was ever offered to nurses on staff." In 2003 a nurse at Catholic Healthcare West (CHW) told me that CHW had also sent recruiters as far away as South Africa and the Philippines to troll for nurses. In Sacramento, nurses who work for CHW facilities have been asked to pick up foreign recruits at the airport, help them navigate the RN licensing process, orient them to their units, and even lodge them in their homes. Yet, they feel the hospital does little to reward the nurses who have worked for years for the system.

Individual nurses may suffer or benefit because of foreign nurse recruitment, but the most serious consequences are felt by the health care systems in those developing countries from which nurses emigrate. The dimensions of nurse recruitment are so great, Mireille Kingma says, that "it's very difficult for the exporting country to fill the gap in their services." Physician-poor countries that depend on nurses for many health care services find there are no nurses available to deliver those services. For example, Hawthorne tells us that in Indonesia, a country in which 80 percent of primary health care services are delivered by nurses, there is a shortage of nurses.

Not only are Western countries taking unprecedented numbers of nurses, Tom Keighley says, they are also skimming off the intellectual and physical cream of the nursing profession in these countries. "This new trend in migration is about selecting a particular group. It's very explicit," says Keighley. "UK hospitals are picking a particular segment of nurses in countries like the Philippines, which have traditionally exported nurses. What we want are people who have been trained to postgraduate level in American health systems in the Philippines. So what we're doing is taking the very best, the next generation of their leadership, out."

The same is true in Africa, Keighley continues. "What we're seeing from African nations is that we're taking the absolute cream, both intellectually and healthwise. This year we've taken 1,200 nurses out of Uganda. Uganda has an HIV rate of 48 percent of population. Believe me, we are not taking HIV-positive nurses. When we take all these healthy nurses in a country so devastated by the HIV epidemic, who will take care of all these sick patients?"

Hawthorne explains that migration is such a cultural expectation in the Philippines that women factor it into their long-term life plans. But there are personal costs these women pay when they decide to move. Many nurses who migrate do so after they've married and had children. According to Hawthorne, a growing literature is documenting how this affects family structure and the nurse herself. "At one level women are increasing their agency and their power. But there's a cost. A lot of women will have children raised by their own mothers. Their husbands won't be faithful. If nurses send money home to their husband, he usually spends it on commodities. So these women lose intimacy and connectedness of family life, and if they decide to return home, they find that all that money has been spent on things like stereo systems or other things—or even other women—and there's nothing left from all their hard work."

The problem of nursing migration is a complex one that various nursing groups are trying to deal with. The Royal College of Nursing, for example, has published a manual of what it considers to be ethical recruitment for employers and RCN negotiators. The International Council of Nurses (ICN) has also published guidelines for ethical nurse recruitment that asks countries to consider the needs of migrant nurses and the needs of the countries from which they emigrate. None of the national or international bodies concerned with nurse migration want to call a halt to international mobility. They realize that nurses function in a global economy and that migration should be an option for those who want to seek new opportunities, new knowledge, and new ways of life. The ICN states that "the fundamental problems which often stimulate nurses' desire to take work in another country—such as poor pay, excessive workloads and violence in the workplace—have not been adequately addressed." The group goes on to say that "the current high level of active international recruitment activity is fuelled by nursing shortages in some developed

382   countries. These destination countries have failed to 'grow their own' and 'keep their own' nurses in sufficient numbers and have used the quick fix of international recruitment, exploiting the existence of push factors, by exerting a 'pull' of better salaries, career opportunities, professional development and improved conditions of employment.

"It is inadequate policy responses by country governments to the fundamental causes of nursing shortages that have been driving the dynamics of aggressive and sometimes exploitive international recruitment. Free trade blocs or agreements may facilitate flows, but these only happen when there is a pull/push imbalance, with the importing country 'pull' being paramount. Recruiting nurses into a dysfunctional health system is at best a short-term solution, and has ethical implications."[30]

Right now governments in many countries, particularly industrialized ones, can afford to ignore these "inadequate policy responses," because they can count on a steady supply of migrant nurses from countries with high birthrates. But what happens when birthrates decline in some of these countries, as they've done in Japan or Singapore? Singapore is dealing with that fact by importing nurses from abroad. Hawthorne describes a fascinating program through which China sends nursing students to bachelor's programs, in Singapore, that are run by Australian schools of nursing. "So Singapore," Hawthorne says, "is the hub and the degree-training body is the Australian university partner. The nurses who are recruited from China pay lower fees in Singapore than they would in Australia. The students use their Mandarin language skills. Singapore meanwhile is providing all the clinical facilities and getting this body of student nurses, whom Singapore relies on and may keep in their nursing work force."

For now, birthrates in Asia are high. "The Philippines look like they'll keep birthrates high for a long time because it's a very Catholic country," Hawthorne continues. "That is what Western nations are relying on. If that ceases to be the case, of course, it will be a very different picture."

Whether we are talking about nurses who migrate from the bedside to a job in advanced practice or nurses who migrate from hospital to hospital, from state to state, or country to country, the issues are the same. Nurse mobility and migration should be an option but it should not be the primary way nurses deal with job-related problems. When it becomes such a popular escape, we should pay close attention to what migrating nurses are telling us about their "home" institutions or homelands. In an effort to lure Filipino nurses to the United States in the mid-1960s, a nurse recruitment agency placed the following ad in a Filipino nursing journal. "Dear Nurse," the ad solicited. "We have placed over 8,000 nurses to different parts of the world. . . . So if you're not happy wherever you are right now, why not take the easy way out and go someplace else.

We can't promise you'll find happiness, but we can help you chase it all **383** over the place."[31]

This ad captures perfectly the appeal of migration and contingent work. To many RNs today, moving around seems to be the only way out. But what are the consequences? Advanced practice, temp and travel agencies, and international recruiters are attracting a new kind of nurse—one who, if he or she had better options, might have stayed at the bedside longer, mentored and encouraged students and new nurses, and shared their wisdom on their units and within their institutions. These nurses might also have joined the fight for better working conditions. Because of their seniority in their institutions, they might have had more influence over other RNs. While advancing their own interests, they would also advance the collective good. Today, however, migratory nursing divides nurses into competing groups and encourages nurses to vote with their feet.

Sean Clarke states it well when he says, "If you're a temporary nurse, you don't have to become part of the political battles or struggles, or even the moral dilemmas that come up in practice. You can numb yourself to it and get yourself through your stint in that particular place. This means that the kind of community that is built on the best nursing units never gets formed. Or the person becomes a free rider on that community and the benefits the permanent staff have created."

While travel, temp, and international recruitment agencies celebrate the myriad possibilities involved in endless job and geographic mobility, underneath the appeals to optimism, they play on a deep and disturbing pessimism. When nurses believe that exit is their only option, they are really expressing their profound sense of defeat. In effect, they are raising a white flag and admitting that the work of caring for the sick is no good, will never be any good, and thus, the only way to adapt is to get in and out as quickly as possible, go for the gold, and work only when you want. This individualistic approach to systemic problems that must be solved collectively is doomed to failure. Nursing the sick is, at heart, a collective activity. It's a 24/7, 365-day-a-year responsibility. Nurses have to be willing to work at night, on weekends, and holidays because patient needs don't stop when the nurse clocks out after a twelve-hour shift. Now that fewer young people are willing to embark on a career that promises only sacrifice, institutions have to offer incentives to make some of the imperatives of nursing work seem worthwhile. Some nurses will willingly work odd hours if they are rewarded and recognized for so doing, and if their needs are accommodated in other ways. To ask nurses to adjust their schedules to patient need and to work longer and harder in chaotic, unpredictable, underfunded settings is asking too much. It's clearly not good for nurses and nursing. And it may be a disaster for patients.

14

Failure to Rescue

Lucy Danforth* was fifty-three when she and her husband Jim* raced to the emergency room of a Massachusetts hospital one night in 2002. Danforth, a nurse, couldn't walk without a walker, had terrible back pain, and a lab test confirmed the presence of bacteria in her bloodstream. She was transferred to an intensive care unit at the Tufts New England Medical Center (NEMC) in Boston because sepsis due to an epidural abscess had produced multisystem failure.

Emily Lowry, an internist whom we first met in Chapter 1, was one of Lucy's oldest friends. When Lucy was transferred to NEMC, Lowry, who lives nearby, became closely involved in her friend's hospital care. Because Lucy was from out of town, she didn't have an admitting doctor who was familiar with either the patient or the details of the case. The service team—the team of physicians who staff the unit and rotate in and out each month—were the doctors in charge. Lowry was thus the only physician who really knew Lucy. Because Lucy and Jim lived about two hours away, Jim couldn't be continually present at her bedside. He had to take care of their children, and he couldn't afford to take a lot of time off work and risk losing his job. With his wife's income in jeopardy, this was particularly important.

Jim made sure Lowry was put on the list of approved visitors (on ICUs only family members and special friends are allowed to come onto the unit). He gave clear instructions that nurses and doctors should talk to Lowry and give her information anytime, night or day.

Lucy stayed on the unit for six weeks. She ended up with severe weakness in all her extremities. Because of the infection to her cervical spinal cord, she was completely paralyzed on her left side. She eventually left the ICU and was transferred to the New England Sinai Hospital and Rehabilitation Center's satellite inpatient unit at NEMC. She was there for a few weeks, and after a short stint at another rehab facility, she was readmitted to the ICU at NEMC and died two weeks later.

The story Emily Lowry tells about her friend's nursing care is a disturbing one. "I've seen great nursing and how it can help patients," Lowry says. "But this was not great nursing. It wasn't even mediocre nursing. It was terrible. You could see how busy these nurses were, how active the unit was, and the patient and everyone else connected with her suffered as a result."

When Lucy first arrived on the ICU, she got good physical care, but the communication was poor, or so Lowry thought as a doctor. It took a week to find a consistent nurse with whom she and Jim could communicate. "With the nurses, every time I visited, I had to explain who I was over and over again. Jim had approved me to receive information. But each time, every single time, I talked to a nurse, I had to explain why it was okay for them to talk to me. It was very painful to have to go through this suspicious questioning, 'Who are you? Why are you here? What do you want?' It was as though there was no unit memory. When you asked a question, it was so impersonal, and they made you feel like a worm. At the end of her stay we finally found a communicative nurse who would give us details and really talk to us. That was so, so important. But it was at the very end."

Things got even worse, she says, when Lucy went to Sinai. Remember, she says, Lucy was totally dependent on nursing care. She could not get up by herself. If she needed to go to the bathroom, the nurses had to come and move her. If she needed to get out of bed, she was lifted by a special device called a Hoyer lift. Two nurses had to manipulate the lift. Supposedly the unit was in the business of rehabilitation, which means you don't let a patient lie around. You get them up, even dressed. But no, they never dressed Lucy.

What was worse, Lowry says, "the nurses made Lucy feel like her needs were irritating to them. If she needed to get up, they would come over and sigh. I heard them, watched them. You had the sense that they had a lot of patients." For four terrible weeks, Lucy endured their sighs and disdain. Lowry and Jim complained. An ombudsman came in. "But," Lowry says, "when we talked to them, they just couldn't see that they weren't doing a good job. Lucy was a nurse, and she'd say, in tears, 'I would never make a patient feel this way.' She was terrified of certain shifts, of being trapped with a bunch of nasty nurses."

Lucy Danforth isn't the only nurse-patient to suffer because nurses are

386 so overextended today. The experience of another nurse, Richard Ferri, is particularly telling. If nurses define their mission as providing holistic care and emotional support, Ferri was their perfect candidate. A nurse practitioner, he had just moved to New York and was a few blocks from ground zero when he watched the Twin Towers disappear from the face of the earth. Almost immediately after, he noticed what he thought was a hemorrhoid, only to find out he had rectal cancer. He was operated on and then only a few weeks later suffered from a collapsed lung. While he was sick, his mother and his aunt, who was, he said, like a second mother to him, died. Ferri, who is HIV positive, was a wreck, both physically and emotionally. As a nurse, he knew just what he needed. Most of all, he required pain management, to help him cope with the agony of rectal surgery and then people cutting into his chest and shoving tubes between his ribs and scarred lungs. But not only that: he also needed a sympathetic person to talk to, and a little human kindness.

He got none of the above.

When he had his rectal surgery, the nurses were so overworked and stressed he worried that they didn't seem to know what they were doing. "They loudly referred to me as the 'guy with AIDS.' When the recovery room nurse asked me how bad my pain was I told her I wanted to die it was so horrible. She just smiled and said, 'That's nice, dear.'"

When he had chest tubes put in and removed, he said, "I had to beg for pain medication. People would come in and ask me how my pain was on a scale of one to ten while I was practically turning blue from the agony, and I'd say, 'Help!' and they wouldn't. One nurse called me a wimp when I begged for morphine while they were slipping the third chest tube in and I could feel it grind against my ribs and the fresh scar tissue. 'Look at your big muscles and you crying like that.'" Ferri groaned and nurses and doctors chatted. "Everyone was so damned stressed out and overworked. All they kept on doing was slipping into survival mode, making sure all the right boxes are checked so the 'standard' would be documented. Screw the patient. No time for that." This happened, Ferri said, at two different Massachusetts hospitals, Cape Cod Hospital and the Massachusetts General Hospital.

Finally, there is the story of Madge Kaplan, then the Boston bureau chief and Health Desk editor for Public Radio's *Marketplace* show, who tells about her father's hospitalization in the winter of 1999. Kaplan's eighty-one-year-old father had a stroke and was sent to a major New York teaching hospital, where he spent a total of three months on its inpatient and rehabilitation units.

The medical aspects of his care, Kaplan explains, were excellent. The nursing care wasn't. "If my father or the three other patients in his room needed to go to the bathroom, if they needed to reposition themselves to eat a meal, if they needed help in adjusting their position in a wheelchair, if they needed help unwrapping utensils to eat a meal, that help was not forthcoming."

It was "tragic," Kaplan says, to watch "these frightened, frail, elderly patients push themselves to the limit of their energy to get someone to pay attention to them, pleading with someone to get a glass of water or to wipe someone up when they had spilled something on their bed."

Kaplan understood that the nursing staff was overwhelmed. "Nurses seemed to have their hands full. So much so that I always came away feeling that the staff seemed tense, stretched, and in no mood to engage with patients and the people visiting them."

Although boosters of market-driven health care insist that "consumers" like Kaplan and her father will vigorously advocate for themselves when they don't get the service they expect, neither complained to hospital administration. Like many people who are sick, vulnerable, and totally dependent, they are loath to alienate those who hold their lives in their hands. "My father was in the institution for several months and continued to get outpatient treatment there," Kaplan says. "He was dependent on people there. He was too nervous about possible repercussions to complain."

In this chapter I am concerned with what happens to patients when nurses confront the problems outlined in the previous chapters. Of the hundreds of stories that patients have told me about the care they have received from harried nurses, I chose Lowry, Danforth, Ferri, and Kaplan for a reason. All of them are savvy health care consumers and then some. Emily Lowry's a physician. Lucy Danforth was a nurse. Richard Ferri is a nurse practitioner. Madge Kaplan is a health care journalist. They know the ropes. The system isn't an alien universe to them. Danforth and Ferri knew precisely the kind of nursing care they needed and mostly didn't get. If these people couldn't get the attention of nurses and the attentive, empathetic care they or their friends or loved ones needed, how can sick people with no health care savvy hope to advocate for themselves? "When you think about it," says Lowry, "it's frightening to imagine being stuck in a hospital with an unkind doctor, but it's even more terrifying to think of being at the mercy of a mean nurse. If you have a mean doctor, you can always complain to the nurse, but if you have a mean nurse, you're completely defenseless."

When I think about the consequences that patients are suffering because of the lack of nurses and nursing care, I always remind myself that

388 we're dealing with sick people, frightened people, difficult cases, relentless need. Sure, nurses and doctors go into their careers with eyes wide open. But sometimes, even on the best of days, they might wish that their eyes were tightly shut. Danforth, Ferri, and Madge Kaplan's father were hard work. Under the best circumstances, nurses may groan at another ring of the bell. But they buck up and do their job. Much of the time, they consider it a welcome challenge. If they don't, they usually put on an act and pretend it's not a burden. But add job stress, too many patients, a nurse's own health problems, and you are likely to get what these patient got—poor care, or even what seems to be a heartless withdrawal from the patient when the patient's needs just won't go away.

Patients notice how busy nurses are. Sometimes they're infuriated. Sometimes they feel sorry for the nurses. Nurses have told me that patients will say that they've noticed how harried nurses are and don't want to bother them—to report, for example, that they've been experiencing chest pain for the past couple of hours. Dana Beth Weinberg's doctoral dissertation, which ultimately turned into *Code Green*, began when her thesis advisor was a patient at the Beth Israel Deaconess Medical Center. She'd expected the nurses coming in and out of her room to be calm and attentive to the needs of their patient. The professor instead found a bunch of frazzled RNs who practically dissolved in tears because of the stresses they experienced. Get over there and see what's going on, Weinberg's advisor suggested to her, and she did.

What the Studies Tell Us

During the 1990s hospital administrators were publicly denying, but privately documenting, that nurses were absolutely on target in their Cassandra-like warnings about the impact of cost cutting on patient care. Thus in 1996 the American Hospital Association sent its members a confidential report entitled "Reality Check: Public Perceptions of Health Care and Hospitals." The report summarized data gathered in focus groups with three hundred patients in twelve states, as well as an opinion survey of another one thousand patients. "Reality Check" said that the "the key indicator that people referred to as a measure of quality of their hospital care was the nurse. . . . When individuals related a positive experience with hospital care and quality, it was always a story about the skill and compassion of caregivers, usually nurses."

The report, however, went on to say that those surveyed "hold a strong belief that skilled nurses are being systematically replaced by poorly trained and poorly paid aides. Their perspective on the 'thinness' of hospital nurse staffing was reflected in a universally mentioned experience: 'If

I hadn't stayed in the hospital room with my mother, child or spouse, they would never have gotten the correct medication or care on time.' People believe the profit motive is behind the reduction in nursing care. They are angry at the reversal in health care priorities this represents."[1]

Dozens of studies and reports have confirmed that cost cutting and hospital restructuring have hardly been a boon for patients in hospitals with dedicated AIDS units or in magnet hospitals. When Linda Aiken and her colleagues analyzed the care of AIDS patients in hospitals with dedicated AIDS units or in magnet hospitals, they documented that "an additional 0.5 nurse per patient day—or an additional nurse for every six patients on each eight-hour shift—would be expected to reduce the likelihood of dying by roughly one-third."[2] In another study, Donna Diers and Cindy Czaplinski found that patients taken care of by nurses who specialized in particular problems cut length of stay and mortality rates.[3] Gil Preuss, at MIT, found that assigning aides to perform nursing activities, like helping patients eat, bathe, and walk or changing sterile dressings, decreases the quality of information that both nurses and doctors receive and leads to medication errors.[4] Harvard professors David Himmelstein and Steffie Woolhandler have done studies of for-profit hospitals, documenting that they skimp on nursing care and that this helps explain some of their poor patient outcomes.[5]

In October 2000 Michael Rie, an anesthesiologist and intensive care physician at the University of Kentucky, presented a quality assurance analysis of ICU readmissions in one university hospital. The data were collected in response to findings that the average length of ICU stay for patients with respiratory problems was longer than that predicted by a nationally accepted benchmark tool. The study found that patients at low risk of death and/or readmission to ICU—who had been discharged to regular hospital floors—were being readmitted at a seemingly elevated rate. Patients with a predicted 10 percent risk of death had an actual mortality rate of 24 percent.

When investigators explored why patients were readmitted to the ICU, they discovered that 80 percent of these patients had potentially preventable ICU readmissions. The problem was they weren't receiving enough basic respiratory care on hospital floors. A plausible inference is that there weren't enough staff in this hospital to suction patients' lungs and help them cough.

Not only was this costing patients their health and sometimes their lives, it was also not cost-effective. In this particular hospital, for example, the nonlabor costs for the ICU readmission of only 79 patients was $1,600,000, or 35 percent of the cost of their entire hospitalization. If labor costs were added to this figure, it would be two to three times as high.[6]

In 1998, Christine Kovner and Peter J. Gergen published a study that

390 found a correlation between nursing care and four adverse events following surgery. These were venous thrombosis or a pulmonary embolism, lung problems (congestion, edema, respiratory insufficiency or failure), urinary tract infections (UTIs), and pneumonia. This study found that better staffing meant fewer of these adverse events.[7] Kovner and Gergen, along with several other researchers, revisited these four postsurgical problems in a 2002 study, where they looked at data on nurse staffing levels in short-term general hospitals in the United States between 1990 and 1996. They examined the same four problems previously studied, trying to refine the results by better controlling for severity of illness. The researchers once again found a positive relationship with nurse staffing.[8]

In 2002 the *New England Journal of Medicine* published an article by Jack Needleman and colleagues that analyzed administrative data from 799 hospitals in eleven states, comprising 5,075,969 discharges of medical patients and 1,104,659 discharges of surgical patients. They asked what the relationship was between nurse staffing and patient outcomes. It turns out that once again the relationship was positive. "A higher proportion of nursing care provided by registered nurses and a greater number of hours of care by registered nurses per day are associated with better care for hospitalized patients." In hospitals where patients were cared for by a higher proportion of RNs, and a lower proportion of licensed practical nurses and nursing aides, medical patients had lower rates of pneumonia, shock or cardiac arrest, and failure to rescue. When patients had both more RNs and more hours of RN care per day, there were lower rates of urinary tract infections and upper gastrointestinal bleeding. For surgical patients, more RNs produced fewer UTIs, and more RN hours of care per day meant a lower rate of failure to rescue.[9] Since patients on both medical and surgical units are at risk for a whole slew of problems including the ones the researchers studied, it clearly makes sense to have more RNs caring for them and to give those RNs the ability to deliver more patient care to each patient each day.

When the Society for Healthcare Epidemiology of America, the Joint Commission on the Accreditation of Health Care Organizations (JCAHO), and the Center for Disease Control's Prevention Epicenters Program joined to sponsor a study on some of the processes involved in infection control in fifty-four ICUs in the U.S. and fourteen other countries, the researchers reported similar findings. Although the study didn't focus exclusively on nurses, adequate staffing had a positive influence on preventing bloodstream infections.[10]

On the topic of infection control, a fascinating article in the *Journal of Trauma* reported as early as 1982 how nurse staffing influences the incidence of serious infections on burn units. Burn victims who have lost their primary barrier to infection, their skin, are very vulnerable to infection. Methicillin-resistant *Staphylococcus aureus* (MRS) has been a serious problem for burn victims, whose ability to fight infection is so severely compromised. Nurses are constantly touching burn victims, and a nurse's hand, when placed on or near a patient's body, is a perfect way to spread infection, particularly during the arduous and often extensive process of changing dressings that may cover as much as 70 percent—or more—of the patient's body.

In this study, the authors found that the risk of patients developing MRS infections was related to nurse staffing on the burn unit. "Staffing of the burn unit with overtime or temporary nurses was associated with increased documentation of MRS transmission," the authors stated. "The occurrence of new cases . . . approximately paralleled the number of overtime hours worked by regular burn unit nurses and the number of shifts worked in the burn unit by nursing personnel assigned temporarily from other hospital areas [i.e., float nurses]. This association was significant . . . and was thought by experienced burn unit nurses to reflect the occasional errors in aseptic technique that most likely occur during periods of fatigue or when personnel are not completely familiar with burn unit routine [in other words, context-dependent expertise]."[11] A number of other subsequent studies have confirmed this relationship between nurse staffing and infection control on ICUs.[12]

When researchers have studied medication errors, another critical problem in hospitals and health care, they again noted the critical role of nurses in preventing errors. One study of 334 medication errors connected to 264 preventable adverse events that took place in two hospitals over six months illuminated the role RNs play. It found that a nurse who has the time to check is the most likely health care worker to discover a medication error made by a physician, by a clerk transcribing the physician's order, or by a pharmacist dispensing that order. In this study almost half of the errors physicians made (think back to Kimberly Hahn and her encounter with the intern) were intercepted before they could harm the patient. "About one-third of transcription and dispensing errors had been intercepted prior to administration, again largely by nurses. Overall, nurses were responsible for intercepting 86 percent of all medication errors made by those in all disciplines." Studies have shown when nurses are distracted by too many interruptions—when, for example, they must take care of too many patients—medication errors are more likely to occur and that overwork and fatigue may also impact error rates.[13]

If nurses are to intercept, or avoid making, medication errors and thus prevent the hospital equivalent of a midair collision, they have to have time to pay attention to these routine hospital events. Their ability to do

392 so can be seriously limited when they have to care for too many patients or deal with too many doctors, other clinicians, and health care workers, not to mention job stress, fatigue, sleep deprivation, and burnout.[14] "To the extent that such interruptions and distractions take place, patient safety is threatened," as the Institute of Medicine succinctly puts it.[15]

Perhaps the most dramatic recent study was conducted by Linda Aiken and her colleagues and published in the *Journal of the American Medical Association*. The researchers pored over the records of 232,342 surgical patients and surveys from 10,184 nurses in Pennsylvania to analyze the link between nurse staffing and increased risk of patients dying after surgery. They also considered separately the impact of staffing on nurse burnout and job dissatisfaction. The nurses worked in 168 different hospitals, and the data reported on were neither unit- nor shift-specific. Nonetheless, the researchers knew that all the nurses surveyed actively cared for patients.

Investigators calculated the average patient load for all the nurses in each hospital and found that for every additional patient in the workload, the risk of the patient dying increased by 7 percent. The more patients the nurses look after, on average, the higher the mortality risk for patients across the whole range of staffing levels in those hospitals. There were hospitals where nurses looked after four patients on average, and hospitals where nurses looked after eight. For every one additional patient per nurse, there was a 7 percent increase in mortality. Adding an extra patient to the nurse's average caseload also increased the risk of job dissatisfaction by 15 percent and the risk of burnout by 23 percent.[16]

"There are a few morals to this story," says researcher Sean Clarke. "Hospitals use nurses at different levels and these variations in levels aren't always in the patient's best interests. We and other researchers are finding that there are differences in patients' risks of having bad outcomes. Not only between the hospitals with the highest and lowest staffing, but also in between the two extremes. Nurse staffing is a public safety issue."

JCAHO issued another set of disturbing findings in 2002. It found that inadequate nurse staffing levels contributed to nearly a quarter of the 1,609 cases of accidental injury or death documented for hospitalized patients since 1997. Nurse-staffing levels contributed to 50 percent of ventilator-related incidents, 42 percent of surgery-related incidents, and 25 percent of transfusion-related incidents. Staffing problems were also related to 25 percent of delays in treatment, 19 percent of medication errors, 14 percent of inpatient suicides, and 14 percent of patient falls.[17]

These studies and many more add statistical rigor and scientific legitimacy to the stories that we have heard in previous chapters, and which health care administrators, politicians, and journalists have often dismissed as merely "anecdotal." To understand better the significance of these studies, however, it's useful to see just how many patients are at risk for the problems these researchers have investigated, as well as some of their potential costs. It's also important to know what nurses do to prevent them, which, in turn, helps us understand why they are needed in hospitals and other settings.

Early Intervention, Warning, and Action

Let's look first at infections. We know that nosocomial (hospital-acquired) infections are one of the greatest risks of illness and its treatment. Studies have shown that urinary tract infections account for up to 40 percent of hospital-acquired infections. Bacteremia—the presence of bacteria in the blood—accounts for a small percent of such infections. Patients who are elderly, women who are menopausal, and those with diabetes are at particular risk for urinary tract infections and bacteremia. These risks are increased with the use of urinary catheters. Sticking a foreign object into the urethra is an absolutely perfect way to introduce bacteria into the bladder, where if unchecked it can migrate to the kidneys and potentially enter the bloodstream.

The first thing a nurse should do about this danger is make sure a patient really needs to be catheterized. Inappropriate use of catheters raises the risk of infection. Here again, patient loads enter into the calculation. If you don't have time to get your patient to the bathroom or give them a bedpan, it's much more convenient to catheterize the patient unnecessarily than to worry about answering her call bell or cleaning up after her if you can't. If the patient does need to be catheterized, the nurse has to use proper hand washing and sterile technique when he inserts a catheter; must know how to manipulate the catheter properly and insert it; and, over the course of a patient's stay, has to keep it clean. He also has to keep an eye on the position of the catheter to make sure the bag doesn't somehow get lifted higher than the patient's bladder (for example, if the foot of the bed where the urine bag is hanging, is jacked up). If that happens urine will spill back into the bladder, rather than exiting from it, causing a real backup problem and another great way to get an infection. Similarly, nurses have to remove urinary catheters when the patient is able to void on their own so that the catheter isn't in use longer than necessary.

Urinary tract infections do not come cheap. Each episode of hospital-acquired urinary tract infection can add an additional $676 to the cost of a hospital stay, while a hospital-acquired bacteremia can add up to $2,836 and may even lead to death.[18] Other cases of infections may occur because

394 of the use of central venous catheters, which are increasingly common in the treatment of patients with cancer, on dialysis machines, and on intensive care units. Infections from central venous catheters, we recall, result in thousands of deaths annually and can add billions of dollars to health care costs. Which is why Jennifer Hawkins, the nurse manager we met in Chapter 12, tried to save her line team.

Let's move on to pneumonias. Just on intensive care units, 20 to 40 percent of patients suffer from hospital-acquired pneumonias. Patients who suffer from these pneumonias have a mean stay of 28.5 days. These patients suffer more complications including shock, renal, respiratory, and heart failure, liver problems, and other infections. Up to 43 percent of ICU patients with pneumonias will die.[19] Nurses help prevent pneumonias by helping patients to cough after surgery, by doing chest physical therapy to move secretions around, by mechanically suctioning the patients' lungs, and by getting them up to move. In stroke patients, they prevent aspiration pneumonias (caused by food going to the wrong place) by making sure a patient can safely feed himself. Patients whose gag reflexes are impaired will not be able to swallow correctly and have to be fed carefully.

Nursing care is also key in the prevention or management of bedsores or pressure ulcers, which are a major problem in hospitals and nursing homes. These deep, gaping wounds result when prolonged pressure, generally on a bony part of the body like a hip or ankle, reduces its blood supply. Hospital and nursing home patients are particularly at risk for pressure ulcers because many are completely or partially immobile, are incontinent or have poor bladder control, or have poor nutrition and impaired mental status. Studies have documented that up to 13 percent of patients in nursing homes and 3 to 11 percent of hospitalized patients are at risk for pressure ulcers. In patients who are between seventy and eighty-nine years old, the incidence of risk jumps to 54 percent. The cost of treating only one pressure ulcer can range from $5,000 to $70,000.[20] Constantly shifting a patient's position, making sure the patient is bathed with moisturizing soaps, cleaning delicate skin gently, and carefully cleaning out washing basins used to bathe patients make an enormous difference. Similarly, nurses must have the time to check that patients are not lying in feces or urine, that they are well nourished, and that they are frequently turned.[21]

Next we come to two other potentially catastrophic risks of hospitalization—venous thromboembolism and pulmonary embolism. These complications result when blood stagnates in the legs of patients who aren't moving enough and eventually forms clots. The resulting deep vein thrombosis (DVT) or blood clot, if not quickly spotted and treated, can lead to a pulmonary embolism and potentially to death. Unless preventive measures are taken, 20 percent of patients undergoing major surgeries may suffer from DVT and 1 to 2 percent will have a pulmonary embolism. Of patients undergoing major orthopedic surgeries, 50 percent are at risk for DVT, with up to 30 percent at risk for pulmonary embolism. Similarly, up to 16 percent of patients hospitalized for general medical conditions may develop DVT. The average length of stay for a hospital readmission for DVT is 13 to 14.9 days. The average cost of treating a three-month episode of DVT is $12,000 for the medications alone.[22]

Moreover, patients who have had blood clots may suffer lifelong side effects. They are at greater risk for having another clot, particularly if they are immobile—say, on a long airplane or car ride. Some, though certainly not all, may develop post-phlebitic syndrome. This happens because the clot has damaged valves in the vein so that they don't close properly when blood isn't moving up toward the heart. The venous scarring and valve dysfunction can cause patients to have swelling in their legs and sometimes a great deal of pain. There's no medication to treat this side effect. A few patients may be at such high risk for another clot that they have to take lifelong anticoagulatory therapy.

To prevent DVT, nurses make sure that patients walk, exercise, wear special stockings, or are administered preventive medications. Because these problems can't always be prevented, nurses are constantly on the lookout for subtle changes in a patient's condition that can indicate a case of DVT or a pulmonary embolism. Their quick action can save lives.

All patients in the hospital are also at risk for medication errors. When patients are injured because of a drug error, malpractice costs go up, length of stay increases, and hospital costs increase—and this list leaves out the patient's suffering. One study estimated that the "annual national cost of drug-related morbidity and mortality . . . was recently estimated at $76.6 billion, with the majority ($47 billion) related to hospital admissions associated with drug therapy or the absence of the appropriate drug therapy."[23]

In 1991 Lucien Leape and his colleagues at Harvard studied adverse events (medication errors and other hospital errors and injuries) suffered by hospitalized patients in New York. Of the patients studied, 3.7 percent experienced adverse events, with the majority suffering adverse drug events (ADEs) or medication errors. According to this study, the patients most vulnerable to medication errors and to adverse effects from medication errors are the elderly, who are the majority of hospitalized patients.[24] In two 1995 studies, researchers found that the ADE rate was 6.5 per admission, with 28 percent of these problems deemed preventable.[25]

When Bates and his colleagues examined this problem again in 1997,

396   they analyzed 4,108 admissions in two Boston teaching hospitals—the Brigham and Women's Hospital and the Massachusetts General Hospital. Not all admissions results include adverse events. The authors found 247 medication errors among 207 admissions. After adjusting for a number of variables—severity of illness, age of patient, case mix of the hospital, estimated length of patient stay in the hospital—they found that each ADE added 2.2 days to the hospital stay and that the increased cost of such an error was $3,244. When it came to preventable errors, the average patient's stay increased by 4.6 days and the total cost increase was $5,857. The estimated costs were $2,595 for all ADEs and $4,685 for preventable ADEs. Based on these figures, the authors estimated that the costs of adverse drug events and preventable adverse drug events in a seven-hundred-bed teaching hospital are $5.6 and $2.8 million respectively.[26]

In another study, researchers found that patients sixty-five and older were almost twice as likely to suffer from adverse drug events than younger patients. For elderly patients, preventable medication errors related to medical procedures were far more common, which led the researchers to suggest specifically that much greater attention be paid to preventing drug errors in the elderly.[27]

When patients are sent home quicker and sicker, home care nurses are the equivalent early-warning and intervention system, or what JCAHO has called "the front line of patient defense." Home care nurses monitor patients' wounds, diet, medication compliance, and their understanding of how to take medications and how to prevent the development of bedsores.[28] The home care nurse is constantly making sure patients are safe on their own and have access to other services like those provided by home health aides and family members, who may be either eager to help but uneducated, reluctant to participate, or even absent. We saw what happened to my friend Joe when his attentive and concerned family wasn't aware of a crucial aspect of his care—helping him walk—and home care nursing was missing. How can nurses provide this vigilance if home care services have been so severely restricted, and if the nurses available to provide care have so little time to spend with patients?

Nurses play a critical role in preventing drug errors in the home when they educate patients about how to take medication. In its highly publicized report *To Err Is Human: Building a Safer Health System*, the Institute of Medicine recommended that clinicians spend much more time with patients reviewing medications and how to take them properly.[29] Again, how can a harried nurse help accomplish what is now becoming a Sisyphean feat? In the hospital, the nurse simply doesn't have the thirty or forty minutes it might take to review carefully how the patient should take his medicine at home, once he's filled the multiple prescriptions he usually receives before leaving the hospital.

Nor may she have much time to attend to patients who are screaming out in pain. When Richard Ferri cried out in pain after his rectal surgery or when a chest tube was pushed into or pulled out of his lungs, he begged for adequate pain medication. He wasn't just being a sissy, as his apparently heartless nurse suggested. Studies have documented that pain is not simply an uncomfortable emotional sensation. It is produced by damage to the tissues following trauma, surgery, or cancer. When that kind of trauma occurs, tissues break down, the metabolic rate increases, blood forms clots, water is retained, and immune function is impaired. Patients in pain may breathe shallowly and suppress coughing. This, in turn, prevents the movement of lung secretions and increases the risk of pneumonia. Because it's too painful to move, some patients won't. This increases the risk of DVT and pulmonary embolism. When patients don't move after surgery, neither the bowel nor the stomach resumes normal functioning. This can lead to severe constipation, bowel obstruction, and aspiration pneumonia.[30]

Nurses are key in evaluating patients for pain. Nurses know that many patients, particularly elderly ones, believe that a stoic attitude toward pain—enduring pain without medication—proves strength of character. They know patients may fear pain medication and its side effects more than pain itself. They know that the fact that a patient does not complain about pain does not mean he or she isn't in pain. Indeed, they are well aware that a patient in pain may deny that pain, and many patients even smile and laugh in an effort to cope with their agony. But if a nurse doesn't have time, he won't be able to manage a patient's pain adequately. When the patients are in pain, they become a greater burden on the already overburdened nurse, who may, like most overstressed people, reconfigure a desperate plea for help as an irritant and turn against the patient rather than helping him.

Energy and Empathy

The stories that began this chapter are distressing. They don't just show nurses on the run. These patients, friends, and family members talk about nurses who seem to be almost callous, if not downright cruel. Did Kaplan, Lowry, and Ferri just happen to come across a bunch of really nasty nurses? Maybe. More likely, they encountered nurses who were burned out. These nurses may have gone home feeling guilty about the fact that

398 they couldn't respond to Kaplan's father and his elderly hospital mates, to Ferri and his pain, to Lucy and her request to go to the bathroom. Not many nurses are going to admit this to an irate patient or family member, an administrator, or an ombudsman inquiring why they aren't being more sympathetic. But when I've talked to RNs, many say they don't feel proud of themselves. They're expected to care—and expect themselves to care—but they simply can't.

As oncology nurse Erica Wilson explained to me, in her cancer clinic nurses are so tightly scheduled that they have no time to process their feelings about their very needy patients. She knows that most of her patients are dealing with a terminal diagnosis and some may die very soon indeed. With great distress, Wilson confessed that she finds her capacity for empathy has decreased. After five or six hours on the job, she doesn't want to learn about another problem a patient has. She just doesn't have the emotional energy to deal with it. As the day becomes more wearing, she finds that she may deal with the relentless "barrage of problems patients have by getting numb." Some nurses have told me they almost don't want to find out that their patients or their families have emotional problems, because they won't have time to deal with them.

In a 2004 study on the care of the dying published in the *Journal of the American Medical Association*, investigators surveyed the family members and friends of 1,578 people who had died from chronic illnesses in 2000. Many of these respondents reported that unless their loved ones were in hospice care, they did not receive physical comfort and emotional support. There was poor communication between caregivers and those they cared for, lack of respect for the dying, little coordination of the care of the dying, and little emotional support for the patient's family.[31] Joan Teno, a Brown University geriatrician and the study's lead investigator, commented that "we're moving toward factory medicine: get 'em in, get 'em out."[32]

We've listened to nurses tell us, "I feel numb," "I can't stop," "I have to move on," "I'm becoming someone I don't like." These statements capture perfectly the emotional numbing and withdrawal that is typical of an acute stress response and its accompanying burnout. The nurse is going to be far too busy fighting or fleeing to come down long enough to calm a distressed patient. While some hospital administrators and health care policy makers seem to believe that the nurse should flit her angel's wings and manifest her saintliness, this is an unrealistic appraisal. As Marco Iacoboni, a neurologist and associate professor of psychiatry and biobehavioral science at UCLA, reminds us, studies suggest that too much stress causes animals to withdraw from one another and to be less empathetic. Studies have shown that humans are more likely to help one another if they believe that they are, in fact, able to do something to help that person. "If you have someone undergoing an extreme stress reaction, what I can see happening is that the empathetic abilities of these individuals will withdraw too," Iacoboni warns. This happens, he told me, because the nurse's brain is reacting in automatic and unconscious ways, and she will find it difficult to control the stress response provoked by the workplace. If she works in an environment where patients are shoved around or ignored, she may well reproduce this aggression.

Even more important in helping us understand how working conditions and empathy interact are studies that illuminate the role neural mechanisms play in empathy. Iacoboni and his co-investigators have used brain-imaging techniques to uncover the fundamental neural mechanisms they believe are key to the production of empathy in humans. They argue that human beings who are particularly empathetic are able to mobilize this response because they are able to subtly imitate the fear, happiness, anxiety, or anger that someone else is feeling. This act of imitation is, these researchers say, "a neurobiological marker of the ability to empathize."[33]

Studies on neuroanatomy and neurophysiology help us understand that empathy—for the nurse or anyone else—is not simply a matter of appropriate upbringing, education, exhortation, will power, virtue, or religious conviction. To be empathetic, it's important to be in the presence of another human being. In the common phrase, you need to walk in his or her shoes so that imitation is triggered. Auditory signals are also effective, Iacoboni says, but visual ones are dominant. The consequences of lack of patient contact may thus be multiple. If nurses don't have time to be with the patient, they obviously can't elicit information from the patient that might help guide their empathetic responses. More crucially, if they can't observe the need or suffering of the patient, it will be difficult for them to engage the neural process that seems to allow them to respond with empathy.

"The main point is that there isn't any such thing as abstract empathy," Iacoboni says. "You really need to be in touch with the patient to empathize with the patient. If the nurses do not have time to be with the patient, that's a major problem because they won't be able to produce empathy without going through this whole neural process."

Iacoboni reaches two conclusions about the nurses' predicament. The first is that "they should not be subjected to such stressful situations because the best way to take care of other people is not to work in stressful working conditions." And the second is that "they should be in touch with their patients all the time. This is because there are some basic neural mechanisms that we can't change. We can't just say okay, this is just a mat-

400 ter of will. There are some objective conditions that make it easier or more difficult to be empathetic and to take care of other people."

Health care administrators today, lulled by traditional images of the saintly nurse, often manage to convince themselves that nurses will somehow be caring and compassionate in spite of all the obstacles strewn in their path. "Most health service managers do not wish to downgrade caring any more than clinicians, but they are compelled to seek efficiency in terms that effectively ignore what is difficult to measure," wrote British physician Julian Tudor Hart and professor of health services research Paul Dieppe in a now famous article in the *Lancet*. These decision makers, Tudor Hart said, often believe that "if they run a tight ship on clinical measures, human support will take care of itself."[34] But understanding the human brain and how it may intersect with nurses' working conditions helps us see why this isn't the case. Caring won't take care of itself in contemporary health care because nurses' brains and physiological circuitry just can't overcome nurses' work environment.

Conclusion:
Changing the Odds

As the nursing crisis and shortage worsens, a variety of high-level summits have been called to consider solutions. At these meetings, participants are invariably exhorted to "push the envelope" and "think outside the box." But it often turns out that all sorts of out-of-the-box solutions—things like union activity, government regulation, safe staffing ratios, universal health care—are off limits. Sitting through these meetings and listening to this or that idea ruled out of order, I've often wondered how nurses can change the odds that work against them when so many potential solutions are excluded from consideration. So far in this book, I've focused on the difficult job conditions, complex professional relationships, and internal group tensions that have rigged the odds to work against nurses. In this concluding chapter, I'd like to assess the pros and cons of some of the various antidotes that have been proposed for the nursing crisis.

We are fortunate to have many working nurses, researchers, academics, union activists, hospital administrators, and health care policy experts who are engaged, all over the world, in exciting efforts to change the culture of nursing through enhancement of nurses' education and workplace author-ity, more relevant nursing research, and effective public advocacy of health care reform. Although it is impossible to discuss all of the "best practices" that have emerged, the ones I discuss are definitely part of the solution. Other initiatives, also described below, are clearly would-be panaceas that fail to address the fundamental problem. Without systemic change, good experiments with alternative models of nursing practice—like the nursing advances developed at the Beth Israel in Boston or in Magnet hospitals—

402 will remain isolated and vulnerable to hospital restructuring and cost cutting. On an individual level, if nurses continue to be treated as interchangeable and disposable units of "production" on a health care assembly line, many more will leave their profession in frustration, regardless of how many "competencies" they develop before dropping out.

Similarly, if we do not add the concept of necessary nursing care to that of necessary medical care, health care policy and funding priorities will never support the kind of nursing that patients need. The public needs to understand the educational process necessary to produce the kind of nurse they assume or hope will answer their call bell, the kind of scientific, technical, medical, emotional, and social knowledge and skills that the nurse calls upon to fulfill her or his mandate to care for the sick, and the organizational and social structures and resources that must be in place if good nurses are to provide good nursing.[1]

Changing the odds for nurses requires that we remember two things about nursing. One is the specificity of the work. As I said earlier, nurses, like doctors and others who work in health care, spend their days with sick, suffering, dying human beings. Even when they are doing public health or health promotion, they are always on the edges of sickness and suffering. Their work is inherently stressful as well as challenging, and any model of nursing work or nursing care delivery has to be built on this fundamental understanding or it will fail. The other is that nursing *is* work—not just a calling, a form of penance, or a hobby. Any change in the reality of nursing—and, eventually, change in how others perceive nursing—must occur in the workplace and radiate out from there. When the role of staff nurses improves within the hospital environment, nursing's professional standing and public image will—with some work—improve accordingly. If RNs don't have time to care for and rescue patients, no amount of PR will convince patients they've gotten good nursing care. When doctors and nurses have more time, doctors may spend some of it listening to and collaborating with nurses. Then and only then will retention *and* recruitment both be possible. Otherwise what we will have is new recruitment followed by failed efforts at retention and another round of frantic societal hand-wringing about the next nursing shortage.

The Case for Safe Staffing Ratios

The first condition for easing the nursing crisis is to assure that the workload of working nurses will not crush them—that they will have the time and the psychological and physical energy to be effective on the job, to empathize with their patients, and to keep them safe from harm. That's why we need safe staffing ratios enacted not just on the state or provincial **403** level, but nationally as well.

Worldwide, the most important example of safe staffing ratios and their positive impact is the Australian state of Victoria. In 2000 the local branch of the Australian Nursing Federation (ANF) won a legislative framework for staffing ratios in all of Victoria's public hospitals. As in California, the ratios themselves were developed through an administrative rule-making process—in this case conducted by Victoria's Industrial Relations Commission. As implemented, the staffing formulas require five nurses to twenty patients on medical-surgical wards, and various ratios for other patient populations. (In Victoria, unlike other states in Australia, no patient care assistants are used in acute care public-sector hospitals.)

Because the ratios mandate five nurses for every twenty patients rather than one for every four, it's possible to take into account the nurses' level of experience and training. "Somebody more senior might have five patients and a more junior nurse might have only three," explains Belinda Morieson, past secretary of the ANF in Victoria. "A nurse who's got someone really sick might have only three patients. It's up to the nurse in charge of the shift to allocate the patients, but there will be five bedside nurses for twenty patients."

Ratios not only give nurses a manageable patient load, they also insure more predictable schedules. "The schedule gets done up six weeks ahead, and therefore you know if you're working on Ward Four-South and you're going to do a morning shift, and you know how many patients you will be looking after," Morieson says. In Victoria, nurses also know that there will be sufficient safe lifting equipment available to handle heavy and immobile patients without injuring themselves, thanks to "no lift" rules that have been implemented in hospitals and other health care facilities.

With its new ratios as the main incentive, Victoria launched a recruitment campaign to encourage nonpracticing RNs to return to the work force. The ANF negotiated a government-paid reentry training program, a thirteen-week refresher course for those who'd let their nursing certificate lapse. In addition, nurses get ongoing support for professional development through a system of guaranteed educational leave time. A part-time nurse receives three paid days off annually to attend seminars and conferences, while a full-time nurse will get five days for this purpose. As news of the ratios and related reforms has spread, four thousand nurses have been recruited back into the work force; there are now few nursing job vacancies in Victoria's public hospitals.

In interviews conducted during a visit to Melbourne in the summer of

404 2003 and in phone interviews afterward, I talked with many Victoria nurses about these developments. Their nearly unanimous opinion was that workplace conditions had changed significantly. One convert was George Mekiel, a former nurse manager and a recent arrival in Australia from the United States, who finds the hospital environment there to be "unlike anything I've experienced in the States." At his new job at the Peter MacCallum Cancer Research Hospital in Victoria, Mekiel found stronger backing for individual career development, far greater collegiality, and an escape from what had become, back home, "an hourly life."

Before the ratios were fully implemented at Austin Health in Melbourne, Rachael Duncan, a neurosurgical nurse, was working part-time and studying. She was routinely assigned six very sick patients on an ordinary section of the floor, and four in its "high-dependency" area. "You left work feeling like a wet rag," she recalled. "There was a very poor skill mix on the floor. A lot of casual [temporary] nurses were making up the numbers. Nursing is always hard work, but you never got ahead, you were always chasing everything. It was very demoralizing. You never felt like you'd done your job. Everyone was stressed—the nurses, the doctors, even the cleaners. Your ability to be civil was pushed to the limit. I copped agro [got complaints] from other nurses all the time, so it was harder to be civil around stressed-out family members of patients who were very sick."

Between May 2002 and the following spring, Duncan finally got a break, but thanks only to her maternity leave. With some trepidation, she returned to work after the birth of her child. The new staffing ratios were now in place. At first, she thought she might be seeing a mirage, experiencing a temporary illusion. "I remember when I came back for those first five shifts. I would leave feeling I'd done my job well. I enjoyed it. I was actually energized when I left work instead of exhausted. Well, maybe I just struck a quiet day, I thought. But no, things had changed." Nurses were taking care of four patients on the regular unit and two in the high-dependency area. "I remain busy," she says. "There are always things to do. But what has changed is that there are other hands and heads to help you. There are just more skilled people around—and more permanent staff instead of casual nurses—to help you when you need it."

Now, when a patient's condition suddenly changes and Duncan has to drop everything to deal with the emergency, there's far more coverage of her other patients. Duncan cites one instance in which she was taking care of four patients, including one who had just undergone brain surgery. Everyone thought he was getting better. Then, unexpectedly, the patient developed a pulmonary embolism. Duncan immediately went into overdrive. She "bagged" the patient—manually helped him breathe—then administered anticoagulatory medicine, and did about a dozen other things

that precluded her checking on her three other patients. "We got the pa- **405**
tient stabilized. I took him up to the ICU and came back down and wrote
up my notes. By the time it was all over, it took about two hours."

Before the ratios, Duncan says, she would have resumed her full patient load, knowing that other patients' medications were missed, their
vital signs not taken, or dressings not changed because there were not
enough coworkers to cover for her. In this case, when she checked on her
other patients, she found that everything had been done and she even had
time to decompress. "You're so knackered after a critical incident like
that. You've just had this huge rush of adrenaline as it's unfolding and you
need to calm down so you can really focus on your other patients. You
need to return to your work slowly. I couldn't do that in the past. Now I
can because I don't just have extra hands to help me, I have hands that
know what to do."

Sanchia Aranda, a professor at the University of Melbourne Graduate
School of Nursing and director of cancer nursing research at the Peter
MacCallum Hospital, believes that staffing ratios make better nursing
possible. Ratios offer the chance "to really prove that nurses make a difference," she argues. "If nurses have enough time, we can take advantage
of this to begin to look at how to really structure nursing work." Aranda
also notes that ratios enable working nurses to contribute far more to systematic tracking of cause and effect in their work, and to apply the critical
findings of nurse researchers. It becomes possible to put research into
practice—actually studying "what happens when you put a particular action in place for a particular problem and get a particular result."

In the spring of 2004 the government of Victoria tried to replace ratios
with the kind of computer data entry acuity systems that are used in the
United States and in private hospitals in Australia. Nurses in the Australian Nursing Federation took "industrial action," closing beds and refusing to work unless ratios were maintained. "Nurses wanted to improve
the ratios in public rural hospitals and public residential aged care facilities," explains Lisa FitzPatrick, the Victoria branch secretary of the ANF.
They also wanted to extend the ratios to day surgery and renal dialysis.
Although they were unable to improve and expand the ratios, they fought
their removal and the ratios remained in place. "The government and directors of nursing don't like ratios," Fitzpatrick says, "because it commits
a budget to nursing." But it is precisely such a commitment, she and others claim, that allows nurses the resources they need to do their work.

In the United States, nurses have also proposed staffing ratios and won
them in California. The California Nurses Association, America's largest
independent RN union, spent a decade lobbying for this goal before
achieving it for the first time anywhere in the United States. In 1999, the

406 governor of California signed a bill which, after much negotiation, implemented nurse-to-patient ratios in all the state's hospitals, as of January 1, 2004. Some ratios are being phased in and others vary according to nursing specialty. For example, nurses on medical surgical units cannot be required to care for more than six patients at a time; after 2005, that number goes down to five patients per nurse. Nurses on labor and delivery floors cannot be assigned more than two patients in active labor or four antepartum; in pediatrics, the ratio will be one to four; in telemetry, one to five (one to four in 2008); and in the ER one to four, with one nurse to two patients in critical care.

At this writing, about thirty other state legislatures in the United States are considering—in the face of fierce industry resistance—similar staffing measures. In my own state, the Massachusetts Nurses Association (MNA) and the Service Employees International Union are lobbying for one such bill, the Act Ensuring Patient Care and Safe RN Staffing. It would mandate minimum RN-to-patient ratios on every unit and floor, eliminate mandatory overtime as a routine staffing mechanism, and establish a system to protect patients who need intense nursing services by mandating more nurses per patient if a patient needs more care.

Some nursing academics are strongly opposed to staffing ratios, joining many nurse managers and hospital administrators who lobby against this reform, wherever and however it is proposed. In 2003 and 2004 representatives of the Massachusetts Organization of Nurse Executives joined officials from the state hospital association in speaking out against ratios.

While generally conceding that staffing levels are a problem that needs to be addressed, such critics make several—sometimes contradictory—arguments. Privately, as we've seen, many nurse managers complain about their loss of freedom to increase the number of nurses working on their units. Publicly, they decry their potential loss of flexibility to move nurses around a hospital as the administration sees fit. They also say the cost of compliance with a legislative mandate will be prohibitive. They argue that ratios will prevent managers from staffing units with an appropriate mix of inexperienced and experienced nurses; that any legislated minimum will soon become a maximum; that nurses will lose control of their practice (as if they have control of it now); and that there won't be enough nurses to meet ratio requirements once they are enacted.

Given the hospital industry's recent track record in the United States, many of these objections seem disingenuous. Over the past decade, hospital administrators—except in some unionized facilities—have had near total flexibility, and thus plenty of opportunity to prove that "voluntary approaches" to minimum staffing are preferable to negotiated or legislated standards. Left to their own devices, few hospitals have let RNs provide more care to fewer patients; instead, they have, in effect, directed them to give less care to more and sicker patients as workloads have increased almost everywhere.

Turning to the critics' objections that merit serious consideration, no safe staffing measure proposed so far would ever prevent nursing managers from assigning more RNs to patients than the minimum ratio specified by law or regulation. Similarly, if hospital nurse managers wanted to meet mandated ratios with a mix of experienced and less experienced nurses, they would be free to do so. Indeed, the bill proposed in Massachusetts includes implementation of a system that would require hospitals to "flex up" to provide additional nursing care if a patient needs it.

Just as state and federal minimum wage laws provide a floor, not a ceiling, having statutory standards for safe staffing won't drive down current levels of care any more than having a minimum wage has meant that each and every worker is paid that. Hospital administrators who argue that ratios will lead to "rationing of care" neglect to mention that they already use patient acuity systems and benchmarking, which are a privately devised method of allocating nursing staff. These internal hospital guidelines dictate how many nursing hours per patient day each patient is allowed. They are sometimes applied on an hour-to-hour basis, not even on the shift-by-shift basis used in safe staffing legislative proposals. Most alarmingly, patient acuity systems and benchmarking gather and apply information about comparative hospital staffing practices, and thus, in today's competitive hospital environment, do indeed drive nursing care down to its lowest common denominator.

The cost argument against staffing ratios reflects concern about similar market pressures. Some hospitals are clearly in dire fiscal straits, while others are flush with money. Regardless of their overall financial condition, hospitals could achieve considerable savings if they reduced the current high and costly rate of turnover—and sometimes absenteeism—among directly employed nurses. Instead, many hospitals are dealing with RN turnover as a fait accompli, while aggravating the trend through their reliance on an increasingly permanent form of "temporary" staffing. One study estimates that the temporary staffing agencies now supplying 5 percent of the nurses who work in hospitals are netting more than $7 billion a year in revenue.[2] This penny-wise but pound-foolish policy has its counterpart in schemes to reduce nursing positions altogether, without taking into account the resulting "collateral damage"—the hidden costs of inadequate nursing care. As I mentioned earlier, a preventable urinary tract infection can add $676 to a hospital stay, a preventable bedsore can cost between $4,000 and $70,000 to heal, and treatment of a preventable blood clot can involve medication expenses of $12,000 or more.

408   There is mounting evidence that work force churn and conversion of
nursing staff into a contingent labor force is both shortsighted and counterproductive. According to a study by the VHA, the rate of hospital
turnover for RNs was 21.3 percent in 2000. The replacement, training,
and other related costs of a nurse leaving can be startlingly high—two to
three times his or her salary. The hospitals must advertise for another
nurse, devote human resource time to screening and interviewing applicants, and, in the meantime, pay overtime or hire travel or temporary
nurses to fill the resulting hole in the staffing schedule. Added to this are
the expenses of lost productivity and "terminal payouts." This means that
if you replace a medical surgical nurse who earns $46,832—the national
average for that position—it will cost the hospital more than $92,442. In
an occupational specialty like oncology or critical care, the total tab is
even higher: $145,000. Multiply the first replacement cost figure by the
total number of RNs departing annually, and a hospital's total "expenditures could amount to as much as $1,969,015 yearly, for the turnover of
medical-surgical nurses alone."[3]

There is mounting evidence that work force churn and conversion of
VHA studies conclude that "high vacancy rates and continuous
turnover of staff are stressing the financial and cultural fabric of health
care providers." High turnover rates of 20 percent or more increase the
average cost per discharge by 36 percent, compared to the costs incurred
by hospitals with low turnover. "At a 100 percent turnover cost factor, a
turnover rate of 20 percent could cost a hospital an average of $5.5 million
a year," the study estimates. In hospitals with such turnover rates, there is
a decreased return on assets. Low turnover leads to a 23 percent return,
high turnover 17 percent. Patients in hospitals with turnover rates of more
than 22 percent have a greater chance of dying and a longer length of stay
(an additional 1.2 days).[4]

Although she doesn't invite government regulation, Cynthia Ambres, a
physician who is executive vice president of Kaleida Health Systems in
Buffalo, agrees that there are sound business reasons for safe staffing ratios. "This is the central issue for nurses who are fighting for their professional lives," Ambres acknowledges. "It would change the whole picture.
One of the biggest issues in nursing is that we have a lot of people out on
disability. Why is that? When I start to talk to nurses who call in a lot and
can't come to work, they say they just can't seem to make it out of their
beds in the morning. They tell me they are worried, when they get up in
the morning, that they may harm someone on the job because they come
to work with a one-to-ten ratio. That's not fun. If you changed that, do
you think there would be so many sick days and people calling in and not
wanting to come to work? One thing funds the other thing. Hospitals that
think they're saving money are really cutting their own throats."

Nevertheless, most nursing managers and some academics remain so **409** opposed to staffing regulations that they continue to offer up voluntary alternatives. Of varying utility, these include consumer education that would supposedly help patients choose hospitals with the best nursing standards; the establishment of state-supported centers that would study the nursing work force; and a series of hospital nursing "report cards" that would score hospitals on nursing care and somehow penalize them through state-imposed fines if patients don't get the care they need.[5] Some of these suggestions might be useful components of an overall solution to the nursing crisis, but they're no substitute for staffing ratios. Nursing research, particularly on what nurses do to prevent costly complications and deliver effective care, can certainly be supportive of workplace initiatives. It will not, by itself, bring about any concrete changes, and it never has. The lag time involved in collecting, interpreting, and publishing data—between three to five years for serious research—is often just too long to capture contemporary reality, much less transform it. As for creating a system of retrospective penalties for hospitals that don't comply with nursing standards, how helpful will that be for patients who have, in the meantime, suffered a preventable complication or even died due to some institutional deficiency? Far better to enact enforceable up-front staffing ratios and penalize those hospitals that fail to comply.

The claims that there aren't enough nurses available now to meet minimum ratio requirements ignore the fundamental connection between retention and recruitment. Nurses are leaving the bedside—and the profession—because of mounting and often unsafe workloads, a condition that also discourages new recruits from entering the field. To the extent that more states, provinces, or nations do enact ratios, they will become a magnet for nurses seeking such relief, thereby exacerbating local shortages elsewhere. Ultimately, this is a problem that can only be addressed through national and international standards—long-term global solutions, rather than shorter-term local ones.

It is tragic that so many nurse managers—at least in the United States—oppose staffing ratios. While ratios can certainly be refined and are not the final solution to the nursing crisis, they are an important tool that managers can use to create stability and predictability in their own working lives and in the units or hospitals they manage. Indeed, they are key to creating a management structure in which mid-level nurse managers manage clinical care, intra- and interprofessional teamwork, and patient safety, not just beds and budgets. And it would help nurse executives at the top of the nursing hierarchy manage care rather than cost or the latest wave of nurse-cutting consultants.

The Magnet Hospital Alternative

While many nurses are campaigning for staffing ratios, others are putting their hopes in a different kind of "magnet"—hospitals throughout North America (and one in the United Kingdom) that have received special designation by the American Nurses Association (ANA) through its American Nurses Credentialing Center (ANCC). Some supporters of the "Magnet hospital" concept view it as a substitute for ratios, others don't. The term "Magnet" was coined in the early 1980s, when researchers for the American Academy of Nursing (AAN), an ANA affiliate, began analyzing hospitals with a good record of nurse retention. The forty-six facilities studied in the original 1983 report were places where nurses, not surprisingly, said they liked to work. These hospitals had low turnover and vacancy rates, although they were located in areas with a lot of labor market competition for nurses.[6]

After the AAN's initial study, forty-one institutions were declared to be Magnet hospitals. More recently, the American Nurses Association has established a subsidiary, the ANCC, to certify additional hospitals for Magnet status, based on the merits of their voluntary applications. The ANCC judges hospitals according to "their ability to meet fourteen standards of nursing care evaluated in a multistage process of written documentation and on-site evaluation by nurse experts—a process similar to JCAHO accreditation."[7] If the hospital is so accredited, it can advertise itself as a certified Magnet hospital. The ANCC charges $9,765 to appraise a 100-bed acute care hospital and $47,250 for a 950-bed acute care hospital. On top of this, there is a $2,500 application fee. These fees do not include the considerable expenditure hospitals must make in allotting staff to prepare for visits from accreditors and to assemble the necessary paperwork. For institutions to keep their accreditation, the process must be repeated every four years.

In its promotional material, the ANCC writes that Magnet status helps hospitals maintain a competitive advantage, recruit the best nurses, improve patient care, attract high-quality physicians and specialists, and reinforce positive collaborative relationships. According to the group's website, "A national survey conducted in March 1999 by Wirthlin Worldwide dramatically illustrates the competitive edge enjoyed by Magnet designated facilities. The survey found that 93% of the public would have more confidence in the overall quality of a hospital" if it had passed the nursing standards required under the ANCC program. Thus, in addition to rating the quality of a facility's nursing care, Magnet designation is supposed to reflect overall quality. Magnet facilities, like the Hackensack University Medical Center in New Jersey, routinely use the designation as a stamp of approval in their marketing. "The Magnet process is incredibly valuable because it helps to validate the programs that you have in place," reports Elaine Graf, "magnet coordinator" for another approved institution, Children's Memorial Hospital in Chicago (Magnet designated in December 2001).[8]

The Magnet movement is certainly an important effort to enhance the value of nursing and improve patient care. But its growth raises a number of questions. First, does nursing really want to emulate the troubled history and conflicts of interests embedded in the JCAHO accreditation process? Second, if the Magnet hospital designation really has the effect of improving patient care, shouldn't the accreditation process be mandatory rather than voluntary? If nursing is critical to all hospitals—if it is the engine of the hospital—shouldn't all hospitals be expected to have the highest standards of nursing care? Would you allow car dealers to sell cars without an engine, or permit people to ride in airplanes in which the safety of the equipment wasn't constantly checked and double-checked? On a voluntary basis, Magnet accreditation may appeal to some hospitals during a nursing shortage. But what happens, the sociologist Dana Weinberg asks, when the shortage ends? Will hospitals maintain their commitment to magnetism when the hiring pressure is off? Or will their nursing programs then succumb to budget cutting, as was the case eventually at the Beth Israel in Boston, one of the original prototypes of a Magnet hospital? While pitching the competitive edge of Magnet status may be a clever marketing strategy, it also has serious ethical implications. Whenever you draw nurses from one hospital to another, you've simply shifted the burden of the nursing shortage to the hospital they came from.

Perhaps the most important question to answer is whether Magnet hospitals can resist broader cost-cutting trends. One nurse I spoke to recently was hired in a Magnet hospital in the Northeast. When she went for her orientation, she was told that nurses had a heavy caseload and barely had time to visit the bathroom. They were expected to deliver trays for meals and do other nonnursing activities. When she called the ANCC to complain, she said she was told that the group couldn't help unless hospital policies violated a state or federal law. A clinical specialist told me about the heavy use of agency nurses and the nursing workload at her recently credentialed Magnet hospital. Although they had "shared governance" and could be on committees that made policy, she said nurses were so burdened it was difficult for them get off the unit to attend such meetings. Since they'd have to play catch-up when they got back to the wards, they didn't volunteer to share in the governance. The hospital had just celebrated Nurses Week 2004, she told me, and there were barely any staff nurses at the party and speeches. "All you saw were the white coats

412 (managers and administrators). Who is Nurses Week supposed to be for?" she asked me.

To have greater industry-wide impact, Magnet standards need to be incorporated into a regulatory framework that applies to all hospitals, and they also must serve as the basis for durable local experiments to improve nursing care delivery. Magnet hospital–type certification and safe-staffing mandates should be complementary tools, not alternatives.

The Question of Work Schedules

With or without ratios, whether or not they work at a Magnet hospital, nurses must have more reasonable schedules in order to improve their working lives. They should not be spending their time on unnecessary paperwork and should have sufficient ancillary help to perform nonnursing activities. They also need some downtime built into their workday or workweek and should not be sent home if there isn't a patient in a bed. Instead, time on the job that is spent learning, or working with other nurses or physicians to improve care, should be viewed as valued work activity.

Most important, predictability in the nurses' work schedule is central. Since nursing work is unpredictable, nurses' schedules shouldn't be as well. They should not be expected, on a regular basis, to sacrifice vacation time, personal time, and sick leave to meet hospital scheduling needs, as unilaterally determined by managers and administrators who rarely make equivalent sacrifices of their own paid or unpaid time off. Predictable nursing schedules should be adjusted to distribute shift and weekend work fairly.

In Western Australia, chief nurse Philip Della was able to improve the retention of permanent staff by addressing the overdependence on temporary agency nurses. Della changed the culture of nursing management (described in Chapter 13) by setting up a central call line for nurse managers who wanted to solve scheduling problems by using temp nurses. Nurse managers would have to justify their decision to use an agency nurse and get permission to call an agency. Agency nurses were no longer given their choice of hospital and shift and could no longer get their schedules weeks in advance. Instead, Della and his team offered the first choice of shift to permanent and in-house casual staff and gave permanent nurses their schedules from four to six weeks in advance. This, says Della, sent a message to permanent staff: you are valued more than temporary replacements. In the last budget year, Della reports, agency costs went down from $55 million to $30 million. In the Australian unionized public system, moreover, no manager can force a nurse to take a day off if the workload is down. Instead, mechanisms allow nurses to take accrued time off if their workload decreases.

Temporary staff aren't the only problem that needs to be addressed, **413** particularly in the hospital sector. There also needs to be a way to adjust workloads for older nurses who no longer have the stamina for running or heavy lifting that they possessed earlier in their careers. These nurses retain vital knowledge and skills that need to be imparted to new nurses in structured mentoring programs. As always, to reap the benefits of nurse longevity, hospitals must first be willing to reward it, as the Washington Hospital Center has done since its 2004 negotiations with Nurses United. Members of that union—1,200 RNs at the largest health care facility in the nation's capital—now have a contract that creates a "reduced work option" for nurses fifty-five or older with twenty-five years of service, enhanced benefits for weekend nurses, an additional day off with pay for senior nurses, and other scheduling or fringe benefit improvements. In Australia, nurses are rewarded for longevity. A nurse who has worked for ten years in the public system (or fifteen years in the private system) gets a three-month paid "long service leave," that is, a fully paid three months off work. Nurses also have the option of taking 80 percent pay for five years and then getting a full year off with full pay. Shift length must also be addressed as an issue, separate from overall scheduling. Under current conditions, many nurses now find the job so uncongenial that they prefer to complete it as soon as possible during the workweek by enduring inhumanly long daily shifts. "Three twelves"—twelve-hour shifts worked three days straight—is additionally appealing because it cuts down on normal commuting time. It also gives nurses, predominantly women, more free time during the remainder of the week for domestic chores, and sometimes even for second jobs outside the home.

With or without union protection, nurses obviously make a distinction between voluntary selection of a "three twelves" schedule and the much more controversial "mandatory overtime" (in the form of management-required hours of work beyond any "basic workday," whether that's defined as an eight-, ten-, or twelve-hour day). Whichever way those extra hours get worked, more nursing-specific research should certainly be done on the resulting impact of regular "overtime" on both nurses and their patients. Occupational health experts who study fatigue in the workplace—as a more general phenomenon—invariably find that after eight hours on the job, whether in mining, manufacturing, or services, workers gradually lose their speed, focus, attentiveness, and awareness of workplace hazards. Accident rate studies in many industries invariably confirm this.

Nursing organizations and their members should be asking themselves much harder questions about the downside of relinquishing the eight-hour day, sixty years after it became the norm throughout society. Do we

414   really want nurses working twelve-hour shifts, particularly when—in the absence of staffing ratios—they are still responsible for six, eight, ten, or even twelve patients? And when we can't be sure that they are only working three twelve-hour shifts per week? In an emergency, would anyone want to depend on a harried, overtired nurse with twelve patients who's in the final hour of a twelve-hour shift in the fourth or fifth consecutive day? Or even worse, working beyond that shift because his or her relief hasn't shown up yet or because he can't get all his work done, even in twelve hours? Changing the management practices and economic conditions that give rise to longer hours is not easy, even for nurses with collective bargaining clout. But allowing the time clock to revert back to workdays more typical of America in the late 1800s or early 1900s can hardly be considered progress!

The Necessity of Better Pay

It's become commonplace for people to insist that money is not the first thing nurses mention when they're asked about solutions to the nursing crisis. While better pay won't compensate for worsening working conditions, it's a crucial complement to improving those conditions. What's needed are not the occasional bribes to convince nurses to work in hostile workplaces—$5,000 or $15,000 sign-on bonuses, or free housing for traveling nurses, or perks for agency nurses, or attractive offers for immigrant nurses. What's needed are decent salaries for all nurses for eight-hour workdays and forty-hour workweeks.

Where will the money come from? Although there are some very good answers to that question, nurses have to stop worrying about asking for too much. Their job is to prove that they're worth the money and to convince the policy makers and politicians to figure out where to get it.

Nurses, like teachers, should be given adequate salaries, adequate raises, as well as longevity pay and scheduled raises that recognize educational attainment. Right now many starting nurses receive the same starting salaries no matter what their graduating degree. Nurses usually get pay raises as they advance in their career, but they very quickly max out in their capacity to earn money and remain at the bedside. According to a salary survey conducted by *ADVANCE for Nurses*, the differentials for education or certification in a nursing specialty (e.g., critical care or oncology nursing) could be significant or minimal, depending on the region of the country. In their survey of more than eight thousand RNs, BSNs earned on average $26.50 an hour, while diploma nurses made $25.65 an hour. When it came to pay differentials for certification, "in some areas, like Delaware or the Carolinas, the difference was dramatic, in other areas

like New Jersey, however, the difference was negligible."[9] One way a **415**
nurse can earn more is to become a manager or an advanced practice
nurse. In each of these cases, she will leave the bedside work of direct
nursing care for the sick.

It's useful to look at teachers' pay scales when considering a different
model. Although teachers should certainly be paid more, their salary
scales, which, in the United States, have been severely limited by the anti-
tax agenda of the Republican right, reflect attempts by school systems to
retain teachers over the long term and keep them in the classroom. In
Massachusetts, to cite only one example, teachers are paid through a series of what are called steps (based on years of service) and lanes (based on
educational advancement). A beginning teacher starts at step one and over
his or her career moves up the ladder with yearly increases. Depending on
the school district, these can be $300 or $400 a year or over $1,000 or
more. Teachers can begin teaching with a bachelor's degree but must,
within a specified period, get a master's degree to keep their jobs. With
this degree, they get a lane raise of $1,000 or more on top of their step
raise. When they pass a national certifying exam, they get another raise.

Then there is usually a series of lanes added to the steps that encourage
teachers to get more educational points. The lanes may include the bachelor's plus fifteen or thirty hours of courses, or the master's plus fifteen,
thirty, sixty, or seventy-five hours. With each additional step and lane, the
teacher remains in the classroom, knowing more and earning more. All
lanes end with the doctorate, which can earn the teacher as much as
$3,000 or more per year. That's on top of step raises and includes any
contractually bargained pay increases. Teachers with doctorates may become department chairs and carry a lighter class load, or curriculum
chairs or vice principals and carry no class load. In the high school my
daughters attended in Arlington, Massachusetts, one of their history
teachers with a PhD was chairman of the history department and taught a
small class load. Assertive teachers' unions that represent the majority of
public school teachers in most American states won all of these steps,
lanes, and raises.[10]

Some hospitals, like those in the Veterans Administration system, are
now giving nurses a salary differential of 3 percent for bachelor's preparation at the starting gate.[11] Some hospitals have tried to initiate programs,
called clinical ladders, which are attempts to give nurses credit for educational and professional advancement and keep them at the bedside. Most
union contracts for nurses guarantee them some sort of differential for
length of service and educational advancement. David Schildmeier, communications director of the Massachusetts Nurses Association, explains
that RNs usually make about $2.50 an hour more as they advance in their

416 education. Because of higher salaries, Schildmeier says, unionized hospitals often have greater retention of their nurses. "One of the problems we face in negotiations is that so many of our nurses are at the top of the pay scale, because they stay in their jobs longer."

Whether it's pay for experience or education or regularly scheduled raises, nurses in nonunion hospitals may not fare as well as their unionized colleagues. "When we go into a hospital that's just been organized, and the nurses suddenly have access to pay information they never had before, we find that their hourly salaries are literally all over the map," Schildmeier adds. "For no rhyme or reason, a nurse with the same length of service and educational credentials may be making $12 an hour less than the nurse she's working next to. Maybe the manager liked the other nurse better. Maybe they were trying to woo her and gave her more money. When we organized one hospital and nurses got their first contract in 2003, we found that the nurses were paid 30 to 35 percent less than nurses at another hospital which was in the same system and practically across the street."

Some nurse educators argue against unions and insist that nurses should continue their education because of the sheer love of learning or to enhance their prestige among their colleagues. The reality is that most people aren't going to devote three or four years of their lives—and thousands of dollars—to getting advanced degrees if there isn't some long-term payoff. Teachers have suffered mightily because of tax cuts and the subsequent cuts on educational expenditures in the United States. They still don't earn as much as other professionals—or even nonprofessionals—with similar educational credentials. Nurses get even less encouragement to learn more and enhance their skills, a problem that is exacerbated by low rates of unionization—17 percent in the United States. Moreover, if hospitals, and by extension our social institutions generally, decide they can do with fewer nurses every decade, this hardly encourages nurses to continue their educational journey. People who fear that a pink slip awaits them every few years will be understandably reluctant to invest in or fight for more education.

The Importance of Education

Education is one of the most important but also one of the most divisive issues among RNs. For over a century, nursing has lacked any single, standardized form of entry into nursing practice. A four-year degree in some sort of university program is standard for most professions and certainly for all other nonphysician health care clinicians. Teachers' unions discovered, long ago, that they could better advance their members' eco-

nomic interests if teachers had a university degree. According to the edu- **417**
cation historian Wayne J. Urban, by the 1970s most two-year teaching degree programs had been discontinued. State teachers colleges switched to
a four-year basic course and, in most states, undergraduate work had to be
supplemented by a master's degree for a teacher to remain employed.[12] In
Massachusetts, for example, teachers can get hired with a BA or BS degree
but must earn their master's within five years.

There have been endless studies and reports, arguing that nurses
should similarly have a full college or university-level education to support their claim to professional status. Dieticians and nutritionists, PTs
and OTs, MDs and social workers—all must have a four-year degree or
more. Dieticians, in fact, are now required to have five years of education.
Why are so many politicians and administrators still relying on the tired
nineteenth-century character of the "overtrained nurse" as they fight
against university education for nurses? Is there such a thing as an overtrained doctor, psychologist, or pharmacist? The idea would be an oxy-
moron. Should the people in a hospital who spend the most time engaged
in direct care of the sick be required to have anything less than the standard professional minimum?

I don't think so. My support for a four-year degree, as a career entry
requirement for all future nurses, is not meant to disparage the work of
the many skilled and experienced RNs who hold three-year diplomas or
two-year associate degrees from community colleges. They perform ad-
mirably and many try valiantly to supplement their education while
they're on the job. But in today's increasingly complex and high-tech
health care world, there is simply too much knowledge to absorb and skill
to master for anyone to do it in just two years.

Nurses who work in hospitals, nursing homes, and other settings
where patients are seriously ill and dependent should ideally have hands-
on residency training in addition to a four-year education. A residency period has been a standard part of doctor training since the 1910 Flexnor report made it a requirement for newly minted medical school graduates.
"For nursing there are no structured residency programs, no standards,
no oversight body to assure that the standards are met, and no funding."[13]
As one nursing school director recently told me, hospitals want schools to
graduate nurses and then have them up and running as soon as they arrive
on a ward, often with little more than a six-week orientation, also not
mandatory. That is absurd, he said. Indeed, it is.

The need for a longer period of formal education, followed by some
form of postgraduate apprenticeship, is a critical one that is being met
elsewhere. In many other countries, nurses are now educated at the university or through programs that link university schools of nursing to

418   community colleges that grant four-year degrees. University education for RNs is the norm in Australia, Portugal, Spain, Iceland, and in most provinces in Canada (two-year nursing schools have been closed in Atlantic Canada). In the United States, nursing academics have been fighting for a four-year standard since 1965. Only one state in the United States, North Dakota, currently requires nurses to have a four-year degree as a minimum educational credential. At the same time, some hospitals are experimenting with residency programs that address the need for postgraduate apprenticeship opportunities. For example, the American Association of Colleges of Nursing and the University Health System Consortium—a ninety-one-member alliance of academic health systems—is experimenting with a one-year residency program for baccalaureate nurses as part of a demonstration project at five academic medical centers.[14]

Australian university programs are more intensely focused on nursing for the entire three-year course of study. In contrast, U.S. baccalaureate nurses generally take two years of arts and science courses and then two years of nursing studies. In Australia, once a nurse graduates, he or she applies for a fourth-year graduate program in a hospital. Like medical residency programs here, these are highly competitive, and slots are apportioned through a computer matching system in which nurses register their selection of programs in ranked order.

During the next twelve months at their assigned hospital, they are rotated through all its different clinical areas. They are paid as graduate nurses and are teamed up with an experienced nurse or preceptor, who works with them on clinical units. Other staff members are assigned to give them additional educational sessions off the units. In the state of Victoria, the government allocates $15,000 per nurse to help pay for the staff time devoted to this graduate year program.

At Victoria's Peter MacCallum Cancer Hospital, the nursing service has total control over the budget for the residency program, which accepts fifteen graduate nurses each year. According to Sanchia Aranda, the Peter MacCallum devotes the equivalent of one and a half full-time positions to the coordination and implementation of the nonclinical time involved in RN residencies. "These people work with graduates outside of the clinical environment for period of time," Aranda explains. "They help them reflect on what they are doing and also these senior nurses will go out and work one-on-one with the nurses themselves." They also work in clinical settings to help them hone their technical skills as they deliver care to patients.

Australian hospitals view this on-the-job training program as a way to recruit nurses who will come to the hospital ready to work after their graduate year. Sioban Nelson, director of the University of Melbourne's **419** School of Nursing, explains that the program was a product of a consensus between government, unions, academics, and managers, all of whom were concerned that graduates of university programs lacked sufficient "work-readiness." Nelson says the unions supported the residency concept because, without it, the presence of unprepared "new grads put an additional burden on their members."

The experience of Australia as well as the United Kingdom offers an interesting contrast to the U.S. model of the advanced practice nursing role. In the United States, a growing number of college and university programs are fast-tracking non-nurses into the profession—as advanced practice nurses with a master's degree—even though their undergraduate training may have had nothing to do with nursing and they may never have worked in health care. The original advanced practice nurses, in contrast, were usually RNs who'd worked for years at the bedside and thus (usually) possessed not only a four-year nursing degree but also considerable practical experience. In Australia and the United Kingdom, the "advanced practice" title is reserved for people who have actually advanced in the *practice* of nursing. That's why Australian nurses who seek to work as nurse practitioners (NPs) must first apply to boards of nursing registration and submit a portfolio proving that they have attained a sufficient level of clinical expertise. They have to document specialist training in a particular field and assemble a dossier of recommendations from interdisciplinary colleagues, who can verify their work background. "There is no direct entry into advanced practice in Australia," Nelson observes. "Just as in medicine, where you can't simply pass a course to become a medical specialist, in nursing here you have to be a nurse first and well established in a clinical field before you can be declared to be advanced in that field." While nurse practitioners in Australia are currently not required to have a master's degree, they are obliged to work toward a master's.

In the United Kingdom, nurses can be recognized as having advanced in practice and become specialists—"nurse specialist" and "consultant" are the terms used in the United Kingdom—only after they have considerable clinical experience as registered nurses. The person applying to move into this category usually has a minimum of three years' experience in practice. Then he will go through a process in an annual review or will apply for a position and the training that goes with it, which often includes an advanced diploma, a master's degree, or a doctorate. "We wouldn't comprehend the system in the United States," says Tom Keighley. "Our belief in Britain has always been that you need a broad understanding and practice in nursing before you specialize. Because if you spe-

420   cialize without it, you will have a more narrow focus and wouldn't be able to provide holistic care."

After years of unsuccessful lobbying for a bachelor's degree as the minimum requirement for entering nursing in the United States, many academics have adopted another approach. The American Association of Colleges of Nursing has been working with some state boards of nursing to codify professional distinctions based on what's called "differentiated practice." Keying its argument to already existing trends in American health care—trends that are not necessarily positive—the AACN states the following:

"As health care shifts from hospital-centered, inpatient care to more primary and preventive care throughout the community, the health system requires registered nurses who not only can practice across multiple settings—both within and beyond hospitals—but can function with more independence in clinical decision making, case management, provision of direct bedside care, supervision of unlicensed aides, and other support personnel, guiding patients through the maze of health care resources, and educating patients on treatment regimens and adoption of healthy lifestyles. In particular, preparation of the entry-level professional nurse requires a greater orientation to community-based primary health care, and an emphasis on health promotion, maintenance, and cost-effective coordinated care."[15]

According to the AACN, nurses with associate degrees "function primarily at the bedside in less complex patient care situations," providing "additional aspects of care, such as teaching patients how to cope with their conditions and to maintain care upon discharge."[16] The AACN believes that creating a tier of "professional nurses"—whether homegrown or fast-tracked from the outside (via the advanced practice nursing programs described above)—will help alleviate the current nursing shortage. In addition, it will provide working nurses with opportunities for career advancement more varied and challenging than just promotions into management. Privately, many nursing school deans confide that they feel postgraduate recruitment of liberal arts majors will create a "brighter" class of nursing students, who haven't yet been socialized into the deferential behavior of nursing culture. Such people will supposedly be better positioned, upon getting their fast-track degrees, to provide superior care and elevate the profile of the profession.

The AACN's proposed solutions raise a number of concerns and questions. The association seems to base its argument for bachelor's preparation on assumptions about the decline of the hospital and the ascension of community health promoted by fans of restructuring. It argues that clinical, scientific, decision-making, and humanistic skills are essential because today's professional nurse "must make quick, sometimes life-and-death **421** decisions; design and manage a comprehensive plan of nursing care; [and] understand patients' treatment, symptoms, and danger signs."[17] But no matter where they work, don't all registered nurses do this to varying degrees? Shouldn't they all have the education necessary to meet such challenges? If patient care will be improved by having better educated nurses at the bedside, shouldn't all nurses be educated to this level?

As we have seen, hospital patients are sicker than ever. They suffer from multiple problems and can destabilize in a matter of minutes. The same is true of patients in nursing homes, rehab hospitals, clinics, and the home. It is usually the person closest to the patient who, if properly educated, will detect an emergency need and be best positioned to intervene in time. Don't all nurses, therefore, need all the skill, knowledge, and authority that could possibly be deployed to succeed in the day-to-day "rescue" work documented by researcher Linda Aiken and her colleagues? "When you look at the real disasters in patient care," says Sean Clarke, "they're not in the technology. It's people not paying attention—due diligence—to basic care."

Today, however, some nursing students, their professors, and advanced practice nurses sometimes seem to disdain the tasks of basic care and even basic nurses. In one meeting of nursing school deans that I attended, I heard nothing but put-downs of "technical nurses." One dean told her colleagues that there will always be a place for such associate degree practitioners who act as "our informed hands and feet." When doctors dispense such backhanded comments, I said to myself upon hearing this, they at least refer to nurses as their "eyes and ears." Now their own colleagues are likening them to their limbs! Other academics, like one professor I spoke to at the University of Utah, explained that advanced practice nurses will function pretty much like physicians.

It's hard to understand how advanced practice nursing can elevate the profile of the profession if these new nurses put down their colleagues who work at the bedside. But this is, at least in the United States and Canada, a disturbing academic subtext. As one professor of nursing recently told me, new four-year graduates enter "at the starting gate probably a little bit less skilled as far as starting IVs and putting in catheters." But BSN degree holders "catch up really fast because that's just stuff you can teach anybody." Besides, she wants them to manage care, not deliver it, and to function as primary care providers who refer patients to MD specialists. "You get very little clinical time in nursing school," Katherine Harris said of her four-year program. "There's a lot about research and nursing theory, which is all very interesting but really doesn't help you in the clinical setting. The attitude of the professors was, 'Don't worry, you

422   won't be one of them [the bedside nurses]—you won't be struggling on the floor. You'll be a manager or advanced practice nurse in no time.'"

Such liberating scenarios beg the question of how effectively someone can manage the work of others when they haven't mastered the skills involved themselves—and even undervalue those skills.

The fact that some nurses disparage the work of the majority of RNs perfectly illustrates political scientist James Scott's point about the tendency of the powerful and the entitled to render the "powerless" invisible. In *Seeing like a State*, Scott points out that elite groups simply fail to "see" or make "legible" the work and lives of those they deem to be subordinate.[18] If a new class of nurses emerges to oversee the activities of technical nurses or aides—and delegates duties to them in the same manner that doctors have long "delegated" to nurses—nursing will only have succeeded in replicating, within its own ranks, status hierarchies inimical to the functioning of real health care teams.

Many of these attitudes of superiority are, in fact, a product of class antipathies within nursing. As the editors of *Enduring Issues in American Nursing* point out, education has always been a "proxy for class" within the profession.[19] If the culture of nursing education becomes permeated with an elitist bias against the basic tasks of the profession, fewer college and university program graduates will be inclined to spend much of their careers in a hospital or other direct care setting, even if working conditions there are improved. As I've said earlier, in my own contact with many nursing school students, I see this trend already developing. Not enough students envision a long-term career in direct care nursing. And that's not just because of current workplace conditions. Many of these students simply look down on bedside care, regarding it as boring, unchallenging, rote work best relegated to doers, not thinkers like themselves.

Regardless of what nurses do with their training—or how they're trained—nursing education remains radically underfunded at a time when it's not getting any cheaper. Federal funding comes through the Nurse Education Act, Title VIII of the Public Health Service Act. Under this legislation in 2001 Congress allocated only $76 million for basic and advanced nursing education and scholarships. In response to the nursing shortage, Congress the next year enacted a special Nurse Reinvestment Act to fund additional tuition subsidies for nursing school students, increase the supply of their teachers, improve nursing care delivery, and recruit new nurses. To accomplish all this, the sponsors of the act originally proposed a first-year allocation of $250 million. Yet Congress ended up devoting only $20 million annually to the program in fiscal years 2003 and 2004.

This level of spending is what Julie Sochalski calls the "equivalent of Post-it notes reminding us of what we should do." In 2002, Sochalski explained, a new program was created to boost funding for medical education in pediatrics, a specialty without any known shortage of practitioners. To support just this one program, Congress allocated almost $280 million among children's teaching hospitals. If there is this kind of funding for training in a single medical specialty, certainly Congress could find sufficient resources to educate the nurses who'll be needed to care for young patients in all those children's hospitals. The medical profession received $7 billion for "direct and indirect graduate medical education to hospitals alone in 2002."[20]

Non-nurses—most of whom will eventually become patients—clearly have an interest in helping registered nurses gain more educational resources. But our social interest in nursing education and its funding depends on the assurance that colleges of nursing will produce people who want to take care of them when they're sick. If a four-year education for registered nurses is desirable, then it has to be because that education will solve the shortage of nursing care, not the inferiority problem of nursing's professional status. Certainly nurses should have the freedom to move into any field or nursing role they choose. But they should do that because they want to, not because hospital conditions or social prejudice, or class antipathy within the nursing profession itself, pushes them away from the bedside and gives legitimacy to hands-off care.

I believe the issue of nursing education needs to be reframed. Nursing academics need to explain far more clearly than they do why nurses need a university education. One recent study, by Aiken and researchers at the University of Pennsylvania School of Nursing, for example, found a correlation between educational preparation and mortality rates in hospitals.[21] Instead of attacking or devaluing nurses with two-year degrees, it would be far more useful to use this kind of data and enlist them as allies in a fight for additional educational resources that would help the bedside nurse be more effective in delivering high-quality patient care. Nursing academics could do this by explaining how the hospital industry and organized medicine have used education as a way to keep nurses relatively powerless and poorly paid. This isn't doctor or hospital bashing, it's simply a statement of the facts as almost every nursing academic knows them and has lived them.

An upgraded education would eliminate invidious distinctions between so-called technical and professional nurses and temper the fragmentation that's taking place within the profession. It's to be hoped that nursing unions would join in this fight because they would understand, as teachers did so long ago, that a university education will help them advance their

424 members' interests, both professional and financial. Some unions would of course assert that now is not the time to engage this battle, that hospitals will just use it to further divide the profession. These are serious concerns. But I would counter that now is the perfect time to engage this issue. We have a nursing shortage of major proportions. Part of it is due to the image of nursing, and that in turn is influenced by constant public confusion about what it takes to be a nurse. Wouldn't it be better for nurses to join together than to create yet another category of nurse and further confuse the public? Unions could be the most powerful lobby for university education for nurses.

The Centrality of Collective Action

In many industrialized countries, a high level of union membership is common. From traditional blue-collar workers to a wide range of white-collar employees, including many professionals (university lecturers, engineers, doctors, and scientists), union membership is the norm. In Britain, even junior managers in private industry are union members. Although union membership has declined in the United States, "organized labor" is remarkably diverse. Nurses may not be aware of it, but many of the highly paid actors and actresses they see on TV and in films are union members, along with many big-name network newscasters and all professional baseball, football, and basketball players.

As a wire service and broadcast journalist and more recently a freelance writer, I've always belonged to a union, whether it was the Newspaper Guild, the American Federation of Television and Radio Artists, or now, the UAW-affiliated National Writers Union. As a result, I've gotten excellent group health benefits, better fees, and contract protection against the kind of arbitrary management decisions that are commonplace in the news business. Like nurse managers who sometimes obscure the fact that they are managers by claiming to be the same as frontline nurses, editors claim to be journalists too. However, most daily newspaper reporters— unlike most nurses I've met—are much clearer about which side their supervisors are on, even at elite media institutions like the *Boston Globe*, the *New York Times*, and the *Wall Street Journal*. When an editor, under pressure from upper management, "lets the profession down" by failing to back a reporter, there's newsroom anger, of course, but rarely—as in the case of nurses—a feeling that we've been betrayed by "one of our own." Similarly, few journalists today look to the impersonal, profit-driven media conglomerates that employ them to uphold professional standards of news gathering and reporting. There are no illusions about newspaper conglomerates being our families. Instead, members of the Newspaper

Guild have turned the union into a leading critic of the corporate prac- **425** tices and priorities that threaten to undermine a free press in the United States.

Under the codes of conduct promulgated by their own organizations, nurses have an ethical obligation to advocate for their patients. This imposes a burden of personal responsibility far greater than that of any reporter to his or her readers because, in a health care setting, lives are at stake. As nurses work for ever-larger employers, including for-profit hospital chains operating on a nationwide or even an international basis, standing up for patients can be a lonely and futile exercise, a David-and-Goliath struggle without the happy ending. Nevertheless, many in American nursing insist that belonging to a labor union is not only unprofessional but somehow irresponsible or inconsistent with nursing's ethical code. Paul and Darlene Clark disagree. Well versed in the realities of American labor law, they argue that it's actually a form of professional suicide to shun union representation, given the difficulty, if not impossibility, of effective patient advocacy in nonunion workplaces, where employee rights and protections are so constricted. "Sending nurses out into a workplace that's just rife with problems, with no sense of how little power and control they are going to have in the work environment," is a formula for failure, Paul Clark contends. "How can you function as a patient advocate if you fail to maximize the influence you can have over patient care in the workplace?"

I asked Mireille Kingma, at the International Council of Nurses, which nursing groups she believes have achieved the most influence over workplace issues and patient care anywhere in the world. Kingma ought to know. She has earned thousands of frequent-flyer miles from crisscrossing the globe and talking to nurses about their work lives. Kingma didn't even have to think for a moment before she answered. Her picks were nurses in heavily unionized Denmark and American nurses as well—but only in those states where strong independent associations and/or AFL-CIO unions have organized many RN collective bargaining units. The common denominator, in both countries, was effective collective action combined with legally sanctioned bargaining rights.

In the United States, organized nurses have been instrumental in lobbying for protections for both themselves and their patients. They have successfully lobbied for mandatory overtime bans in six states: Oregon, Washington, New Jersey, Maryland, Minnesota, and Maine. Unions like the Service Employees International Union (SEIU) and those in the ANA have been in the forefront of the fight to force hospitals to use safe needle technology and thereby reduce life-threatening needlestick injuries. As noted previously in this chapter, organized nurses in California lobbied

426   for and won the premier safe staffing legislation in the United States, after their counterparts in Australia convinced state parliamentarians in Victoria to implement the first ratios anywhere in the world.

American Nurses Association members—particularly those affiliated with its collective bargaining arm, the United American Nurses (UAN)—have also sought legal protections for health care whistle-blowers, in both Congress and state legislatures. Far stricter laws or regulations have long required social workers, teachers, and day care providers to be "mandatory reporters" of suspected abuse or neglect that they discover among children and old people. In contrast, all the proposed whistle-blower initiatives in health care make whistle-blowing optional, leaving it up to the conscience of individual providers who will, at least, be better protected against management retaliation.[22]

Keeping the retaliation option open may or may not be the hidden agenda of hospital administrators, but their industry's opposition to whistle-blowing laws—in any form—has been fierce. It took the Massachusetts Nurses Association, which left the ANA in 2001, three years to win its whistle-blower protection campaign. After much publicity about Barry Adams's ordeal as a nurse fired for vocal patient advocacy, an MNA-backed bill was finally passed in Massachusetts in 1999. It protects health care workers who complain to corporate higher-ups or to public bodies (i.e., some kind of government agency), as long as they've first gone through lower-level hospital channels to no avail. The MNA has also successfully used the new law to protect nurses who speak to the media after their patient safety complaints have fallen on deaf ears. A more limited statute, backed by the New York State Nurses Association and several other unions, went into effect in New York in 2002. It allows health care workers who have "faced retaliation to seek reinstatement or restitution in court." Courts can impose a civil fine on employers found guilty of violating the law and can issue an injunction to prevent further management retaliation.

Some form of whistle-blower legislation has now been adopted in sixteen American states. The SEIU has also sought to incorporate whistle-blower provisions—for workers who report unsafe staffing situations or illegal instances of forced overtime—in a variety of proposed bills related to safe staffing and mandatory overtime. In Canada, there are few statutory whistle-blower protections, but most collective bargaining agreements contain "professional responsibility" clauses, which allow RNs to raise patient care issues with their employer without fear of retribution.

Unions have also been very proactive on the issues of pay equity and workplace violence.[23] The Swiss Nurses Association, and the Fédération des infirmiers et infirmières du Quebec (FIIQ) have based their "compar-

able worth" campaigns on analyses of how nursing pay and job responsibilities rank against those of other workers in the public sector. The FIIQ
has initiated an impressive program to deal with the problem of gender
discrimination experienced by their members. On the subject of workplace violence, we recall the role the union played when Anne Dolan's
hand was injured. This is part of a larger program the FIIQ has initiated
to try to return civility to the workplace. At the Royal Victoria Hospital in
Montreal, the Nurses Union of the McGill University Health Centre has,
for example, printed and distributed several thousand sets of pocket-sized
cards designed to help nurses deal with hostile work environments and
threats of physical violence. One card is a two-by-four-inch pink checklist
that reads as follows:

> I am empowering myself to eliminate violence in the workplace.
> 1. I take a deep breath; I trust myself.
> 2. I tell the person: "I do not accept this behavior" and give them the
>   red card.
> 3. Report the incident to the hotline [a call-in number the union has
>   established].
> 4. Inform your union representative.

The "red card," like a referee's warning card for fouls during a soccer
game, is intended to curb improper conduct. Nurses are encouraged to
hand the card to a doctor, a patient, a patient's family member, a supervisor, or even a coworker in situations involving verbal abuse, disrespect, or
threats. The card politely reminds any offender that their "behavior is inappropriate as per the MUHC (McGill University Health Centre) policy
for the prevention of violence at work."

Ro Licata, president of the union, explains the rationale for developing
this "carding" system. "Nurses often have a difficult time confronting
threatening or abusive behavior. By giving them these cards, we give them
some way to deal with it that doesn't force them to confront it all by
themselves. And we back them up, when they do, with follow-up investigations and complaints to management."

When I told a friend who's a physician about this program, she smiled
and said, "God, I'd love to have one of those cards to give to Dr.——,"
and she mentioned the name of a difficult colleague. "Just card 'em, what
a great idea."

There are multiple reasons why creative, innovative responses to workplace problems that empower working nurses are more achievable in
Canada or Scandinavia than in the United States. There is less tension
and conflict, and more collaboration and mutual respect, among unions,

428 professional associations, nurse managers, and academics in societies where all are functioning within the framework of the public sector or a publicly funded national health care system. In the United States, market-based health care has exacerbated organizational fragmentation and labor-management differences. Often, groups who should be natural allies, such as nursing educators and the working nurses they train, end up being at odds with each other, even though some of their objective interests are the same. For example, both Canadian and U.S. unions play an important role in making it financially possible for nurses to continue their professional education. As part of their overall contract bargaining, the unions negotiate tuition reimbursement assistance for nurses who want to continue their schooling while working—a commitment that hospitals would otherwise be free to drop at any time, based on budgetary considerations.

Even in Canada, however, it took much hard work by key leaders to weld together a unified network of nursing organizations. By the early 1990s, there was, at the federal and provincial level, a profusion of nursing entities—regulatory boards, unions, academic organizations, and professional associations—all claiming to speak for all of nursing. This often duplicative, sometimes discordant chorus made it easier for health care policy makers and legislators to shrug off key nursing concerns.

In 1997 Mary Ellen Jeans, who was then executive director of the Canadian Nurses Association (CNA), felt nurses had to come together in one room and agree on a set of common goals, so these could be pursued more effectively. Kathleen Connors, president of the National Federation of Nurses Unions, joined Jeans in seeking to create better relationships after years of tension between their two organizations. Along with other interest groups, they began holding a series of annual meetings called the National Nurses Forum.

The involvement of collective bargaining representatives was particularly significant because they had separated themselves from the CNA, two decades before, following a legal challenge to the Saskatchewan Association of Registered Nurses. That challenge was based on the claim that a mixed organization of working nurses and managers was not permitted under Canadian labor law. The Supreme Court of Canada upheld the plaintiffs' concern about "management domination," which led to the creation of separate collective bargaining and professional association entities throughout the country.

According to Connors, the National Nursing Forum has led to greater coordination and mutual understanding. "Nurse academics didn't appreciate that nurses' unions actually bargain additional money for people on the basis of academic preparation. They'd say to us, 'Why don't you get more money for people who advance in their education,' and we said, **429** 'Well, we do, it's called an academic allowance.'" Leaders and members of nursing unions also changed their minds about the value of nursing research. "Because of people getting together, nurse unions have come to rely much more on nurse researchers when we argue for a variety of things—like skill mix and staffing ratios."

Looking at the United States from north of the border, Connors is dismayed not only by the disorganization and powerlessness of nonunion nurses here. She finds the fragmentation and fractiousness of union "sisters and brothers" to be equally disheartening. In Canada, there is usually only one nurses' union per province. In most cases, that union represents both RNs and LPNs. These nurses come together, at the federal level, in the National Federation of Nursing Unions, which has no counterpart in the United States. Instead, many different—often competing—organizations represent American nurses. Some are in the AFL-CIO, others are outside of it. In the past, competition for members often took the form of raiding existing units, until the collective bargaining arm of the American Nurses Association became the United American Nurses and affiliated with the AFL-CIO as well. In another positive development, two bitter adversaries in California, the California Nurses Association and the SEIU, recently patched up their long-standing differences and agreed to wage complementary, rather than competitive, membership recruitment drives. Elsewhere, however, past policy differences and hard feelings from old organizing rivalries or ANA chapter defections have morphed into long-term hostility and suspicion.

There have probably been enough "nursing summits" called already in response to the nursing crisis. But, if anyone wants to organize another, it could have the concrete goal of creating a Canadian-style National Nursing Forum here as well. Union members and officers, leaders of nursing specialty organizations, and deans and professors of nursing schools could all be invited to bury the hatchet for a day or two, and not leave the room until enough old baggage has been jettisoned to forge some kind of common program, a minimum agenda for working together in the interests of nurses and their patients.

Reconciling Doctors with Nurses

When medical experts discuss the epidemic of medical errors and injuries in the health care system, they often consider the actions taken by other high-risk industries—nuclear power, the airlines, and forest fire fighters, for example. Accidents or injuries, most conclude, are often due to human error, and human error usually involves failed or faulty communication

430   between workers. This is often due to barriers created by hierarchical power relationships, by failures in leadership and decision making, and by the fact that people have little if any education in how to communicate effectively and negotiate in conflict situations. Because so few nurses and physicians have training in conflict resolution and genuine intra- or inter-disciplinary communication, some of the solutions adopted in these industries are crucial to resolving dysfunctional nurse-doctor relationships.

Take the airline industry. While not a perfect match, nurses and doctors and others in health care have a lot to learn from the bridges built between pilots, copilots, and flight engineers and between the cabin crew and ground crew. Pilots are a lot like doctors. They are not touchy-feely communicators. They usually deny the impact of stress and fatigue on performance and are not particularly accepting of the idea that someone without the "right stuff"—like a flight attendant—might have useful information or a relevant concern. As a result, the people without the right stuff—or some whose stuff isn't quite right enough (copilots, for example)—have either been silenced or silence themselves in an emergency.

Increasingly concerned with the costs of crashes and the safety of passengers, the airline industry has worked with safety experts to develop Crew Resource Management trainings (CRM). Initially, these trainings, which have different names depending on the airlines, targeted only pilots. They have since been expanded to include flight attendants and other crew members.

Among other things, in some airlines pilots and other members of the team are given what is called a CRM tool kit, a cue card that carries advice on how to create effective communication: "Be clear, avoid ambiguous terms. Be specific—avoid the 'hint and hope.' Be concise—say only enough to convey the message. Be timely—say it now, if it needs saying. Do 3 Things: Stop talking and listen. Abandon your idea if the other is better. Be assertive if required."

The tip sheet also gives suggestions for requesting feedback—describe what happened from your point of view to start a discussion; ask for reactions and perceptions; ask, what if anything could be done to make that happen? There is also a section titled "Recognize Red Flags." People are warned about talking without listening, being too rushed, and imparting ambiguous or confusing information. The tool kit recommends an idea that is particularly useful in conflict situations. Ask the other person, "What would you be comfortable with?"

I recently spoke with Michael Hirsch, who has been a pilot for thirty years and has worked with a major commercial airlines for the past fourteen. I asked Hirsch about his view of CRM. He was effusive in his praise of the program. "The program itself has increased a level of understanding and cooperation among the crew at both ends of the airplane," he **431** said.

As an example, he told me that during a recent trip a flight attendant called him, as first officer, to report that while they were taxiing toward the runway, she was hearing a very unusual noise in one of the engines. Even though they had left the gate and were ready to depart, she persisted in relaying her concerns. As Hirsch, the flight attendant, and the captain continued to discuss the problem, "she just kept sticking to the facts," he said, "repeating that the noise was really unusual. So we brought the aircraft back to the gate. What she had heard was an unusual pneumatic sound, and upon returning to the gate the mechanics found a crack starting in the compressed air section of the engine. So the crack was found before it became a problem. After we got back to the gate and changed airplanes, the captain told the passengers what had happened and praised the flight attendant for her vigilance. Public praise goes a long way. It's communication that keeps the plane in the air and the passenger alive," Hirsch concluded.

Susan Bianchi-Sand has an interesting perspective on the airline industry and its relevance to nurse-physician relationships. Bianchi-Sand was a flight attendant with United Airlines for thirty years and was president of the Association of Flight Attendants for seven. Now she's national executive director of the United American Nurses, the union arm of the ANA. Bianchi-Sand remembers when flight attendants were considered "sky girls," and communication between the pilot and flight attendant consisted largely of instructions (the pilot telling the flight attendant how he liked his coffee and when to serve it), social chitchat, and sexist comments made by the pilot.

That changed when the airline industry got more serious about safety. "Everyone began to recognize that people make errors, that no one can analyze their own actions all by themselves, and that you needed more voices that were heard," Bianchi-Sand explains. Interestingly, she also notes that concern for safety coincided with a union campaign designed to change the image of the flight attendant from "fly girl"—"Hi, I'm Cheryl, fly me"—to safety professional. The combination made a great deal of difference. "What has changed is that there is now a high-level professional exchange about what each group of people knows about the upcoming flight and their respective job."

Although Bianchi-Sand left the airline industry four years ago, Barbara Servis, a flight attendant with United Airlines, says the same is true today. The government affairs chair for Local 27 of the Association of Flight Attendants, she usually flies as purser, which means that she's in charge on board the aircraft. At United, she says, both the cabin crew and pilots go

432   through a version of CRM called Command Leadership Training. Servis says that while there are still tensions between pilots and the cabin crew, the program has made a difference, in some instances a big one. Pilots are now trying to be more attentive and communicative. Prior to these training sessions, for example, if they had information about a flight delay or problem, they used to keep it to themselves, leaving the flight attendants to field questions from increasingly irate passengers who wanted to know why the plane hadn't landed or left the ground. Now they are more willing to share it with the cabin crew and even passengers. As one of those passengers, I've noticed that some pilots are positively chatty these days. Maybe some people don't like it, but as a nervous flyer, I find it immensely reassuring to know they're still alive up there.

Servis says that most pilots today understand the concerns of the crew and are more supportive of them. "When the pilots come on board and the captain does his briefing either with me as the purser or the entire flight attendant crew, nowadays more often than not he will say to us, 'We don't leave this gate until you are happy with everything on board this aircraft, that means the people, the galley equipment, your emergency equipment. If you have a problem, you let us know. We don't leave the gate until you're happy.' That is a welcome change.

"If I have issues among the cabin now, I have the training to go to them and say, 'Look, this isn't working out, this is what we need to do.' Before, we never did that kind of thing. Now that we've all had that kind of training, the communication between the cockpit and the cabin is better than ever. If I want someone taken off the aircraft and we haven't left the gate yet, and I go up there and say, 'The guy's drunk, he's abusive,' nine times out of ten they will back me up. Or if we're in the air and a passenger is out of hand and he hits a flight attendant or hits another passenger, I want to know that when I take this to the cockpit they're not going to say, 'Well, let me know what happens.' I want them to say to me, 'All right, I'm putting this plane on the ground, depending on where we are, and I'll have the authorities meet this aircraft.' And they usually do."

Servis says that when she has a disagreement with a pilot about a safety issue, she feels that the combination of this training and her union make it possible for her to both express it and, if necessary, act to protect herself and her passengers. "You can get somebody down to the aircraft if you have a disagreement about safety." If a captain or copilot were to hit a flight attendant, the captain or pilot would be disciplined and possibly prosecuted. "That's illegal," says Bianchi-Sand, "it's not tolerated."

What Hirsch, Bianchi-Sand, and Servis describe is an attempt to take safety seriously. Indeed, aviation safety experts like Robert Helmreich at the University of Texas in Austin make clear that the way into issues of hierarchy and authority is through the route of safety.[24]

Although it will take some work to figure out how to replicate the airline industry model in health care, what is clearly needed is a version of team management. The rationale includes civility and collegiality, but it is fundamentally about keeping patients safe. Systematic, respectful team communication is the only way to do this.

If we want real interdisciplinary teamwork, then doctors and nurses and other clinicians should receive some education in communication, conflict resolution and negotiation skills. This kind of training would be much more effective if doctors and nurses were educated and trained together throughout their professional lives—during their initial training, in refresher courses, and through workplace contact. In nursing and medical schools, educational opportunities abound and should become standard operating procedure. Should doctors and nurses dissect cadavers together or learn anatomy and physiology in the same classroom? Probably not. But there are many ways in which they could learn together. In both nursing and medical school, lessons in patient communication are now highly valued. But how can nurses and doctors communicate with patients if they can't communicate with each other? These parts of the curricula are a perfect place to introduce interdisciplinary learning. So are courses or modules that deal with special subjects. At the University of Toronto since 2002, Judith Watt Watson, a professor of nursing, and Judith Hunter, a professor of physical therapy, and an interprofessional team of professors and experts from six faculties (dentistry, medicine, nursing, occupational therapy, pharmacy, and physical therapy) have developed a special interprofessional training curriculum on pain management. For four days each year students hear lectures on pain research and management. They break down into small groups with interprofessional leaders in which they review the case of a patient who is in pain and develop a plan of care. The work takes place in the lecture hall, but students also work together on-line.

In France, when I met with Bernard Charpentier, the head of the organization for directors of medical faculties in France and dean of the medical school at Kremlin-Bicetre Hospital in Paris, he described a program that has existed for more than fifteen years in all French medical schools. During the second year of a six-year training—the year in which they go onto the hospital wards—all French medical students spend four weeks following a nurse and an aide. "This is the first time they are seeing the patient in bed, and it should not be with an MD, because the doctors have only a very quick contact with the patient. Nurses are on the ward and very close to the patient, so this is a good way to give students a view of

434 their future, to learn by watching people who are with the patient, at the bedside, day and night," Charpentier explains. "When a student is unable to have a good approach to the patient, we see it early in this kind of program," he adds. "It also helps students understand the hospital hierarchy and how it works."

In hospitals in France, doctors also do rounds with nurses, and the head nurses and nurses involved with direct patient care are included. "If we stop treatment, we ask all the nurses. We ask everyone, the family, the patient, everyone involved in this big decision. Every three months there is a big meeting of the ward council. By law, these councils must exist and there are elections to choose who will be on them. Councils include physicians, nurses, nursing assistants, secretaries, and other clinical and hospital staff. We define objectives, discuss problems, and talk about medical students and whether they have any problems."

Although relationships between French physicians and nurses may be problematic, a medical student at Cremlin-Bicetre told me that her view of nurses had changed because of this program. The daughter of two well-to-do professionals, she had the conventional view of nursing as second-class and second-choice work (in France some students who don't pass the medical school entrance exam go into nursing instead). After shadowing nurses, she recognized how demanding and challenging their job is. "I didn't realize they had so much responsibility," she told me, "that they make so many decisions, that the doctor is there so rarely." (Nurses in France, by the way, don't have a university education.)

More interdisciplinary learning is also taking place in the United States. Some four-year schools of nursing share educational opportunities with medical students. In advanced practice training, nurses have much more contact with medical students, residents, and physicians. The AACN and the American Association of Medical Colleges are working on joint educational opportunities. All of this is an important first step. Because more than half of nurses are graduates of two-year nursing schools, these nurses also need to learn to practice better with doctors, and doctors and doctors-in-training need to learn to communicate better with them.

Cynda Rushton and her physician colleague Michael Williams have been conducting interdisciplinary training programs at Johns Hopkins to teach doctors and nurses about communication at the end of life. Through a grant from HRSA, they have developed an innovative educational model using actors to portray family members who are dealing with brain death and are considering organ donation. The interdisciplinary model is a powerful tool to create an environment of respect for and appreciation of quality end-of-life care.

Some nursing educators argue that nurses with BSNs or master's de-

grees will be the communication pipeline between "professional" and **435**
"technical" nurses and doctors. A recent story in the *Boston Globe* reported
on a new phenomenon that arose after the hours that medical residents
work were restricted. Nurse practitioners are now employed to supplement the work of medical residents and even oncologists and cardiologists. The NPs and MDs in the article discuss how nurse practitioners
have "moved beyond general nursing." Physicians, the article reported,
respect these nurses, consult with them, and consider them to be valuable
members of the health care team. The problem with these developments
is that no one ever reports on greater physician respect for, or collaboration with, the thousands of generalist or even specialist nurses who work
in hospitals and other health care institutions.

With all due respect to this group of nurses, when doctors communicate only with an elite, this doesn't necessarily help patients. What if there
are no advanced practice nurses on-site when a disgreement or communication problem arises between so-called lower-level RNs and MDs? Or
what happens if doctors communicate crucial information only to a "professional" nurse because they've assumed that the "technical" nurse isn't
bright enough to receive it and lacks the critical thinking and decision-
making skills to process it? Finally, will nurses with higher degrees share
information and collaborate with "technical nurses," or will they, like
physicians, tacitly exclude such nurses from the consultation and decision-
making process that is at the heart of teamwork?

Whether it be with their peers or with physicians, nurses often contend
that they are more collaborative and collegial than MDs. The reality is
that many nurses also need training in teamwork that includes how to
communicate with team members at every level of the occupational ladder. Most of the education nurses receive in communication centers on
patient-nurse communication, not nurse-doctor or nurse-team communication. We've heard that doctors often feel nurses are ineffective in expressing their concerns. Similarly, nurses may be no more willing to listen
to their so-called inferiors—the LPN or aide (or associate degree
nurse)—than doctors are willing to listen to RNs. Learning how to delegate and supervise in the current environment does not necessarily mean
learning how to communicate respectfully with others. If the silos are to
be shattered, they should all come down, not just a select few.

One way to do this would be to introduce the kind of program I participated in when I first began to write about nursing in the late 1980s. Developed by the Beth Israel Hospital's nursing department, it was called
"Nurse for a Day." The program invited "influence makers" to spend the
day with a nurse and help her take care of patients, handing her linens,
helping give a bed bath, and so forth. Although I'd been in the hospital for

436 a story I'd written on nursing for the *Boston Globe*, this was different, and I'll never forget helping the nurse give a bath to a 103-year-old man with poop on his head. When the Beth Israel launched the collaborative care unit to study nurse-doctor collaboration, doctors on the unit were also nurses for a day. In fact, the collaborative care model, one that worked before it was arbitrarily dismantled, is an excellent one that should be dusted off and used wherever possible.

Nurse-for-a-day programs, however, could be expanded to include many more health care workers. Doctors could shadow nurses, LPNs, aides, pharmacists, social workers, dieticians and nutritionists, and any other relevant personnel, and these health care workers should do the same, as should nurses and other clinicians. Nurses, for example, think they understand the doctor's work life. But their understanding from afar is not the same as seeing things from the physicians' perspective. Some of the most important players to include in such job shadowing experiments would be hospital administrators and health policy experts. How can insurance company executives, government bureaucrats, and hospital administrators (and these include VPs of patient care services) understand what clinicians and health care workers experience if they never get a dose of their contemporary reality?

When it comes to abusive doctors, there are a number of programs in existence to try to retrain physicians with behavioral and emotional problems. Most hospitals have policies on the books about abusive workers. Some are taking more active measures to deal with disruptive physicians or other problem workers. These programs and measures, however, have to be well publicized, and management has to be serious about implementing sanctions or therapeutic or remedial programs to help such clinicians. Many medical societies have programs for troubled physicians. Larry Harmon, the clinical psychologist we met earlier, is codirector of the Physicians Development Program in Miami. The program evaluates, educates, and monitors physicians and nurses and other health care professionals who exhibit disruptive behavior in the workplace. Harmon developed a program that surveys the nurses, supervisors, and other colleagues with whom the physician most often works. These surveys, which provide what Harmon calls a "consensus measure of disruptive behavior and hostile work environment," are presented to the physician and hospital administration and used to develop a behavior contract with the doctor, while follow-up surveys continue to monitor the doctor's behavior. Another interesting program is run by the applied medical anthropologist John Henry Pfifferling and his Center for Professional Well-Being in Durham, North Carolina. In order to make these programs work, however, nurses have to know about them, and they must be willing to come forward about problem physicians. If they are in unions, they need to **437** contact their union about the problem or encourage those unions that don't deal assertively with the issue to do so.

These are obviously big changes. But what look like little changes can make a big difference. Hospital administrators, for example, are key in initiating or supporting changes in the hospital environment that put nurses—or any other so-called subordinate staff member—at a disadvantage. Why, in so many hospitals, are notes containing vital information placed in a patient's chart under a section called Doctor's Orders? That's the question Christine R. Kovach and Sarah Morgan ask in a recent article. They argue, quite correctly, that language signals intent. Is this way of looking at the world useful? Is "order" the proper word here? Do nurses, pharmacists, physical therapists, or nutritionists really want to be ordered about? And how about the patient? Do I want to be given orders with which I must comply? Can't we come up with a better word? Kovach and Morgan suggest "Request for Services" as a section in the patient's chart. That's certainly a beginning.[25]

Since language means a lot, it would be important for nurses and doctors to start using the same language when they write their notations in the charts and speak about their work. Isn't it time to recognize that nurses are constantly making medical diagnoses in their daily work? Not just advanced practice nurses, but all nurses. Obviously, there's a difference in the kind of diagnostic work that physicians do—say, in making an initial diagnosis or diagnosing ongoing problems. The notion that nurses don't also diagnose a variety of conditions and problems is ludicrous, however. As is this rigid division between medical and nursing diagnosis. It's as if mathematicians told physicians that numbers and mathematical terms belonged to them alone and that, if they want to talk about equations or subtraction and multiplication and other calculations, they'll have to find another language. Surely some clever regulator or policy maker can figure out a way to distinguish between the kind of diagnoses physicians make and those that nurses make and participate in, while simultaneously acknowledging the role RNs play in medical diagnosis and treatment.

This, of course, raises the issue of the language of nursing diagnosis. Here I have even more questions. As it is currently constructed and taught, is this the best way to account for nurses' work? Or does it subtly discount that work by couching it in terms that no one else can possibly understand, should they even decide they want to?

Discourse, costume, forms of address, signs, and symbols are very evocative. In this regard nurses, doctors, and others in health care need to find a comfortable form of address that is applied equally to all, conveys

438   courtesy, and explains function. Everyone should either be on a first-name basis in their mode of address and introduction or should use last name and title. What individual clinicians use as a form of address with patients is a separate negotiation.[26] If this means that nurses give up their notion that caring and closeness requires a form of address without titles and last names, thank god for that. It's about time that nurses buried Nurse Ratched and left her fate to the movie buffs. It would also be a lot more productive if nurses professionalized their appearance rather than their jargon. When I was getting a colonoscopy a couple of years ago, I was understandably nervous about the procedure. I didn't find it at all reassuring to be greeted by a middle-aged woman in hearts-and-flower scrubs who introduced herself with "Hi, I'm Bobby. I'll be taking care of you today. Follow me." Who was she? A nurse? What was her last name? How could she be held accountable or responsible for anything? When a nurse dressed in crisp khaki pants, a nice tee shirt, a neat hair cut, and with her name tag clearly displayed approached me, repeated her name and title, held out her hand, and told me how she would help me through the procedure, I practically leapt out of bed to embrace her.

Finally, there is the issue of whether the nurse is publicly presented as part of the patient care team. Earlier I mentioned the plaque in my children's pediatrician's office that listed the names of all the doctors who worked with the practice and omitted those of the nurses. The nurses' names should be added to the list. The doctors might object that if they do that, it will start a stampede. Why stop at nurses? What about the names of the nursing assistants, the secretaries, the social workers? Why not? It's a big wall.[27]

These sorts of advances are very important to the public. How nurses negotiate their relationships with doctors can have a significant impact on anyone who is sick and vulnerable and in need of medical and nursing attention. Whether their ways of dealing with difficult doctors or medical biases and prejudices are effective is a public matter, not a private issue or one that concerns only nurses and doctors.

The Nursing Image

No matter what solution to the nursing shortage they advocate, what organization or union they belong to, or even what country they live in, most nurses agree that the profession needs a new image. They believe this new image should capture contemporary realities and help the public, the media, and the political and health care community understand the critical role of nurses. To present this new image, dozens of organizations, foundations, governments, hospitals, and other groups have designed public relations or recruitment campaigns. They have urged their mem- **439** bers or employees to tell their stories and have lobbied governments, foundations, and hospital associations for money to fund public service announcements and advertisements that would attract new candidates to the profession.

All of this is certainly essential to helping the public better understand the work of nurses. But the image campaigns are not enough. Developing public relations campaigns to recruit nurses can be very productive if, at the same time, institutional actors are urged to do their share in promoting nursing work. In the United States, for example, some of the scarce funds going to the Nurse Reinvestment Act and similar state initiatives are earmarked for hospital and health care associations that want to promote a better image of nursing. But why should taxpayer money be spent on recruitment or public service ads when hospitals could be doing so much more through the routine work of PR staff? Such staff are in daily contact with the media. They should be pitching nursing stories on a routine basis and working with heads of nursing departments, who in turn should be consistently educating and updating them on the work nurses do in their institutions. They should then be trying to educate the media and to transform their view of nursing. Sigma Theta Tau International has done some useful work in this area, as has the Royal College of Nursing in Britain. University medical centers should be doing what schools like the University of Pennsylvania, the University of California at San Francisco, the University of Washington, and many others are doing— that is, pitching nursing research and innovations in nursing practice to the media. Nursing unions should also put this on their agenda. All should be urging the creation of nurse-for-a-day programs and making sure that the hospital, medical center, and university PR staffs are some of the first to participate. Then perhaps they will understand what it is they are trying to sell and finally grasp that it's indeed worth selling. Journalists would also make excellent candidates for such workplace encounters.

In our book *From Silence to Voice*, Bernice Buresh and I have detailed myriad strategies that nurses can use to promote their work. We believe the most important thing that employers, educators, and representative groups can do is encourage nurses to talk about their work and teach them how to do it in a credible and compelling manner. We've seen that nurses are still socialized to fear talking about their work and exposing critical problems. This reluctance will not necessarily be overcome by producing a new generation of nurses with advanced degrees. When I was working on Part One of this book, one of these "new" nurses I spoke with insisted I make up a pseudonym for him because he was so nervous about

440 expressing any public reservations about the state of doctor-nurse relationships. This in spite of the fact that his experiences took place seven years ago. He was a graduate student who was embarking on a career in nursing research and academia. Why was he so nervous? I asked. "Well, it's just so frowned upon to talk about this kind of thing," he said, adding that nursing culture is very harsh, that dissent is little tolerated. To continue this kind of cultural socialization puts nurses at a huge disadvantage when they are finally invited to a table with doctors, lawyers, administrators, and policy experts who have been trained to speak more assertively and directly confront disagreements and conflicts of interests between different players. Individual assertiveness training only goes so far in helping nurses overcome their long socialization in silence. Nursing schools and organizations might consider teaching nurses debating skills—as well as negotiating and mediation skills—that would help them more comfortably navigate and engage in constructive conflict. This would help nurses understand how the rules of conversation and confrontation differ in various settings.[28]

Updating the image of nursing will involve applying some critical thinking to the sentimentalized virtue script that nurses so often rely on today. As I mentioned earlier, nursing campaigns and individual nurses' comments about their work rely heavily on some of the following mantras: We're always there to care for you. Nursing—the most noble profession. Lifting spirits, touching lives. Nursing—an expertise of the heart. Nursing—the heart of health care. These scripts are rarely amplified with information about the importance of nursing knowledge and the lifesaving function of nursing action. One reason so many Nurses Week slogans seem so safe and conventional may be that their logos are plastered on tote bags and coffee mugs and banners that hospitals are asked to purchase to either display or distribute to nurses as gifts. Would hospitals be as interested in purchasing and distributing mugs and other paraphernalia that deliver a hard-nosed message about the critical role nurses play and how irreplaceable they are?

Some campaigns and groups try to expand our understanding of nursing by presenting nurses in a variety of roles and by taking on traditional stereotypes of nurses. In the United States, nurse Sandy Summers started a website, the Center for Nursing Advocacy, that monitors the image of nurses, encourages better understanding of nursing, and rallies nurses to protest media stereotyping. Diana J. Mason, editor in chief of the *American Journal of Nursing*, has published and heavily promoted articles that document the cutting-edge care delivered by nurses and that analyze troubling issues such as nurse-physician relationships.

Nurses for a Healthier Tomorrow, a venture spearheaded by Sigma

Theta Tau International, seeks to "reposition nursing as a highly versatile **441** profession where young people can learn science and technology, customer service, critical thinking and decision-making."[29] In order to convince the public that nursing is not what it thinks, the campaign initially seemed almost to shun nurses who work at the bedside or in direct care. Profiles of nurses focused on a nurse who had become a CEO of a hospital, a policy maker, or a manager. Since then, the promotional efforts have expanded and include a greater variety of nurses, many of them giving direct care.

In some instances, it seems almost as if the scientific studies that nursing research produces and the PR campaigns that nursing organizations mount are running on parallel tracks that never cross. Consider, for example, *Nursing: The Ultimate Adventure*, a video produced by the National Student Nurses' Association for junior and senior high school students. The video advertises nursing as an exciting career. It tells us that nurses learn a lot and make a big difference. One of nursing's major attractions, according to the video, is that it rewards the nurse with big doses of public affection. Beverly Malone, at that time president of the American Association of Nurses, declares: "The public loves me as a nurse and they don't even know my name, but if I say I'm an RN, there's affection and warmth and an experience that means so much to me." She is then followed by a young woman who advises that "if you really want a job where people will love you," you should choose nursing.[30]

When nurses use this virtue language to describe their work, Sioban Nelson and I argue, they create a feedback loop that constantly reinforces nineteenth-century stereotypes. "Through this feedback loop nurses send virtue messages to other professionals, members of the public, patients, and the media. These groups, in their turn, broadcast these messages to an even wider public and then back to nursing."[31]

We can see this feedback loop at work in one of the most highly publicized and expensive media and recruitment campaigns of the last decade. In 2002 the Johnson & Johnson pharmaceutical company launched its Campaign for Nursing's Future. The company spent over $20 million on brochures to promote nursing and on television advertising spots and videos. In one video, nurses talk about their work, and another presents patients' perspectives on the profession. The company also hosted fund-raising dinners to raise money for nursing education and established a website where a group of nurses describe why nursing makes a difference and what is so special about the profession. All of the materials that the campaign produced were vetted by a nurse advisory committee.

While this is an important validation for nursing, one that a great many nurses have applauded, many of the messages are extremely problematic.

442   All the Johnson & Johnson materials feature the right mix of men and women, blacks, whites, Asian Americans, and other ethnic groups. The brochures are fairly straightforward and proclaim that nurses make a difference. It is in the TV spots and videos and on the website that the virtue script emerges fully. These are accompanied by jingles. On one TV spot and the recruitment video, it's the following:

> There are some who live for caring with all they have to give
> There are some who have comfort to share
> They dare to care
> They dare to cry
> They dare to feel
> They dare to try
> They dare to be, at the end of the day,
> More than they were the day before
> There are some who find their treasure inside a grateful smile
> There are some who will always be there
> There are some who make the journey just to find out who they are
> There are some who have the courage to care
> There are some who dare to care.[32]

On the video presenting patient perspectives, it goes like this:

> You're always there when someone needs you
> You work your magic quietly
> You're not in it for the glory
> The care you give comes naturally
> You take my hand
> Touch my life
> When I need you.[33]

On the recruitment video, one nurse comments that "the art and science of medicine combined with awesome nursing care can perform miracles." With no mention of either the art or science of nursing, and such heavy doses of sentimentalized caregiving, one is catapulted back into the nineteenth century, where nursing was depicted as either angelic or miraculous. Indeed, in this video nursing is often reduced to the typical stereotype of hand-holding. "Nursing is powerful work," one voice-over tells us. "Not many professions offer you the chance to touch lives and make a difference the way nursing does." She is then followed by a male nurse who defines the power of nursing as follows:

"Being a nurse is about holding someone's hand. Being a nurse is about giving a really good shot to a six-year-old who's terrified. It's about putting an ice pack and making it better on someone . . . or getting the wrinkles out of the back of a sheet that's causing someone to be uncom- **443** fortable who has to lay on the bed. They don't have any other place to go. They have to be there. And sometimes just rubbing someone's back is the answer to all their prayers."

On the website some nurses go into more detail about the difference nursing care makes. Others repeat some of the same clichés: nurses are the "doctor's eyes and ears"; nurses experience the gratitude in patients' eyes.

These media scripts represent a repackaging of the nineteenth-century virtue script in twenty-first-century production values. By sticking to the virtue script, the Johnson & Johnson campaign and many other nurse recruitment campaigns also deliver a highly gendered message. While some of the nurses are men, one has to ask how many men will be drawn to sentimentalized images of nursing work. Nursing has remained stubbornly female, inching down from 97 percent to the 95 percent mark but never attracting a significant influx of men. Medicine, on the other hand, is now more than 50 percent female. This certainly has to do with money and status. But it may also have to do with the fact that nursing consistently presents itself in terms that reproduce gender stereotypes that would not appeal to many men—or to modern women for that matter.

A look at how the Army Nurse Corps advertises nursing work is relevant here. In the Army Nurse Corps, about 36 percent of nurses are men. In promotional materials, both women and men are depicted as doing tough, challenging work in difficult conditions. Nurses are shown as masters of technology and humanitarian missions. One might object that the military's promotional literature and images is gendered in a different way. That may be so. But it seems to be working.[34]

Through its images, songs, and commentary, the Johnson & Johnson campaign and many others tend to emphasize emotion more than intelligence and skill. Doctors, on the other hand, advertise their work as cutting edge, as lifesaving, health saving, and even money saving. Do they dare to care? Indeed they do, through advances in palliative care, women's health care, and geriatrics, among others. Nurses here are self-sacrificing ("You're not in it for the glory") and silent ("You work your magic quietly"). Their caregiving doesn't seem to depend on education and experience ("The care you give comes naturally"). When nurses are asked to define their work, they talk about making a difference, but how they do this is not well articulated.

I was surprised, for example, at the imprecision in the seven-minute patient perspectives video. Patients had a chance to help us understand what nurses actually did to help them survive and thrive. But again, the emphasis was on nurses' emotional work, on their comfort and support. A

444   woman who was on an ICU with a brain tumor talked about the nurse as a source of solace and truth telling but never supplemented the picture with the incredible technical mastery that surely kept the patient alive moment by moment. A woman talked about how nurses enter a room and notice everything, like whether a window was open, but didn't mention all the catastrophes the nurse prevented. Only one young man, who witnessed a school nurse do CPR on a basketball court, talked about what nurses do to save lives. Throughout this video, a woman's voice singing in the background kept repeating the mantra that nurses are "Unsung heroes . . . I sing a song of praise to you."

Nurses may relish this kind of attention, but reliance on virtue scripts may have serious political ramifications. What happens to the nurse who no longer wants to be silent, who wants a little recognition, not to mention well-deserved glory? What happens if they speak for themselves and ask for a raise? Do they risk loss of this kind of public support and trust because they are no longer altruistic and devoted caregivers? What kind of students will this version of nursing attract? Will someone who doesn't want to be an "unsung hero" be drawn to the career? Will new recruits be disappointed and leave when they discover they don't have time to give a massage, or when they find themselves dealing with very sick patients who aren't grateful for their work?

In a period of cost cutting, it's imperative that caring be described in a clear and concrete language that explains precisely why the nurse-patient relationship and clinician-patient trust are so important and demonstrates precisely how the knowledge and skill of nurses protect patients from danger and risk.

Changing the public image of nursing isn't easy and will be impossible if working conditions don't change. The best way to alter the image is to build on a solid foundation. That means helping the public understand the complexity of bedside, direct care nursing, and then moving out from there. To illustrate how this can be done, consider how the British Columbia Nurses Union pitched nursing in a PR campaign in the spring of 1997. A nurse is standing smiling at a patient's bedside, as he is about to begin eating his hospital meal. The ad copy reads:

> He thinks he's having a conversation about the hospital Jell-O. She's actually midway through about 100 assessments. In the seconds it takes to reach the bedside, a Registered Nurse will have made over 100 assessments.
>
> Any one of which could mean the difference between recovery and tragedy.

Take away direct patient care from Registered Nurses and vital **445**
knowledge affecting the health of the patient is lost.

Nurses are doing vital work. It's that simple. While rethinking our
regional health care system, it is vital to strengthen the role of Registered Nurses, the most comprehensively trained nurses in the system.

Registered Nurses are not an adjunct to our evolving health care
system, they are at the very hub of it. Making sure they keep direct
patient contact is critical to the quality of our health care system.

While they may not be specialists in green Jell-O, when it comes to
health care, Registered Nurses are irreplaceable.

For the biennial meeting of the International Council of Nurses in
2000, the Danish Nurses Association commissioned a photographer,
Soren Svenson, to take pictures of Danish nurses doing their routine
daily work. The pictures are remarkable for their candor, tact, and emotional resonance. With the exception of some shots of well-child visits,
most of the nurses Svenson photographed are taking care of sick and
vulnerable human beings. They are assisting at complex surgeries, monitoring patients on ventilators, helping patients in hip-high casts, giving
medication and food to elderly patients at home, and witnessing and alleviating the despair and loneliness of patients in mental hospitals. We see
nurses attending to people with their legs pinned, their bodies crumbling, and their souls bared. The DNA exhibit helps us look at some difficult images without flinching and captures the uncomfortable realities
of the human condition that nurses deal with every day. Accompanying
the exhibit were concise descriptions of what nurses do. Nothing fancy,
nothing gussied up, just the facts of routine care and the difference it
makes.

When I thought of this exhibit and reflected on the studies I've cited in
this book, I decided to take a crack at rewriting one of the comments a
nurse made for the Johnson & Johnson video. Nursing is indeed powerful. But I'd suggest that being a nurse is quite different from the claims of
this particular video. I would have the nurse say this:

"Being a nurse is about saving patients' lives. Being a nurse is about
making sure a patient doesn't develop a fatal complication after surgery.
It's about paying attention to the smallest but most significant details.
Like smoothing out the wrinkles on a sheet so a patient doesn't develop
an excruciating and costly bedsore. Sometimes by sitting and talking to
someone, I find out the most important things, like whether patients understand how to take their medications, whether they have support at
home, and whether they are frightened and anxious."

Universal Health Care

One of the best ways in which nurses can enhance their public image is to fight for some form of universal health care in the United States, and to continue to fight privatization schemes in countries that already have some form of single-payer national health system. More money for nursing education, for adequate nursing staff, for nursing education, for better pay, and for interdisciplinary collaboration, these all depend on an end to the chaos of market-driven health care and a stable way of financing health care delivery that really controls wasteful spending. Similarly, the future of nursing in countries with tax-supported universal health care will depend on fending off efforts to privatize public health care systems and rejecting attempts to introduce the waste that is so rampant in the United States. Judging by the problems we've seen outside the United States, a universal health care system offers no guarantee that nursing will be adequately valued and funded. But it is one of the necessary but insufficient conditions for ending the crisis. If, along with the implementation—or protection—of publicly funded universal health care, the image and education of nurses is addressed and problems in the provision of care and physician-nurse relationships are remedied, this will go a long way to solving the nursing crisis.

This book cannot outline all the advantages and forms of universal health care systems that exist in the world. Suffice it to say that if America finally decides to join the rest of the industrialized world in giving all citizens access to health care services, there are numerous models to choose from. Almost every other industrialized country in the world has better health outcomes and spends less money per capita on health care than the United States. Indeed, the United States unarguably excels in one area—spending more on health care than any other nation on earth, while giving less care to increasingly large segments of its population.

Some form of publicly funded universal health care is critical for nurses for several reasons. First and foremost, it allows nurses to fulfill their obligation as patient advocates. It's hard to advocate for patients who have no access to services or whose access is restricted by Byzantine insurance rules designed to deny them needed care. In this kind of advocacy, nurses not only help their patients, they help themselves when they become patients. Today, many RNs are afraid to leave their jobs because they fear the loss of job-related health care. Many RNs who would like to retire early because they can't take the physical strain are unable to do so, not only because they need a paycheck but because job loss means loss of health insurance. While RNs in other industrialized countries face a host of problems, this is not one of them.

Universal health care is also critical because we will be unable to secure **447** enough money to pay nurses what they deserve, and staff hospitals and health care institutions with sufficient numbers of RNs, if we can't eliminate the staggering amount of clinical and administrative waste in the U.S. health care system. Alan Sager, professor at Boston University School of Public Health outlines the sorry facts. The United States spends about 50 percent of its health care dollars—that's 50 percent of $1.8 trillion—on clinical waste (unnecessary medical care, defensive medicine, incompetent care), administrative waste (advertising, marketing, and profit), excessively priced pharmaceuticals and durable medical equipment, and outright theft. For example, pharmaceutical costs in the United States are 67 percent higher than in Canada and 78 percent higher than the average in seven wealthy nations.

If waste were squeezed out of the system, Sager and others argue, more money would be available for needed clinical care. "Health care, unlike education, housing, and the environment, is the easiest problem to fix in the United States. It's the only problem on which we already spend enough. We don't need more money, we just need to recycle dollars, and spend sanely instead of insanely."

Some form of single-payer system would, Sager continues, allow us to identify which hospitals and which emergency rooms and other services are needed to protect the health of the public. A government interested in safe and effective health care for all would guarantee that as long as they are efficiently operated, needed hospitals would stay open and have enough money to provide high-quality care.

By eliminating competing insurance plans, universal health care would potentially liberate RNs from the enormous amount of paperwork that is generated by the confusing welter of companies and their conflicting rules. It would also liberate them from the frustrating job of scrounging services for people who are uninsured, fighting for services that are denied to people who are insured, and finally being the enforcers of a system that often limits needed care. Indeed, we could add more nurses to the patient care work force if we recycled nurses who are discharge planners (i.e., who negotiate with insurance companies about the patient handoff) and utilization reviewers in hospitals or insurance companies—retrieving them from cost/profit management to some form of care.

The most positive aspect of universal health care is that it would create some form of health care stability. As we've seen, hospital budgets in the United States are so unstable and unpredictable that administrators lurch from crisis to crisis with their eye firmly fixed on short-term profit. They are willing marks for whatever quack remedy or financial silver bullet the latest hotshot consultant advertises. Universal health care would give hos-

448 pitals a stable budget that would allow them to plan for the long term, says Bruce Vladeck. He is professor of health policy and geriatrics at the Mount Sinai School of Medicine in New York, and from 1993 to 1997 he was the administrator of the U.S. government's Health Care Financing Administration, the agency that runs Medicare. According to Vladeck, "Some kind of universal health care system would presumably have some mechanism to make certain that hospitals got paid for everybody they took care of, and they would be less susceptible to short-term swings in patterns of insurance coverage and in the number of uninsured people who show up at their door. That would give them substantially greater certainty about their budget, if not more money. You'd have a mechanism to negotiate down drug and medical equipment prices and some mechanism for negotiating hospital prices. After some period of time it would presumably be a relatively stable mechanism, as it is in most of those countries that have universal health insurance."

Nurses are singularly situated to fight for universal health care and educate the public about the need for a long-term solution to our health care crisis. A number of groups in the United States, like Physicians for a National Health Program, are advocating some form of universal health care system. Several nursing unions—the California Nurses and Massachusetts Nurses Associations, and nurses in the Communications Workers of America in Buffalo—have been vocal advocates of national health care. The American Nurses Association is on record supporting some form of single-payer universal health care system, but does little member or outside education about the issue. Other nursing unions and nursing organizations, although certainly not all, have understood the need for such a fundamental change.

Some nurses privately admit that there is really no other way to solve the nursing crisis or any of the other problems that plague the system. But they insist that a single-payer system is a dream that is not politically feasible. Nothing could be further from the truth. As many acknowledge, our system is crumbling and needs a total overhaul. Nurses certainly need to be part of a solution on which the integrity of their profession will depend. The nurse practitioner movement grew out of the passage of Medicare and Medicaid in the sixties. Imagine how many more nurse practitioners and advanced practice nurses we'd need if forty-four million Americans weren't excluded from basic primary care services. Imagine how many nurses we could afford if that wasted 50 percent of $1.8 trillion—that's $900 billion—were liberated to provide needed care.

Summing Up

Whether we are discussing styles of discourse, debating about staffing ratios and education, or pondering how to define nursing for the public, the central question has to be this: How are we going to find enough people willing to deliver hands-on care to very sick people in a world in which women have new occupational options, men still fail to see the challenge in nursing, and people are living longer with more chronic and acute needs? As we project future health care needs, we must produce enough nurses to care for sick people, to teach nursing students, and to conduct nursing research. We need to factor in the recognition that even under the best of circumstances, nurses will move around, change jobs, and even go into other fields. We particularly need to recognize the enormous burden of caring that will arise in a world in which people live longer and sicker with all sorts of illnesses and disabilities, some of which we can't even imagine today (after AIDS and SARS, who knows what will be next?). In industrialized countries, people are demanding intensive treatments well into their eighties, sometimes even into their nineties.

In a world in which birth rates are plummeting in many countries, we can't afford to construct nursing as women's work or to view basic nursing work as something that requires little education, intelligence, or expertise. Neither can nurses. We need to help the world understand the complexity and consequences of seemingly trivial nursing "tasks" as we move on to create new categories of nurses who will practice outside traditional nursing roles. We can't afford to produce a kind of hands-off care that will reinforce the medical grip on the public imagination and entrench the idea that only those who are doing "medicine" deserve advanced education, better pay, and significant control over their work and collegial relationships. Solutions to the nursing crisis, or shortage, won't work if what they really solve is the maldistribution of physician services and misallocation of financial resources that go to physician reimbursement.

Of course we need well-educated, experienced people in nursing. Of course we need nurses who work in a variety of different roles and settings—in the community, in public health, in primary care. But we also need them in operating rooms, where they create the environment in which surgery is possible and where they can warn us when a surgeon is incompetent, or so overworked that he is a danger to his patients. We need them to help us take care of unstable patients in hospitals, in our homes, and in psychiatric institutions, clinics, schools, nursing homes, and rehabilitation facilities.

Believe me, if you're sick today, no matter where you are cared for, you want the person who gives you a bed bath, feeds you, helps you walk, or

450   teaches you about the twelve different medications you're supposed to take, to be the best educated, most experienced, and most satisfied nurse you can find. You want this nurse to be able to work with doctors and to challenge and negotiate with them. You want hospitals to give them more voice, more authority, and better pay, workloads, and schedules. You want the media to write about what they do, not about why they are no longer doing it. And you want their culture to be supportive, to encourage voice not silence, and to cope with inevitable intraprofessional divisions without being devoured by them. This is why, as I said earlier, my mantra has become "Retention and recruitment." If you can retain your work force, then you can recruit new additions to it. If you cannot, shortage-plagued areas in nursing will remain what they are today, a revolving door of attraction and repulsion that endlessly reproduces the dilemmas I have described. That isn't good enough for patients today and it certainly won't be good enough for the millions of people who will depend on nursing care tomorrow and in the years to come.

Notes

Introduction

1. Versions of this story appeared as "Thinking like a Nurse, You Have to Be a Nurse to Do It," *Nursing Inquiry* 9, no. 1 (2002): 57–61; and "Outpatient . . . and Out of Luck?" *Revolution* 1, no. 1 (January/February 2000): 19–21.
2. American Hospital Association, "The Hospital Workforce Shortage: Immediate and Future," *Trend Watch* 3 (2001).
3. Julie Sochalski, "Nursing Shortage Redux: Turning the Corner on an Enduring Problem," *Health Affairs* 21, no. 5 (2002), 157.
4. California Nurses Association, "RNs Deride Governor's Health Care Vetoes, Rejection of Safe Lift Policies, Hospital Closure Bills Put RNs, Patients at Risk, Says Calif. Nurses Assn.," press release, September 23, 2004.
5. Linda H. Aiken et al., "Nurses' Reports on Hospital Care in Five Countries," *Health Affairs* (May/June 2001): 43–53.
6. Sochalski, "Nursing Shortage Redux," 159.
7. Albert O. Hirschman, *Exit, Voice and Loyalty: Responses to Decline in Firms, Organizations, and States* (Cambridge: Harvard University Press, 1970).
8. James C. Scott, *Seeing Like a State: How Certain Schemes to Improve the Human Condition Have Failed* (New Haven: Yale University Press, 1998), 316–317.
9. *New York Times*, crossword puzzle, January 16, 2003.
10. See Suzanne Gordon, *Life Support: Three Nurses on the Front Lines* (New York: Little, Brown, 1996).

1. Manufacturing the Dominant Doctor

1. U.S. Department of Health and Human Services, Public Health Service, Agency for Health Care Policy and Research, *Acute Pain Management: Operative or Medical Procedures and Trauma* (Rockville, MD: Department of Health and Human Services, 1992), 11.
2. Leonard Stein, "The Doctor-Nurse Game," *Archives of General Psychiatry* 16

452

(1967): 699–703; Leonard Stein, David Watts, and Timothy Howell, "The Doctor-Nurse Game Revisited," *New England Journal of Medicine* 322 (1990): 546–549.

3. Alan H. Rosenstein, "Nurse-Physician Relationships: Impact on Nurse Satisfaction and Retention," *American Journal of Nursing* 102, no. 6 (June 2002): 26–34.

4. Joint Commission on the Accreditation of Health Care Organizations, "Health Care at the Crossroads: Strategies for Addressing the Evolving Nursing Crisis" (report, JCAHCO, 2002), 12.

5. Fédération des infirmières et infirmiers du Québec (FIIQ), "A Policy to Counter Violence at Work" (report, Montreal, 2002).

6. FIIQ, "Research Report on Violence against Nurses in the Workplace," A95-CF-IV-D7 (report, 1995), 18.

7. Daniel Chambliss, *Beyond Caring: Hospitals, Nurses, and the Social Organization of Ethics* (Chicago: University of Chicago Press, 1996), 75.

8. John E. Heffner, "Letter from the MUSC Medical Director," in *The Many Faces of Nursing* (Charleston: Medical University of South Carolina, 2002), 5.

9. Denise Webster, "Medical Students' Views of the Role of the Nurse," *Nursing Research* 34 (1985): 315.

10. Chambliss, *Beyond Caring*, 77.

11. As Eliot Freidson has written, it is the "organization of the immediate work environment . . . and the pressures of the situation" that shape professional identity and interprofessional relationships.

12. D. C. Aron and L. A. Headrick, "Educating Physicians Prepared to Improve Care and Safety Is No Accident: It Requires a Systematic Approach," *Quality and Safety in Health Care* 11 (2002): 171.

13. Robert C. McKersie, "In the Foothills of Medicine" (unpublished).

14. Lillian Rubin, *Intimate Strangers: Men and Women Together* (New York: Harper and Row, 1984).

15. Deborah Tannen, *Gender and Discourse* (New York: Oxford University Press, 1994), 23, 22.

16. For a more extensive discussion of this problem, see Bernice Buresh and Suzanne Gordon, *From Silence to Voice: What Nurses Know and Must Communicate to the Public* (Ithaca: Cornell University Press, 2000).

17. T. M. Luhrmann, *Of Two Minds: The Growing Disorder in American Psychiatry* (New York: Alfred A. Knopf, 2000), 93.

18. Timothy McCall, "Impact of Long Working Hours on Resident Physicians," *New England Journal of Medicine* 318 (1988): 775–778.

19. June J. Pilcher and Allen L. Huffcutt, "Effects of Sleep Deprivation on Performance: A Meta-Analysis," *Sleep* 19 (1996): 323.

20. Ibid., 318–326; Judith S. Samkoff and C. H. M. Jacques, "A Review of Studies Concerning Effects of Sleep Deprivation and Fatigue on Residents' Performance," *Academic Medicine* 66 (1991): 687–693.

21. Aron and Headrick, "Educating Physicians," 168.

22. J. Bryan Sexton, Eric J. Thomas, and Robert L. Helmreich, "Error, Stress, and Teamwork in Medicine and Aviation: Cross-Sectional Surveys," *British Medical Journal* 320 (2000): 745, 746.

23. SUPPORT principal investigators, "A Controlled Trial to Improve Care for Seriously Ill Hospitalized Patients: The Study to Understand Prognoses and Preferences for Outcomes and Risks of Treatments (SUPPORT)," *Journal of the American Medical Association* 274 (1995): 1591–1598.

24. Bernard Lo, "Improving Care near the End of Life: Why Is It So Hard?" *Journal* **453**
    of the American Medical Association 274 (1995): 1634–1636.
25. Aron and Headrick, "Educating Physicians," 170.
26. Atul Gawande, *Complications: A Surgeon's Notes on an Imperfect Science* (New York:
    Picador, 2002), 57.
27. "Report of the Manitoba Pediatric Cardiac Surgery Inquest: An Inquiry into
    Twelve Deaths at the Winnipeg Health Sciences Centre in 1994," Provincial
    Court of Manitoba, May 2001, 356.
28. Sally Satel, *PC, M.D.: How Political Correctness Is Corrupting Medicine* (New York:
    Basic Books, 2000), 79, 95.
29. Andrew Abbott, *The System of Professions: An Essay on the Division of Expert Labor*
    (Chicago: University of Chicago Press, 1988), 65–66.
30. Aron and Headrick, "Educating Physicians," 168.
31. Arthur M. Magun, letter to the editor, *New York Times*, December 23, 2002, A26.
32. Steven G. Friedman, "Anyone in the O.R.?" *New York Times*, June 10, 2003, A27.

2. Designing the Doctor-Nurse Game

1. For a detailed elaboration of this history see Roy Porter, *The Greatest Benefit to
   Mankind: A Medical History of Humanity* (New York: W. W. Norton, 1997);
   Guenter B. Risse, *Mending Bodies, Saving Souls: A History of Hospitals* (New York:
   Oxford University Press, 1999); Paul Starr, *The Social Transformation of American
   Medicine* (New York: Basic Books, 1982); Charles E. Rosenberg, *The Care of
   Strangers: The Rise of America's Hospital System* (New York: Basic Books, 1987).
2. M. Jeanne Peterson, *The Medical Profession in Mid-Victorian London* (Berkeley:
   University of California Press, 1978), 5.
3. Ibid., chaps. 3, 4.
4. Susan M. Reverby, *Ordered to Care: The Dilemma of American Nursing 1850–1945*
   (Cambridge: Cambridge University Press, 1990), 26.
5. See Peterson, *Medical Profession*, chap. 4; Starr, *Social Transformation*, 87.
6. Thetis M. Group and Joan I. Roberts, *Nursing, Physician Control, and the Medical
   Monopoly: Historical Perspectives on Gendered Inequality and Roles, Rights, and Range
   of Practice* (Indianapolis: Indiana University Press, 2001); Judith Moore, *A Zeal for
   Responsibility: The Struggle for Professional Nursing in Victorian England, 1868–1883*
   (Athens: University of Georgia Press, 1988); Reverby, *Ordered to Care*, 47–48.
7. Peterson, *Medical Profession*, 184–185.
8. Ibid., 186–187.
9. "Sex in Mind Education," *Lancet*, May 9, 1874, 663.
10. Ibid., 664.
11. "Medical Women," *Lancet*, March 11, 1876, 398.
12. "Skilled Nursing," *Lancet*, January 13, 1877, 62.
13. *Times* (London), October 18, 1880, 9.
14. J. Braxton Hicks, "On Nursing Systems," *British Medical Journal*, January 3, 1880,
    11.
15. Peterson, *Medical Profession*, 183.
16. Katrin Schultheiss, *Bodies and Souls: Politics and the Professionalization of Nursing in
    France, 1880–1922* (Cambridge: Harvard University Press, 2001), 19.
17. Ibid., 52.
18. Ibid., 21, 23.
19. Ibid., 7.

454

20. John H. Packard, "On the Training of Nurses for the Sick," *Boston Medical and Surgical Journal* 95, no. 20 (1876): 577. This journal was the forerunner of the *New England Journal of Medicine*.

21. Ibid.

22. "The Reciprocal Relations of the Nurse and the Physician," editorial, *Boston Medical and Surgical Journal* 121, no. 17 (1889): 417.

23. W. Gilman Thompson, "The Overtrained Nurse," *New York Medical Journal* 83, no. 17 (1906): 845.

24. "Woman as Doctor and Woman as Nurse," *Lancet*, August 17, 1878, 227.

25. Thompson, "Overtrained Nurse," 846.

26. Ibid.

27. Moore, *Zeal for Responsibility*, 105–111.

28. "Reciprocal Relations," 417.

29. Karen Buhler-Wilkerson, *No Place like Home: A History of Nursing and Home Care in the United States* (Baltimore: Johns Hopkins University Press, 2001), 46.

30. Ibid., 98, 109, 110.

31. "Woman as Doctor," 227.

32. Ibid.; Packard, "Training of Nurses," 574.

33. Schultheiss, *Bodies and Souls*, 95, 31.

34. "Guy's Hospital," *Times* (London), December 21, 1886, 8.

35. Schultheiss, *Bodies and Souls*, 104, 93.

36. Sioban Nelson, *Say Little, Do Much: Nursing, Nuns and Hospitals in the 19th Century* (Philadelphia: University of Pennsylvania Press, 2001), 123.

37. Buhler-Wilkerson, *No Place like Home*, 110.

38. Rosenberg, *Care of Strangers*, 235.

39. Reverby, *Ordered to Care*; Rosenberg, *Care of Strangers*.

40. Nelson, *Say Little, Do Much*.

41. Margarete Sandelowski, *Devices and Desires: Gender, Technology, and American Nursing* (Chapel Hill: University of North Carolina Press, 2000), 72.

42. Thompson, "Overtrained Nurse," 845.

43. Sandelowski, *Devices and Desires*, 71.

44. Ibid., 75.

45. Ibid., 90.

46. Ibid., 64.

47. Ibid., 2.

48. Ibid., 87.

49. Julie Fairman and Joan Lynaugh, *Critical Care Nursing: A History* (Philadelphia: University of Pennsylvania Press, 1998), 5, 11.

50. Sandelowski, *Devices and Desires*, 127.

51. Ibid., 112.

52. Eliot Freidson, *Profession of Medicine: A Study of the Sociology of Applied Knowledge* (Chicago: University of Chicago Press, 1988), 17, 69.

53. Suzanne Gordon, "Necessary Nursing Care," *Nursing Inquiry* 7 (2000): 217–219.

54. Freidson, *Profession of Medicine*, 69.

55. Fred E. Katz, "Nurses," in *The Semi-Professions and Their Organization: Teachers, Nurses, Social Workers*, ed. Amitai Etzioni (New York: Free Press, 1969), 56, 58.

56. Ibid., 59, 60, 64, 70.

57. Rosenberg, *Care of Strangers*, 235.

3. The Disruptive Medical System

1. Bureau of Justice Statistics, *Workplace Violence, 1992–1996*, special report, July 1998, NCJ 168634, www.ojp.usdoj.gov/bjs/pub/ascii/wv96.txt.
2. Fédération des infirmières et infirmiers du Québec, "Research Report on Violence against Nurses in the Workplace" (Montreal, 1995), 18, 19.
3. International Labour Organization, "Violence at Work," *Travail*, no. 26 (September 1998).
4. Anne Federwisch, "Occupational Hazard: Nurses Are Susceptible to Workplace Violence at the Hands of Strangers and Co-Workers," *NurseWeek*, April 23, 2001, www.nurseweek.com/news/features/01–04/violence.asp.
5. Alan H. Rosenstein, "Nurse-Physician Relationships: Impact on Nurse Satisfaction and Retention," *American Journal of Nursing* 102 (2002): 31.

4. Fatal Synergy

1. Murray Sinclair, *The Report of the Manitoba Cardiac Surgery Inquest: An Inquiry into Twelve Deaths at the Winnipeg Health Sciences Centre in 1994* (Winnipeg: Provincial Court of Manitoba, 2001).
2. Institute of Medicine, *To Err Is Human: Building a Safer Health System* (Washington, DC: National Academy Press, 1999), 1.
3. D. C. Aron and L. A. Headrick, "Educating Physicians Prepared to Improve Care and Safety Is No Accident: It Requires a Systematic Approach," *Quality and Safety in Health Care* 11 (2002): 168.
4. J. H. Silber et al., "Hospital and Patient Characteristics Associated with Death after Surgery: A Study of Adverse Occurrence and Failure to Rescue," *Medical Care* 30 (1992): 615–629.
5. Sinclair, *Manitoba Inquest*, 113; hereafter cited by page number in the text.
6. For a fuller description of the campaign to help the nurses, see Bernice Buresh and Suzanne Gordon, *From Silence to Voice: What Nurses Know and Must Communicate to the Public* (Ithaca: Cornell University Press, 2000), 203–205.
7. Gabriel Scally, "Eerie Parallels between British, Canadian Inquests into Infant Deaths," *Canadian Medical Association Journal* (2001), http://www.cma.ca/cmaj/cmaj_today/2001/07_26.htm.
8. See Sue Burr, "Making a Difference," *Nursing Management* 8 (2001): 6–10.
9. Statement of Patricia Dorothy Fields, in *The BRI Inquiry into Pediatric Cardiac Services in Bristol, 1984–1985*, WIT O154 0008 (Bristol Royal Infirmary Inquiry, 2001).
10. Ibid., WIT 0085 0003.
11. Ibid., WIT 0132 0012.
12. This quotation and those following are from pages 5–32 of the inquiry transcripts, http://www.bristol-inquiry.org.uk/evidence/transcripts/day59.htm.
13. Patricia Benner, Christine A. Tanner, and Catherine A. Chesla, *Expertise in Nursing Practice: Caring, Clinical Judgment, and Ethics* (New York: Springer, 1996).
14. Ibid., 282–283.
15. Ibid., 283.
16. Ibid.
17. For this account I am indebted to Peter Heffner, an attorney for Lynch and Lynch who prepared the case. Heffner spoke with me at length and provided a summary of the facts in the case, as the plaintiffs presented them.

456   18. Sinclair, *Manitoba Inquest,* 355.

19. Ibid., 134.

20. Ibid., 357.

21. Benner, Tanner, and Chesla, *Expertise in Nursing Practice.*

5. Making Matters Worse

1. Kenneth B. Schwartz Center, fact sheet, Boston, December 9, 2003.

2. Deborah Tannen, *Gender and Discourse* (New York: Oxford University Press, 1994), 21.

3. Guenter B. Risse, *Mending Bodies, Saving Souls: A History of Hospitals* (New York: Oxford University Press, 1999), 73–74.

4. Sioban Nelson, "From Salvation to Civics: Service to the Sick in Nursing Discourse," *Social Science and Medicine* 53 (2001): 1217–1225; Sioban Nelson, "Entering the Professional Domain: The Making of the Modern Nurse in 17th Century France," *Nursing History Review* 7 (1999): 171–188.

5. Sioban Nelson, *Say Little, Do Much: Nursing, Nuns, and Hospitals in the Nineteenth Century* (Philadelphia: University of Pennsylvania Press, 2001), 17–19.

6. Colin Jones, quoted in ibid., 19.

7. Deidre Wicks, *Nurses and Doctors at Work: Rethinking Professional Boundaries* (Buckingham, UK: Open University Press, 1998), 55.

8. Ibid., 51, 52.

9. Laurel Thatcher Ulrich, *A Midwife's Tale: The Life of Martha Ballard, Based on Her Diary, 1785–1812* (New York: Vintage, 1990).

10. Wicks, *Nurses and Doctors,* 52, 53.

11. Nelson, *Say Little, Do Much,* 123.

12. Ibid.

13. Isabel Marcus, "Dark Numbers: Domestic Violence, Law, and Public Policy in Russia, Poland, Romania, and Hungary" (unpublished manuscript).

14. Mary C. Sullivan, ed., *The Friendship of Florence Nightingale and Mary Clare Moore* (Philadelphia: University of Pennsylvania Press, 1999).

15. For a full account of this activity see Sioban Nelson and M. Patricia Donahue, *Nursing: The Finest Art,* 2nd ed. (Saint Louis, MO: Mosby, 1996).

16. Janet Horowitz Murray, *Strong-Minded Women and Other Lost Voices from 19th Century England* (New York: Pantheon Books, 1982), 4.

17. Colleen Hobbs, *Florence Nightingale* (New York: Twayne, 1997), 79.

18. Ibid.

19. Murray, *Strong-Minded Women,* 5.

20. Risse, *Mending Bodies,* 367.

21. Richard Sennett, *The Fall of Public Man* (New York: Alfred A. Knopf, 1977), 23.

22. Sioban Nelson, "Hairdressing and Nursing: Presentation of Self and Professional Formation in Colonial Australia," *Collegian* 8 (2001), 28–31.

23. Susan M. Reverby, *Ordered to Care: The Dilemma of American Nursing 1850–1945* (Cambridge: Cambridge University Press, 1990).

24. Charles E. Rosenberg, *The Care of Strangers: The Rise of America's Hospital System* (New York: Basic Books, 1987), 235.

25. "Skilled Nursing," *Lancet,* January 13, 1877, 62.

26. Margarete Sandelowski, *Devices and Desires: Gender, Technology, and American Nursing* (Chapel Hill: University of North Carolina Press, 2000), 176.

27. Michael Beebe, "Operation Comeback," *Buffalo News,* October 10, 1999, A1.   **457**

28. Darlene Clark and Paul Clark, personal communication.

29. Wicks, *Nurses and Doctors,* 5.

30. Adele W. Pike, "Moral Outrage and Moral Discourse in Nurse-Physician Collaboration," *Journal of Professional Nursing* 7 (1991): 351–362.

31. Ibid., 351.

32. Arlie Hochschild, *The Managed Heart: Commercialization of Human Feeling* (Berkeley: University of California Press, 1983).

33. Patricia A. Potter and Anne Griffen Perry, *Fundamentals of Nursing* (New York: Mosby, 2001), 311, 314.

34. Anne Gardner et al., "Don't Call Me Sweetie," *Collegian* 8 (2001): 32–38.

35. Daniel Chambliss, *Beyond Caring: Hospitals, Nurses, and the Social Organization of Ethics* (Chicago: University of Chicago Press, 1996), 87.

6. Dropped from the Picture

1. Jean-Jacques Deutsch and Françoise Doumayrenc, *Je sais qui nous soigne* (Paris: Magnard, 2000), 19, 18.

2. Philip A. Kalisch and Beatrice J. Kalisch, *The Changing Image of the Nurse* (Reading: Addison-Wesley, 1987), 3.

3. Kaiser Family Foundation, "Documenting the Power of Television: A Survey of Regular ER Viewers about Emergency Contraception," www.kff.org/womens health/1358–ers.cfm.

4. Joseph Turow and Rachel Gans, "As Seen on TV: Health Policy Issues in TV's Medical Dramas," report to the Kaiser Family Foundation (Menlo Park, CA, 2002), 1.

5. Dominique de Saint Mars, *Max va à l'hôpital* (Paris: Calligram, 1993).

6. Charlotte Roederer, *L'hôpital* (Paris: Gallimard, 2000).

7. Michael Bond and Karen Jankel, *Paddington Goes to the Hospital* (London: HarperCollins, 2001).

8. Ronne Randall, *Nurse Nancy* (London: Ladybird Books, n.d.).

9. *Jeanine the Nurse Paper Doll* (Mineola, NY: Dover, 2000).

10. Fred Rogers, *Going to the Hospital* (New York: Putnam and Grosset, 1988).

11. Alice K. Flanagan, *Ask Nurse Pfaff, She'll Help You!* (New York: Children's Press, 1997).

12. Kim Watson, *A Trip to the Hospital* (New York: Simon Spotlight, 2001).

13. Beatrice and Phillip Kalisch traced the portrayal of nursing from the mid-nineteenth century to the late twentieth centuries in fiction, drama, news media, television, radio, and movies. They found that nurses appear as angels of mercy, Girl Fridays (either physicians' helpmates or love interests), heroines at home and at war, postwar wives and mothers, sixties sex objects, or fearsome figures (Kalisch and Kalisch, *Changing Image,* 2).

14. Charles Dickens, *Martin Chuzzlewit* (New York: Penguin, 1968), 374, 378.

15. Ibid., 479.

16. Kalisch and Kalisch, *Changing Image,* 14–15.

17. Ken Kesey, *One Flew over the Cuckoo's Nest* (New York: Penguin, 1962).

18. Joseph Heller, *Catch-22* (New York: Simon and Schuster, 1955); John Irving, *The World according to Garp* (New York: Pocket Books, 1976); Samuel Shem, *The House of God* (New York: Delta, 1978).

458   19. Shem, *House of God*, 154.

20. Anna Quindlen, *Black and Blue* (New York: Random House, 1998).

21. Diane Johnson, *Health and Happiness* (New York: Fawcett Crest, 1990), 7.

22. Robin Cook, *Fatal Cure* (New York: G. P. Putnam's Sons, 1993).

23. Susan Reverby's *Ordered to Care*, Diedre Wicks's *Nurses and Doctors at Work*, and Janet Calman's *Sex and Suffering* are notable examples of books that are not written by nurses and that take nursing seriously.

24. Joseph Turow, *Playing Doctor: Television, Storytelling, and Medical Power* (New York: Oxford University Press, 1989), 26.

25. Ibid., 37, 93–94.

26. Ibid., 93.

27. Kalisch and Kalisch, *Changing Image*, 176.

28. Turow and Gans, "As Seen on TV," 4.

29. Ibid., 16, 15.

30. British Columbia Nurses Union, "Z95.3 Agrees to Stop Airing Commercial That Denigrates Nurses," September 29, 2004, http://www.bcnu.org/News_Releases_2004/NR_039_2004.htm.

31. Anita Singh, " 'Naughty Nurses' TV Drama to Be Remade in U.S.," September 21, 2004, http://news.scotsman.com/latest.cfm?id=3527233.

32. Stephen King, *Misery* (New York: Signet, 1987).

33. Suzanne Gordon, *Prisoners of Men's Dreams* (New York: Little, Brown, 1986).

34. In an op-ed in the *New York Times*, February 23, 1991, titled "The Feminist Disdain for Nursing," the nursing professor and historian Ellen D. Baer discusses how nurses feel when their successful female friends scorn their work and try desperately to rehabilitate them.

35. We are reminded here of Sioban Nelson's work on the nursing nuns in the West of the United States as described in *Say Little, Do Much* (Philadelphia: University of Pennsylvania Press, 2001).

36. For a longer discussion of this play, see Suzanne Gordon, "Doctors' Brains," *Nation*, July 26/August 2, 1999, 32–34.

37. Tony Kushner, *Angels in America. Perestroika* (New York: Theater Communications Group, 1992), 20.

38. Ibid., 26–27.

39. Peter Baida, *A Nurse's Story, and Others* (Jackson: University Press of Mississippi, 2001), 3–35.

40. Echo Heron, *Pulse* (New York: Ivy Books, 1998).

41. Anne Perry, *The Face of a Stranger* (New York: Ivy Books, 1990).

42. Anne Perry, *The Sins of the Wolf* (New York: Ballantine Books, 1994), 325, 326.

7. Missing from the News

1. *New York Times*, January 5, 2004, A21.

2. "About Mass General," www.mgh.harvard.edu/about.html.

3. Harbor-UCLA Medical Center, www.humc.edu; UCLA Medical Center, www.ucla.edu.

4. "About MSH," www.mtsinai.on.ca/AboutUs/default.htm.

5. Here's what the American Association of Nurse Anesthetists says about the little-known history of the Mayo Clinic. The earliest existing records documenting the anesthetic care of patients by nurses were those of Sister Mary Bernard, a Catho-

lic nun who assumed her duties at St. Vincent's Hospital in Erie, Pennsylvania, in 1887. The most famous nurse anesthetist of the nineteenth century, Alice Magaw, worked at St. Mary's Hospital in Rochester, Minnesota. That hospital, established by the Sisters of St. Francis and operated by Dr. William Worrell Mayo, later became internationally recognized as the Mayo Clinic. Dr. Charles Mayo conferred upon Alice Magaw the title of Mother of Anesthesia for her many achievements in the field of anesthesiology, particularly her mastery of the open-drop inhalation technique of anesthesia utilizing ether and chloroform and her subsequent publishing of her findings.

Together, Dr. Mayo and Ms. Magaw were instrumental in establishing a showcase of professional excellence in anesthesia and surgery. Hundreds of physicians and nurses from the United States and throughout the world came to observe and learn their anesthesia techniques. Alice Magaw documented the anesthesia practice outcomes at St. Mary's Hospital and reported them in various medical journals between 1899 and 1906. In 1906 one article documented more than 14,000 anesthetics without a single complication attributable to anesthesia (*Surgery, Gynecology and Obstetrics* 3 [1906.]: 795, http://www.aana.com/about/history.asp).

6. "Doctor for a Day," *Children's News* (Children's Hospital, Boston), May 23, 2003.

7. Heather Giles, "Florence Nightingale: The History of Nurses Week," http://www.countryjoe.com/nightingale/nursesweek.htm.

8. Bernice Buresh, Suzanne Gordon, and Nica Bell, "Who Counts in News Coverage of Health Care?" *Nursing Outlook* 39 (1991): 204, 205.

9. Ibid., 208. In 1997, Sigma Theta Tau, the international honor society of nursing, also published a study—the Woodhull Study on Nursing and the Media—about health care's invisible partner. Nursing students at the University of Rochester looked at some twenty thousand articles that appeared in newspapers and magazines during the month of September 1997. The study concluded, once again, that nursing was underrepresented in news coverage.

10. Bernice Buresh and Suzanne Gordon, *From Silence to Voice: What Nurses Know and Must Communicate to the Public* (Ithaca: Cornell University Press, 2000), 98.

11. Wirthlin Worldwide, "Myths and Misperceptions about Aging and Women's Health: Initial Findings" (National Council on Aging, 1997).

12. Sandra G. Boodman, "Nursing a Lousy Image: RNs Blame Crisis on TV's ER," www.washingtonpost.com/wp-dyn/articles/A53866–2003Nov17.html.

13. Nancy Dickenson-Hazard, "New Harris Poll Is Sobering Wake-Up Call for Profession," *Excellence in Clinical Practice* 1, no. 4 (October 2000): 2.

14. Siobhan McDonough, "Fifteen Nurses Honored for Risking Lives to Save Others," *Boston Globe*, September 24, 2002, A20.

15. Bill Taylor, "Angel in Our Midst," *Toronto Star*, February 9, 2002, T1.

16. Milt Freudenheim, "Nurses Treading on Doctors' Turf," *New York Times*, Week in Review, November 7, 1997, 5; Ron Winslow, "Nurses to Take Doctor Duties, Oxford Says," *Wall Street Journal*, February 7, 1997, A3.

17. Alicia Change, "Hospitals Auction Nursing Shifts Online," *Boston Globe*, December 28, 2003, A28.

18. "How Much Do I Hear for This Nurse?" *Business Week*, December 8, 2003, 14.

19. Robert D. McFadden and Robert Hanley, "Nurse Accused of Slaying Patient Reportedly Admitted 30 Killings," *New York Times*, December 16, 2003, A1.

20. "On the Trail of Nurses Who Kill," editorial, *New York Times*, December 21, 2003, A8.

460

21. In a *New York Times* article by Mary Cadwalader, Claire Fagin, and Donna Diers ("Becoming a Nurse: Two Views, 1900 and 2000," November 7, 2000), the accompanying art showed three faceless nurses in caps.

22. Becky Mollenkamp, "Nurses Wanted," *Better Homes and Gardens*, September 2001, 232.

23. Kirk Johnson, "Demanding a Diagnosis, and Surviving Anthrax," *New York Times*, December 3, 2001, A1, B7.

24. Jean Gordon, "A Positive Childbirth," *Jackson (MS) Clarion-Ledger*, February 1, 2004, 1F–2F.

25. For example, consider Sharon Lerner, "Medical Students Go beyond Books to Learn about Activism," *New York Times*, December 2, 2003, D5.

26. Donald G. McNeil Jr. "In Ethiopia's Malaria War, Weapons Are the Issue," *New York Times*, December 9, 2003, D5.

27. Sarah Boseley, "Dying of Neglect by the Pharmaceutical Giants," *Guardian Weekly*, January 1–7, 2004, 5.

28. Leslie Eaton, "A Fireball, a Prayer for Death, Then an Uphill Battle for Life," *New York Times*, October 17, 2001, A1, B12.

29. Ben Macintyre, "Paralysed Superman Actor Fights for Life," *Times* (London), June 1, 1995; "Star Breaks Neck in Fall," *Australian*, June 1, 1995; Salatheia Bryant, "Reeve Urges Home Care Workers to Help Patients Recapture Lives," *Houston Chronicle*, August 28, 1996, A27; Geraldine Bedell, "Interview: You'll Believe a Man Can Walk," *Observer*, February 9, 2003, 3.

30. Denise Grady, "To the U.S., in a Slim Bid for Separate Cribs," *New York Times*, August 18, 2002, A1; Steve Rubenstein, "First Self-Contained Heart Implanted," *San Francisco Chronicle*, July 3, 2001, A1.

31. Irene Wielawski, "Post-9/11 Training Helped Save Lives at Club Fire," *New York Times*, March 3, 2003, A20.

32. *USA Today*, health topics index, http://www.usatoday.com/news/health/healthindex.htm, January 2, 2004.

33. Jane E. Brody, "Premature Births Rise Sharply, Confounding Obstetricians," *New York Times*, April 8, 2003, D5.

34. NIH, news release, http://www.nhlbi.nih.gov/news/press/01–09–10.htm.

35. Will Dunham, "Doctors See Fatal Delays in Heart Attack Cases," *Boston Globe*, September 11, 2001, A25.

36. George Anders, *Health against Wealth: HMOs and the Breakdown of Medical Trust* (Boston: Houghton Mifflin, 1996), 102.

37. Raja Mishra, "Adriana's Trial: A Young Life Interrupted, an Experiment Begins," *Boston Globe*, April 28, 2002, A1, A15.

38. Raja Mishra, "A Cancer Patient's Longest Wait," *Boston Globe*, April 29, 2002, A8.

39. Raja Mishra, "Balancing Benefits and Risks," *Boston Globe*, April 30, 2002, A10, A11.

40. "ICU," http://abcnews.go.com/onair/icu/.

41. Doug Donaldson, "Worry-Free Hospital Stays," *Better Homes and Gardens*, September 2004, 262.

42. Christopher Reeve, *Still Me* (New York: Random House, 1998), 38–39.

43. Ibid., 104.

44. Christopher Reeve, *Nothing Is Impossible* (New York: Random House, 2002), 7, 60–61.

45. Trisha Meili, *I Am the Central Park Jogger* (New York: Scribner's, 2003), 29.

46. Ibid., 60, 64.   **461**
47. Ibid., 68, 69.
48. Ibid., 71.

8. Unavailable for Comment

1. For a more detailed discussion on nurses' concerns about public exposure see Bernice Buresh and Suzanne Gordon, *From Silence to Voice: What Nurses Know and Must Communicate to the Public* (Ithaca: Cornell University Press, 2000).
2. Sioban Nelson and Suzanne Gordon, "The Rhetoric of Rupture," *Nursing Outlook*, in press.
3. Madge Kaplan, address, annual meeting of the American Academy of Nursing, Washington, DC, November 19, 1999.
4. Echo Heron, *Tending Lives: Nurses on the Medical Front* (New York: Fawcett Columbine, 1998).
5. Carmelle M. Bellefleur, "Retain Those Recruits," *Advance for Nurses*, September 16, 2002, 24.
6. Erving Goffman, *The Presentation of Self in Everyday Life* (New York: Doubleday, 1959), 10, 2.
7. Ibid., 12–13.
8. Buresh and Gordon, *From Silence to Voice*.
9. E-mail message to author. See http://www.nsna.org; "USA Films Announces Nurse Betty Scholarship Fund," http://public.gvc.edu/nsa/betty.html.
10. All three of these justifications are interesting. Consider the issue of violence. There is a great deal written about how to protect workers from workplace violence. Strategies include teaching workers how to identify a potentially violent patient/client or coworker, training them how to manage and diffuse violence, and hiring extra security personnel. Nowhere have I read anything about not giving one's last name or title as a means of successfully preventing or dealing with violence in the workplace. Indeed, giving one's first name and appearing porous and infinitely accessible would seem to make nurses more targetable than, say, doctors, who establish distance between themselves and the patient by using last names and titles.

    As to privacy, this is an even more fascinating claim. One of the core components of professionalism is accountability—professing to or standing up for what one does and taking responsibility for one's professional judgments and actions. Unlike the jobs of clerks or janitors, what a professional—particularly one whose actions can be a matter of life or death—does is so consequential that we want to ascertain the individual's full identity. That way, accountability and responsibility are easy to determine. While in principle a professional has a right to personal privacy, he or she has relinquished the right to professional privacy by claiming the status of professional. Thus it is peculiar that "professional leaders" would support—rather than rigorously oppose—any suggestion or action a nurse takes that would make it difficult to determine her individual identity. After all, policemen, who are likely victims of physical violence on the job, always have to display and give their full name and badge number. Since serious media exposure can change this image of anonymity and transform it into one of professional legitimacy and accountability, it may be no accident that hospital nurse managers seem to do so little to transform their institution's view of the nurse and promote efforts

462

that would make it more difficult for them to pursue the kinds of policies described in the next section.

In fact, a number of nurses have told me that they have tried to adopt a more professional form of introduction—for example, "Hello, I'm Nurse Jane Smith"—and have insisted that their last names be included on the assignment board. But their managers—not fellow nurses—have been resistant to this change in professional presentation and status.

11. Holistic health care is a "system of comprehensive or total patient care that considers the physical, emotional, social, economic, and spiritual needs of the person, the response to the illness, and the impact of the illness on the person's ability to meet self-care needs." In essence it involves the mastery of many skills and a great deal of knowledge, which, in the care of the sick, can be turned into "halfism"—the part the doctors don't want to do.

12. At a college in the Northeast, nurse practitioner students and their professor seemed quite distressed when I tried to get them to talk about the medical knowledge an NP inevitably must amass if he is to give effective primary care. "But we give holistic care," the students argued. When I asked why they felt that the holistic approach excluded the medical, they repeated that the holistic approach was the core of their work. The suggestion that they could combine the two and thus double their appeal to the public was viewed not as an addition but as a drawback. One nurse, practically in tears, said, "But for years we've been trying to argue for our work. We've finally found a niche, which is holism, and you're telling us not to talk about that." As if talking about a nurse practitioner's medical knowledge denigrates the nurse's relational connection to the patient.

13. *Info Nursing* 34, no. 1 (April/May 2003).

14. According to the ICN website, "The symbol is meant to characterize the caring, knowledge and humanity that infuse the work and spirit of nursing. The white heart is also a unifying symbol for nurses globally. White was selected because it brings together all colours, demonstrating nursing's acceptance of all people. White also has a world-wide association with nursing, caring, hygiene and comfort. The heart shape communicates humanity and the central place that nursing has in quality health care" (http://www.icn.ch/whiteheart.htm).

9. Mangling Care

1. Institute of Medicine, *Keeping Patients Safe: Transforming the Work Environment of Nurses* (Washington, DC: National Academy Press, 2004), 71.

2. American Hospital Association, "American Hospitals in Midst of Workforce Shortage," press release, June 5, 2001.

3. U.S. Bureau of Labor Statistics, "Number of Nonfatal Occupational Injuries and Illnesses Involving Days Away from Work by Selected Occupation and Industry Division," table 3, 2002, http://www.bls.gov/news.release/osh2.t03.htm.

4. U.S. Bureau of Labor Statistics, "Lost-Worktime Injuries and Illnesses: Characteristics and Resulting Time Away from Work," 2002, http://www.bls.gov/news.release/osh2.nr0.htm.

5. Daniel Chambliss, *Beyond Caring: Hospitals, Nurses, and the Social Organization of Ethics* (Chicago: University of Chicago Press, 1996), 16–17.

6. Robert Kuttner, *Everything for Sale: The Virtues and Limits of Markets* (New York: Alfred. A. Knopf, 1997), 128.

7. David U. Himmelstein and Steffie Woolhandler, *The National Health Program* **463**
Book (Monroe, ME: Common Courage Press, 1994), 236.

8. Kuttner, *Everything for Sale*, 128.

9. David Himmelstein and Steffie Woolhandler, *Bleeding the Patient: The Consequences of Corporate Healthcare* (Monroe, ME: Common Courage Press, 2001).

10. For a more thorough discussion of the problems of managed competition, see Himmelstein and Woolhandler, *Bleeding the Patient;* Kuttner, *Everything for Sale;* and Theta Skocpol, *Boomerang: Clinton's Health Security Effort and the Turn against Government in U.S. Politics* (New York: W. W. Norton, 1996).

11. Kuttner, *Everything for Sale*, 138.

12. H. S. Luft, "How Do Health-Maintenance Organizations Achieve Their 'Savings'?" *New England Journal of Medicine* 298 (1978): 1336–1343.

13. For a more detailed discussion of this phenomenon, see Suzanne Gordon and Timothy McCall, "Healing in a Hurry," *Nation*, March 1, 1999, 11–15.

14. Uwe Reinhardt, "Spending More through 'Cost Control': Our Obsessive Quest to Gut the Hospital," *Health Affairs* 15 (1996): 145–154.

15. Himmelstein and Woolhandler, *Bleeding the Patient*, 120–121.

16. Reinhardt, "Spending More," 147.

17. Institute of Medicine, *Keeping Patients Safe*, 78.

18. Reinhardt, "Spending More," 148.

19. Liz Kowalczyk, "Surge of Patients Taxes Hospital Resources," *Boston Globe*, September 22, 2002, A1.

20. Michael Hammer and James Champy, *Reengineering the Corporation: A Manifesto for Business Revolution* (New York: Harper Business, 1993).

21. James O'Shea and Charles Madigan, *Dangerous Company: Management Consultants and the Businesses They Save and Ruin* (New York: Penguin, 1997), 10–11.

22. Leah Curtin, "Unsafe at Any Price," *Nursing Management*, September 7, 1993.

23. Institute of Medicine, *Keeping Patients Safe*, 40.

24. Darlene Clark and Paul Clark, interview with author.

25. Taylor's theories were used by Henry Ford to automate his assembly line. Knudsen worked for Chevrolet. Leffingwell applied scientific management to the service industries in the 1920s. For a full description see Simon Head, *The New Ruthless Economy* (New York: Oxford University Press, 2003).

26. Ibid., 6, 8.

27. See Himmelstein and Woolhandler, *Bleeding the Patient;* Head, *New Ruthless Economy;* Kuttner, *Everything for Sale;* George Anders, *Health against Wealth: HMOs and the Breakdown of Medical Trust* (Boston: Houghton Mifflin, 1996), among many others.

28. Head, *New Ruthless Economy*, 23.

29. "WORCS Consulting and Software," http://www.healthworcs.com.

30. http://www.trendcare.com.au/products_l.html; http://www.vanslyck.com/about vsa.html.

31. Head, *New Ruthless Economy*, 42.

32. George Anders, "Nurses Decry Cost-Cutting Plan That Uses Aides to Do More Jobs," *Wall Street Journal*, January 20, 1994, B1, B6.

33. American Nurses Association, "Registered Nurse Virginia Trotter Betts Named to Key U.S. Department of Health and Human Services Position," press release, February 23, 1998.

34. www.tpogassociates.com/reference/2004/TimVita2004.pdf.

464 35. "Tim Porter-O'Grady Associates," http://www.tpogassociates.com/.

36. Ibid.

37. Tim Porter-O'Grady, "Working with Consultants on a REDESIGN," *American Journal of Nursing*, October 1994, 33, 34.

38. Ibid.

39. Ibid., 34–35.

40. Ibid., 35.

41. Ibid.

42. Ibid.; italics added.

43. Ibid., 33–34, 37.

44. Suzanne Smith Blancett and Dominick L. Flarey, *Reengineering Nursing and Health Care: The Handbook for Organizational Transformation* (Gaithersburg, MD: Aspen, 1995), xv.

45. Ibid., 409, 412.

46. Ibid., 11, 12.

47. Ibid., 81–82, 253.

48. Ibid., 411–412.

49. Peter I. Buerhaus, "Nursing, Competition, and Quality," *Nursing Economics* 10 (1992): 21–29.

50. Peter I. Buerhaus and Douglas O. Staiger, "Managed Care and the Nurse Workforce," *Journal of the American Medical Association* 276 (1996): 1492, 1493.

51. Ibid.

52. Edward O'Neil and Janet Coffman, eds., *Strategies for the Future of Nursing: Changing Roles, Responsibilities, and Employment Patterns of Registered Nurses* (San Francisco: Jossey-Bass, 1998), 4, 5, 6.

53. Ibid., 215, 216.

54. Mike Bury, "Illness Narratives: Fact or Fiction?" *Sociology of Health and Illness* 23 (2001): 275.

10. The New Nursing Universe

1 Institute of Medicine, *Nursing Staff in Hospitals and Nursing Homes: Is It Adequate?* (Washington, DC: National Academy Press, 1996), 81–86.

2. Ibid., 86.

3. Institute of Medicine, *Keeping Patients Safe: Transforming the Work Environment of Nurses* (Washington, DC: National Academy Press, 2004), 77.

4. Ibid., 40, 41.

5. Institute of Medicine, *Nursing Staff*, 102. The document continues: "Hospitals vary widely in the levels of training they provide to these personnel. Barter and colleagues (1994) found that 99 percent of the hospitals in California reported less than 120 hours of on-the-job training for newly hired ancillary nursing personnel. Only 20 percent of hospitals required a high school diploma. The majority of hospitals (59 percent) provided less than 20 hours of classroom instruction and 88 percent provided 40 hours or less of instruction time."

6. Ellen D. Baer, Claire M. Fagin, and Suzanne Gordon, *The Abandonment of the Patient: The Impact of Profit-Driven Care on the Public* (New York: Springer, 1996), 35.

7. Institute of Medicine, *Keeping Patients Safe*, 45.

8. The Institute for Health and Socio-Economic Policy.

9. American Hospital Association, *Hospital Statistics* (Chicago, 2003).

10. Minnesota Nurses Association, "Will Care Be There?" press release, October 17, **465** 1999.

11. See Institute of Medicine, *Keeping Patients Safe*, 41.

12. For more information on these risks and costs see A. T. Artigas, S. B. Dronda, and E. Chacon Valles, "Risk Factors for Nosocomial Pneumonia in Critically Ill Trauma Patients," *Critical Care Medicine* 29 (2001): 304–309; J. Carlet, "Dying from or with a Nosocomial Pneumonia in the Intensive Care Unit?" *Critical Care Medicine* 29 (2001) 2392–2394.

13. Two excellent articles on this subject C. H. Lyder et al., "Quality Care for Hospitalized Medicare Patients at Risk for Pressure Ulcers," *Archives of Internal Medicine* 161 (2001): 1549–1554; and J. V. Agostini, D. I. Baker, and S. T. Bogardus, "Prevention of Pressure Ulcers in Older Patients: Making Health Care Safer: A Critical Analysis of Patient Safety Practices," http://www.ahrq.gov/clinic/pt safety/chap27.htm.

14. Suzanne Gordon, "Nurse Interrupted," *American Prospect*, February 14, 2000, 28.

15. Staff Nursing—Staff RN and LPN Jobs," http://www.ultimatenurse.com/ubbthreads/showflat.php?CAT=&Number=5148&Main=4769#Post5148, March 11, 2004.

16. Institute of Medicine, *Keeping Patients Safe*, 38.

17. Barbara R. Norrish, "The Impact of Hospital Restructuring on the Work of Registered Nurses" (PhD diss., University of California–Berkeley, 1999).

18. Melissa Earl, Marguerite Jackson, and Leland Rickman, "Improved Rates of Compliance with Hand Antisepsis Guidelines: A Three Phase Observational Study," *American Journal of Nursing* (March 2001): 26–33.

19. Atul Gawande, "On Washing Hands," *New England Journal of Medicine* 350 (2004): 1283–1286.

20. Carole Levine, ed., *Always On Call: When Illness Turns Families into Caregivers* (New York: United Hospital Fund, 2000), 9–11.

21. Institute of Medicine, *Keeping Patients Safe*, 202.

22. Ibid., 203.

23. Ibid., 204.

24. Michael Smith, "Mandatory Overtime and Quality of Life in the 1990s," *Journal of Corporation Law* 21 (1996): 599–622.

25. American Nurses Association, "On-line Health & Safety Survey," September 2001, www.nursingworld.org/pressrel/2001/pr0907b.htm, 29–30.

26. Robert Steinbrook, "Nursing in the Crossfire," *New England Journal of Medicine* 346 (2002): 1764.

27. American Nurses Association, "On-line Survey," 26.

28. Robert M. Schwartz, *Your Rights on the Job: A Practical Guide to Employment Laws in Massachusetts* (Boston: Labor Guild of Boston, 2000).

29. "Nurses Collect Back Wages," *Boston Globe*, June 13, 2004, G2.

30. Julie Sochalski, "Nursing Shortage Redux: Turning the Corner on an Enduring Problem," *Health Affairs* 21, no. 5 (2002): 161–162; Steinbrook, "Nursing in the Crossfire," 1759.

31. Sochalski, "Nursing Shortage Redux," 162.

32. Simon Head, *The New Ruthless Economy* (New York: Oxford University Press, 2003), 13–14.

33. David Koeppel, "Nurses Bid with Their Pay in Auctions for Extra Work," *New York Times*, June 6, 2004, sec. 10, p. 1.

466 **11. Nurses on the Ropes**

1. Linda H. Aiken et al., "Hospital Nurse Staffing and Patient Mortality, Nurse Burnout, and Job Dissatisfaction," *Journal of the American Medical Association* 288 (2002): 1990.

2. Peter D. Hart Research Associates, "The Nurse Shortage: Perspectives from Current Direct Care Nurses and Former Direct Care Nurses" (report, April 2001).

3. Julie Sochalski, "Nursing Shortage Redux: Turning the Corner on an Enduring Problem," *Health Affairs* 21 (2002): 159, 161, 160.

4. Ibid., 160–161.

5. Claire M. Fagin, "When Care Becomes a Burden: Diminishing Access to Adequate Nursing," *Milbank Reports*, February 2001.

6. Donna Diers, *Speaking of Nursing: Narratives of Practice, Research, Policy and the Profession* (Sudbury, MA: Jones and Bartlett, 2004), 1.

7. Paul Duke, "If ER Nurses Crash, Will Patients Follow?" *Newsweek*. February 2, 2004, 12.

8. Ibid.

9. Charles E. Cavagnaro III, "Nurse Ratios Harm Hospitals," *Boston Globe*, March 2, 2004, A15.

10. Karen Higgins, letter to the editor, *Boston Globe*, March 8, 2004.

11. Nightingale's goal was not to *empower* (a concept she would have not even recognized) the ordinary nurse. If she fought for a female sphere of influence for nursing, it was for nursing management. The ordinary nurse would be subject to the physician's and the matron's orders. As she wrote in 1855, "Bind the *Superintendent* by every tie of signed agreement & of honor to strict obedience to her Medical Chief. . . . But let all his orders to the Nurses go through her. I mean, of course, not with regard to the medical management of the Patients, but with regard to the placing & discipline of the Nurses. . . . *I* am under his (the Principal medical Officer's) direction. *They* are under mine." Martha Vincinus and Bea Nergaard, eds., *Ever Yours, Florence Nightingale* (Cambridge: Harvard University Press, 1990), 122–123.

12. Barry Adams, "My Turn: Protecting Our Patients," *Newsweek*, November 16, 1998, 17.

13. For an account of the campaign around Adams and whistle-blower protection, see Bernice Buresh and Suzanne Gordon, *From Silence to Voice: What Nurses Know and Must Communicate to the Public* (Ithaca: Cornell University Press, 2000), 196–200.

14. Urs Weyermann, "Testing the Law: Swiss Nurses Go to Court to Fight for Equal Pay," *International Nursing Review* 50 (2003): 1–2.

15. Darlene Clark and Paul Clark, personal communication.

16. Jean Ann Seago and Michael Ash, "Registered Nurse Unions and Patient Outcomes," *Journal of Nursing Administration* 32 (2002): 148.

17. Ibid., 150.

18. Claire M. Fagin, Ellen D. Baer, and Suzanne Gordon, *The Abandonment of the Patient: The Impact of Profit-Driven Care on the Public* (New York: Springer, 1996), 38.

19. Robert Steinbrook, "Nursing in the Crossfire," *New England Journal of Medicine* 346 (2002): 1759.

20. American Nurses Association, "Nursing World Health and Safety Survey," September 2001, http://www.nursingworld.org/surveys/hssurvey.htm, 10–14.

21. U. Lundberg, "Stress Responses in Low-Status Jobs and Their Relationship to Health Risks: Musculoskeletal Disorders," *Annals of New York Academy of Science* 896 (1999): 162–172.

22. American Nurses Association, "Nursing World Health and Safety Survey," 8–16. **467**
23. Sean P. Clarke, Douglas M. Sloane, and Linda H. Aiken, "Effects of Hospital Staffing and Organizational Climate on Needlestick Injuries to Nurses," *American Journal of Public Health* 92, no. 7 (2002): 1115–1119.
24. Sean P. Clarke et al., "Organizational Climate, Staffing, and Safety Equipment as Predictors of Needlestick Injuries and Near-Misses in Hospital Nurses," *American Journal of Infection Control* 30 (2002): 207.
25. American Nurses Association, "Nursing World Survey," 20, 18.
26. Joel J. Hillhouse and Christine M. Adler, "Investigating Stress Effect Patterns in Hospital Staff Nurses: Results of a Cluster Analysis," *Sociology of Science and Medicine* 45 (1997): 1781.
27. Ibid.
28. C. Maslach, W. B. Schaufeli, and M. P Leiter, "Job Burnout," *Annual Review of Psychology* 52 (2001): 397–422.
29. NIOSH, "Stress," http://www.cdc.gov/niosh/stresswk.html.
30. Ibid., 4.
31. Ibid.
32. Ibid., 6.
33. Shigeru Sokejima and Sadanobu Kagamimori, "Working Hours as a Risk Factor for Acute Myocardial Infarction," *British Medical Journal* 317 (1998): 775–780.
34. Robert M. Sapolsky, *Why Zebras Don't Get Ulcers: An Updated Guide to Stress, Stress-Related Diseases, and Coping* (New York: W. H. Freeman and Company, 1998), 42.
35. When one researcher studied the impact of social stress on rodents, for example, he found that "the sympathetic nervous system is particularly activated in a socially subordinate rodent that is vigilant and trying to cope with a challenge. In contrast, it is the glucocorticoid system that is relatively more activated in a subordinate rodent that has basically given up on coping. Studies of stressed or depressed humans have shown what may be a human analogue of that dichotomy. Sympathetic arousal is a relative marker of anxiety and vigilance, while heavy secretion of glucocorticoids is more a marker of depression." Ibid., 35–36.
36. Hillhouse and Adler, "Investigating Stress Effect Patterns," 1787.
37. In his book on the crisis of the clergy in the Catholic Church, the former priest and professor of sociology Richard A. Schoenherr sets the controversial issue of priestly celibacy in an intricate matrix of social, organizational, and demographic forces that has produced a shortage of men willing to become Catholic priests. Some of the forces at play include the rise of feminism and its challenges to patriarchal structures, a decline in clerical control and rise of lay participation in the Church, a shift from dogmatism to pluralism, changing ideas about human sexuality, and less social emphasis on altruism and more on tangible material rewards for specific individuals. Although one reason for this shortage stands out—celibacy—it becomes the lightning rod for other social changes.
38. Steinbrook, "Nursing in the Crossfire," 1759.
39. Barbara R. Norrish, "The Impact of Hospital Restructuring on the Work of Registered Nurses" (PhD diss., University of California–Berkeley, 1999), 57–58.

12. No Nurse Left Behind

1. Dana Beth Weinberg has told in great depth the story of the once great Beth Israel Hospital nursing department and its decline. Dana Beth Weinberg, *Code*

468   *Green: Money-Driven Hospitals and the Dismantling of Nursing* (Ithaca: Cornell University Press, 2002).

2. Institute of Medicine, *Keeping Patients Safe: Transforming the Work Environment of Nurses* (Washington, DC: National Academy Press, 2004), 38–39.

3. For a more detailed account of Fergus's experiences, see my question-and-answer article, "Be More Efficient at the Expense of Patient Care," *Boston Globe*, January 2, 2000, C3.

4. Institute of Medicine, *Keeping Patients Safe*, 131.

5. Joyce Clifford, *Restructuring: The Impact of Hospital Organization on Nursing Leadership* (Chicago: Jossey-Bass–AHA Press, 1998).

6. Institute of Medicine, *Keeping Patients Safe*, 132.

7. Ibid., 132, 133.

8. Saint Sanjay, Richard H. Savel, and Michael A. Matthay, "Enhancing the Safety of Critically Ill Patients by Catheter-Related Infections," *American Journal of Respiratory, Critical Care Medicine* 165 (2002): 1476.

9. Institute of Medicine, *Keeping Patients Safe*, 133–136.

10. Ibid., 134–135.

11. Barbara R. Norrish and Thomas G. Rundall, "Hospital Restructuring and the Work of Registered Nurses," *Milbank Quarterly* 79 (2001): 69.

12. American Association of Colleges of Nursing, "Nursing School Enrollments Continue Steady Climb," AACN survey, December 21, 1994.

13. American Association of Colleges of Nursing, "While Demand for RNs Climbs, Undergraduate Nursing Enrollments Decline," press release, March 1999.

14. American Association of Colleges of Nursing, "Nursing Shortage Fact Sheet," http://NursingPower.Net/index2.html.

15. American Association of Colleges of Nursing, "Faculty Shortages in Baccalaureate and Graduate Nursing Programs: Scope of the Problem and Strategies for Expanding Supply," May 2003, http://www.aacn.nche.edu/Publications/White Papers/Faculty Shortages.htm.

16. American Association of Colleges of Nursing, "Accelerated Programs: The Fast-Track to Careers in Nursing," *Issue Bulletin*, August 2002.

17. Linda H. Aiken et al., "Educational Levels of Hospital Nurses and Surgical Patient Mortality," *Journal of the American Medical Association* 290 (2003): 1617–1623.

18. Nursing World, "Registered Nurses Rank Number One in Job Growth," press release, February 12, 2004; American Association of Colleges of Nursing, "Faculty Shortages," 1.

19. American Association of Colleges of Nursing, "Faculty Shortages," 2–3.

20. Ibid., 6, 3.

21. Ibid., 7.

22. Ibid., 6.

23. Ibid., 5.

24. Kathleen Dracup, "State of the School" (lecture, University of San Francisco, February 27, 2004).

25. Linda H. Aiken et al., "Nurses' Reports on Hospital Care in Five Countries" (May/June 2001), 43, 46.

26. Ibid., 48, 50–51.

27. Linda Diebel, "10 Questions for a SARS Inquiry" *Toronto Star*, June 8, 2003, A1.

28. Registered Nurses of Ontario, *Survey of Casual and Part-Time Nurses in Ontario*, Toronto, May 2003, 23.

29. Thomas A. MacWilliam, "Strategic Planning Committee Canadian Association

of Schools of Nursing: Trends and Issues in Health and Nursing" (Ottawa, **469**
March 2003), 10s.

30. Statement of Patricia Dorothy Fields, "The BRI Inquiry into Pediatric Cardiac Services in Bristol 1984–1985," WIT O154 0008.

31. Royal College of Nursing, "Nursing Shortages Will Jeopardise NHS Modernisation Unless Government Delivers on Spending Review, Says RCN," press release, February 19, 2002.

32. James Buchan, Tina Parkin, and Julie Sochalski, "International Nurse Mobility: Trends and Policy Implications" (report, World Health Organization, Geneva), 23.

33. E. M. Chiarella, *The Legal and Professional Status of Nursing* (Edinburgh: Churchill Livingstone, 2002), 282.

34. Ibid., 283, 285.

35. Ibid., 285.

36. Ibid., 286.

37. Gillian Considine and John Buchanan, "The Hidden Costs of Understaffing: An Analysis of Contemporary Nurses' Working Conditions in Victoria" (Australian Nursing Federation), 3.

38. Ibid., 4.

39. "Aged Care: Time to Stop the Exodus," *Australian Nursing Journal*, May 8–10, 2001.

40. Mireille Kingma, "Human Resources Annual Report," International Council of Nurses, doc. A53/23 and A53/INF Doc. 13 (2000).

41. Ibid., doc. A54/28 (2001).

13. Management by Churn

1. Institute of Medicine, *Keeping Patients Safe: Transforming the Work Environment of Nurses* (Washington, DC: National Academy Press, 2004), 74.

2. Harriet Davidson et al., "The Effects of Health Care Reforms on Job Satisfaction and Voluntary Turnover among Hospital-Based Nurses," *Medical Care* 35 (1997): 634.

3. Lonnie Golden and Eileen Appelbaum, "What Was Driving the 1982–88 Boom in Temporary Employment? Preference of Workers or Decisions and Power of Employers?" *American Journal of Economics and Sociology* 51 (1992): 473–494.

4. Jackie Krasas Rogers, *Temps: The Many Faces of the Changing Workplace* (Ithaca: ILR Press, 2000).

5. Alan Sager, personal communication, April 26, 2004.

6. Simon Head, *The New Ruthless Economy* (New York: Oxford University Press, 2003).

7. "InteliStaf Travel," http://www.flyingnurses.com/AboutUs.html.

8. "Jobs with Staying Power," *U.S. News and World Report*, March 8, 2004, 68–69.

9. "Cross Country TravCorps," http://www.crosscountrytravcorps.com/index.jsp.

10. Institute of Medicine, *Keeping Patients Safe*, 75.

11. Richard Saltus, "Patients Suffer as Agency Shields Troubled Hospitals: Patient's Death Leads to Change at the Brigham," *Boston Globe*, Metro/Region sec., February 16, 1996.

12. Leah Curtin, "JCAHO to Certify Supplemental Staffing Agencies: An Interview with Laure Dudley of JCAHO and Frank Shaffer of Cross Country Health Care," *Journal of Clinical Systems Management*, http://www.crosscountrytravcorps.com/content.jsp?type=jcaho_news.

470 13. Michael J. Berens and Bruce Japsen, "Patients Suffer as Agency Shields Troubled Hospitals," *Chicago Tribune*, November 10, 2002, C1.

14. Ibid.

15. Scott Allen, "Silencing Debate on the Nursing Shortage," *Boston Globe*, March 30, 2004.

16. David Schildmeier, personal communication.

17. Katharine Levit et al., "Health Spending Rebound Continues in 2002," *Health Affairs* 23, no. 1 (January–February 2004), exhibit 7.

18. Institute of Medicine, *Keeping Patients Safe*, 42, 43. In this study the IOM notes that other industries have found that using contingent workers produces higher accident rates and "is associated with labor management relations when contingent workers are used in an attempt to bypass labor-management conflicts." The International Atomic Energy Agency, for example, proposed that when an organization replaces permanent staff with contract workers, it is a "symptom of incipient weaknesses in the organization's safety culture. While hiring contract personnel has some benefits to the employer, it often comes at the expense of safety—either directly as a result of lower contractor standards or indirectly as a result of effects on permanent employees" (75–76).

19. Catherine Ceniza Choy, *Empire of Care: Nursing and Migration in Filipino American History* (Durham, NC: Duke University Press, 2003), 188.

20. Ibid., 111.

21. Fiona Armstrong, "Migration of Nurses: Finding a Sustainable Solution," *Australian Nursing Journal*, September 11, 2003, 25.

22. James Buchan, Tina Parkin, and Julie Sochalski, "International Nurse Mobility: Trends and Policy Implications" (report, World Health Organization, Geneva).

23. Armstrong, "Migration of Nurses," 25.

24. Choy, *Empire of Care*, 187.

25. *Australian Nursing Journal* 11, no. 6 (December 2003/January 2004), 50.

26. Public Services International, *Women and International Migration in the Health Sector: Final Report of Public Services International's Participatory Action Research 2003* (Ferney-Voltaire, France: Public Services International, 2003).

27. Internationally recruited nurses pay up to £2,000 to care for patients, April 22, 2000, http://www.rcn.org.uk/news/display.php?ID=46&area=Press.

28. Choy, *Empire of Care*, 186.

29. Joseph Berger, "From Philippines, with Scrubs," *New York Times*, November 24, 2003, A20.

30. International Council of Nurses, "New International Study Shows Working Conditions the Major Factor in Nurse Migration," press release, June 28, 2003.

31. Choy, *Empire of Care*, 59.

14. Failure to Rescue

1. American Hospital Association, "Reality Check: Public Perceptions of Health Care and Hospitals," confidential report from Dick Davidson to AHA member CEOs, 1996.

2. Linda H. Aiken et al., "Organization and Outcomes of Inpatient AIDS Care," *Medical Care* 37 (1999): 760–772.

3. Cindy Czaplinski and Donna Diers, "The Effect of Staff Nursing on Length of **471** Stay and Mortality," *Medical Care* 36 (1998): 1626–1638.

4. Gil Preuss, "Sharing Care: The Changing Nature of Nursing in Hospitals" (Washington, DC: Economic Policy Institute, 1998).

5. David Himmelstein and Steffie Woolhandler, *Bleeding the Patient: The Consequences of Corporate Health Care* (Monroe, ME: Common Courage Press, 2001), 129–134.

6. Suzanne Gordon, "Nurse Interrupted," *American Prospect*, February 14, 2000, 30.

7. Christine Kovner and Peter J. Gergen, "Nurse Staffing Levels and Adverse Events Following Surgery in U.S. Hospitals," *Image: The Journal of Nursing Scholarship* 100 (1998): 315–321.

8. Christine Kovner et al., "Nurse Staffing and Postsurgical Adverse Events: An Analysis of Administrative Data with a Sample of U.S. Hospitals, 1990–1996," *Health Services Research*, June 2002.

9. Jack Needleman et al., "Nurse Staffing Levels and the Quality of Care in Hospitals," *New England Journal of Medicine* 346 (2002): 1715–1722.

10. S. B. Kritchevsky et al., "Impact of Hospital Care on Incidence of Bloodstream Infection: The Evaluation Processes and Indicators in Infection Control Study," *Emerging Infectious Diseases* 7 (2001): 193–196.

11. Paul Arnow et al., "Control of Methicillin-Resistant *Staphylococcus aureus* in a Burn Unit: Role of Nurse Staffing," *Journal of Trauma* 22 (1982): 954–959.

12. Jerome Robert et al., "The Influence of the Composition of Nursing Staff on Primary Bloodstream Infection Rates in a Surgical Intensive Care Unit," *Infection Control and Hospital Epidemiology*, January 2000, 12–17; Archibald Lennox et al., "Patient Density, Nurse-to-Patient Ratio and Nosocomial Infection Risk in a Pediatric Cardiac Intensive Care Unit," *Pediatric Infectious Disease Journal* 16 (1997): 1045–1048; Scott K. Fridkin et al., "The Role of Understaffing in Central Venous Catheter-Associated Bloodstream Infections," *Infection Control and Hospital Epidemiology*, March 1996, 150–158.

13. Institute of Medicine, *Keeping Patients Safe: Transforming the Work Environment of Nurses* (Washington, DC: National Academy Press, 2004), 35–36, 45, 46.

14. Norrish and Rundall's concept of cumulative workload is critical for understanding the difficulties involved here. See Barbara R. Norrish and Thomas G. Rundall, "Hospital Restructuring and the Work of Registered Nurses," *Milbank Quarterly* 79 (2001).

15. Institute of Medicine, *Keeping Patients Safe*, 45.

16. Linda H. Aiken et al., "Hospital Nurse Staffing and Patient Mortality, Nurse Burnout, and Job Dissatisfaction," *Journal of the American Medical Association* 288 (2002): 1987–2041.

17. Joint Commission on Accreditation of Healthcare Organizations, "Health Care at the Crossroads: Strategies for Addressing the Evolving Nursing Crisis" (report, 2002). Anne Barnard, "Casualties Tied to Gaps in Nursing," *The Boston Globe*, August 7, 2002, A1.

18. Saint Sanjay, Richard H. Savel, and Michael A. Mattay, "Enhancing the Safety of Critically Ill Patients by Reducing Urinary and Central Venous Catheter-Related Infections," *American Journal of Respiratory and Critical Care Medicine* 165 (2002): 1475–1479.

19. Antonio Tejada Artigas et al., "Risk Factors for Nosocomial Pneumonia in Critically Ill Trauma Patients," *Critical Care Medicine* 29 (2001): 304–309.

472   20. Courtney H. Lyder et al., "Quality of Care for Hospitalized Medicare Patients at Risk for Pressure Ulcers," *Archives of Internal Medicine* 161 (2001): 1549–1554. Joseph V. Agostini et al., "Prevention of Pressure Ulcers in Older Patients," in *Making Health Care Safer: A Critical Analysis of Patient Safety Practices*, Evidence Report/Technology Assessment, No. 43. Agency for Health Care Research and Quality.

21. Susan Skewes, "Skin Care Rituals That Do More Harm Than Good," *American Journal of Nursing* 96 (1996): 32; Courtney Lyder, "Pressure Ulcer Prevention and Management," *Journal of the American Medical Association* 289 (2003): 223–226.

22. Jennifer Kleinbart et al., "Prevention of Venous Thromboembolism," in *Making Health Care Safer*. DeLissovy et al., "Cost for Inpatient Care of Venous Thrombosis: A Trial of Enoxaparin vs. Standard Heparin," *Archives of Internal Medicine* 160 (2000): 3160–3165. John A. Heit et al., "Relative Impact of Risk Factors for Deep Vein Thrombosis and Pulmonary Embolism," *Archives of Internal Medicine* 162 (2002): 1245–1248.

23. D. W. Bates et al., "The Cost of Adverse Drug Events in Hospitalized Patients," *Journal of the American Medical Association* 277 (1997): 307–311.

24. T. A. Brennan et al., "Incidence of Adverse Events and Negligence in Hospitalized Patients: Results of the Harvard Medical Practice Study," *New England Journal of Medicine* 324 (1991): 370–376.

25. D. W. Bates et al., "Incidence of Adverse Drug Events and Potential Adverse Drug Events: Implications for Prevention," *Journal of the American Medical Association* 274 (1995): 29–34; L. L. Leape et al., "Systems Analysis of Adverse Drug Events," *Journal of the American Medical Association* 274 (1995): 35–43.

26. Bates et al., "Cost of Adverse Drug Events."

27. E. J. Thomas and T. A. Brennan, "Incidence and Types of Preventable Adverse Events in Elderly Patients: Population Based Review of Medical Records," *British Medical Journal* 320, no. 7237 (2000): 741–744.

28. Institute of Medicine, *Keeping Patients Safe*, 34.

29. Institute of Medicine, *To Err Is Human: Building A Safer Health System* (Washington, DC: National Academy Press, 1999: 169–170).

30. U.S. Department of Health and Human Services, Agency for Health Care Policy and Research, *Acute Pain Management: Operative or Medical Procedures and Trauma*, Clinical Practice Guideline, no. 1. (Rockville, MD, 1992).

31. J. M. Teno et al., "Family Perspectives on End-of-Life Care at the Last Place of Care," *Journal of the American Medical Association* 291 (2004): 88–93.

32. Alice Dembner, "Too Little Respect Seen for the Dying," *Boston Globe*, January 7, 2004, A1.

33. Laurie Carr et al., "Neural Mechanisms of Empathy in Humans: A Relay from Neural Systems for Imitation to Limbic Areas," *Proceedings of the National Academy of Sciences* 100 (2003): 5497–5502.

34. Julian Tudor Hart and Paul Dieppe, "Caring Effects," *Lancet* 347 (1996): 1607.

Conclusion: Changing the Odds

1. Suzanne Gordon, "Necessary Nursing Care," *Nursing Inquiry* 7 (2000): 217–219.

2. Joint Commission on Accreditation of Healthcare Organizations (JCAHO), "Health Care at the Crossroads: Strategies for Addressing the Evolving Nursing Crisis" (report, 2002), 19.

3. Bonnie L. Atencio, Jayne Cohen, and Bobbye Gorenberg, "Nurse Retention: Is It **473** Worth It?" *Nursing Economics* 21 (2003): 262–268.

4. Ibid. See also VHA, "The Business Case for Work Force Stability Study Summary," November 11, 2002.

5. In an article opposing the ratio bill proposed by the Massachusetts Nurses Association, Richard T. Moore, Massachusetts state senator, argued that a better alternative to staffing ratios would be to give loans and financial aid to new nurses, mandate hospitals "to file descriptions of their staffing plans with the state," establish hospital nursing performance measures (hospitals will pay fines if they are violated), and fund a Center for Nursing that will study nursing issues. Richard T. Moore, "Time to Heal the Nursing Issue," *Boston Globe*, April 6, 2004.

6. Joan Gleason Scott, Julie Sochalski, and Linda Aiken, "Review of Magnet Hospital Research: Findings and Implications for Professional Nursing Practice," *Journal of Nursing Administration* 291 (1999): 9–19.

7. Linda H. Aiken, Donna Havens, and Douglas, M. Sloane, "The Magnet Nursing Services Recognition Program: A Comparison of Two Groups of Magnet Hospitals," *American Journal of Nursing* 100 (March 2000): 26–36; Margaret L. McClure and Ada Sue Hinshaw, *Magnet Hospitals Revisited: Attraction and Retention of Professional Nurses* (Washington, DC: American Nurses Publishing, 2002). American Nurses Credentialing Center, *Profiles in Excellence: Highlighting Organizations Awarded Magnet Status*, 1994–2001 (Washington, DC: ANCC, 1994).

8. "Benefits of Magnet Recognition," http://www.nursingworld.org/ancc/magnet/benes.html.

9. Timothy A. Mercer, "2002 Salary Survey Results," *ADVANCE for Nurses*, http://nursing.advanceweb.com/Common/editorial/editorial.aspx?CTIID=1216&SEC=PRC.

10. Arlington and Randolph Education Association salary scales, April 2004.

11. Cathy Rick, personal communication, October 2001.

12. See also Marjorie Murphy, *Blackboard Unions: The AFT and the NEA 1900–1980* (Ithaca: Cornell University Press, 1990).

13. JCAHO, "Health Care at the Crossroads," 30.

14. Ibid., 31.

15. American Association of Colleges of Nursing, "The Baccalaureate Degree in Nursing as Minimal Preparation for Professional Practice" (Washington, DC, December 2000), 3.

16. Ibid., 4.

17. American Association of Colleges of Nursing, "AACN Position Statement: The Baccalaureate Degree in Nursing as Minimal Preparation for Professional Practice" (Washington, DC, 2000).

18. James C. Scott, *Seeing like a State: How Certain Schemes to Improve the Human Condition Have Failed* (New Haven: Yale University Press, 1998), 12–13.

19. Ellen D. Baer et al., eds., *Enduring Issues in American Nursing* (New York: Springer, 2001).

20. Personal communication; also U.S. House Labor, HHS Committee, "Labor–Health & Human Services–Education and Related Agencies," p. 12.

21. Linda H. Aiken et al., "Educational Levels of Hospital Nurses and Surgical Patient Mortality," *Journal of the American Medical Association* 290 (2003): 1617–1623.

22. What is perhaps most interesting about U.S. whistle-blower legislation is that it

474   may not go far enough. Workers can be protected if they blow the whistle on unsafe practices that jeopardize patients. But they are not *required* to expose those practices. Contrast this with laws that protect elders and children from abuse and neglect. People who work with elders and children are legally considered to be mandatory reporters. According to George Annas, a health law expert at the Boston University School of Public Health, people who work with these vulnerable populations are required by law to report suspected or actual cases of abuse and neglect. If a case of abuse or neglect is uncovered and the mandatory reporter failed to report it, he or she can be held legally liable if it is proved that public exposure could have prevented further harm.

All across the United States, and the globe, health policy experts insist they are trying to protect patients from harm—from medical errors and injuries, from arrogance or ignorance, from failures in communication and from interprofessional disintegration. Yet, most do not apply the same standards to the sick that are applied to those who are vulnerable yet healthy. Perhaps that should be the next step in a global effort to build a genuine commitment to patient care.

23. Many other organizations like the International Council of Nurses and the American Association of Critical Care Nurses have put out position statements about violence in the work place.

24. Robert L. Helmreich, "The Evolution of Crew Resource Management Training in Commercial Aviation," *International Journal of Aviation Psychology* 91 (1999): 19–32.

25. Christine R. Kovach and Sarah Morgan, "Doctor's Orders: Rethinking Language and Intent," *Journal of Nursing Administration* 33 (2003): 563–564.

26. For a more lengthy discussion of this issue see the discussion of naming practices in Bernice Buresh and Suzanne Gordon, *From Silence to Voice: What Nurses Know and Must Communicate to the Public* (Ithaca: Cornell University Press, 2000).

27. Of course doctors will argue that secretaries and other personnel come and go. Some do, some don't. Doctors are also movable objects and leave practices after a short time. The point is that key staff members who have been around for a long time should be described as members of the team.

28. In her book *Gender and Discourse* Deborah Tannen analyzes the way different cultures engage in conversational discourse. People who disagree with others or interrupt them frequently may be considered aggressive. In fact, these high-involvement speakers are actually showing engagement with and respect for their interlocutors. Their interruptions and disagreements indicate that they believe that the person they're talking to is strong enough to handle conflict and counterargument.

29. "Facts about the Nursing Shortage," http://www.nursesource.org/facts_shortage .html.

30. National Student Nurses Association, *Nursing: The Ultimate Adventure*, VHS (New York, 2000).

31. Sioban Nelson and Suzanne Gordon, "An End to Angels and Hearts," *American Journal of Nursing*, in press.

32. "Television Advertising 2002 and Nurse Recruitment," *The Campaign for Nursing's Future*, VHS (Johnson & Johnson, 2002).

33. "Patient Perspectives," *The Campaign for Nursing's Future*, VHS (Johnson & Johnson, 2002).

34. U.S. Nurse Corps brochure (September 2002); U.S. Nurse Corps, "You Can Help Others and Help Yourself," certified registered nurse anesthetist brochure (April 2002).

Index